SEXUAL ATTITUDES

SEXUAL ATTITUDES
myths & realities

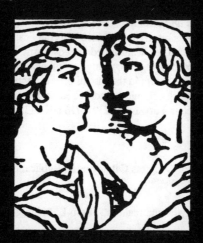

Vern L. Bullough, R.N., Ph.D.
& Bonnie Bullough, R.N., Ph.D.

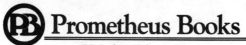 Prometheus Books

59 John Glenn Drive
Amherst, NewYork 14228-2197

To our granddaughter, Jamie Bullough-Latsch

Published 1995 by Prometheus Books

99 98 97 96 95   5 4 3 2 1

Library of Congress Cataloging-in-Publication Data

Bullough, Vern L.
    Sexual attitudes : myths and realities / Vern L. Bullough and Bonnie Bullough.
        p.   cm.
    Includes bibliographical references and index.
    ISBN 0-87975-949-6
    1. Sex customs—History. 2. Sexual ethics—History. I. Bullough, Bonnie.
II. Title.
HQ12.B873   1995
306.7′09—dc20   94-47645
                                                                         CIP

Printed in the United States of America on acid-free paper.

Contents

Introduction   7

1. Why the Hostility to Sex?   11

2. Alternative Views of Sexual Activity   29

3. "Unnatural" Sex   47

4. Masturbation   67

5. Sex and Gender   85

6. Menstruation   107

7. Contraception   125

8. Abortion   147

9. Infertility, Impotence, and Artificial Insemination   159

10. Pornography and Obscenity   183

11. Prostitution   203

12. Homosexuality, Sex Labeling, and Stigmatized Behavior   229

13. Sex in a Changing World   251

Index   269

Introduction

Sex research has been, and in many ways remains, a taboo area. There are many reasons for this. One is simply a carryover from the Victorian era, that certain topics, sex among them, were not proper for public discussion. A result of this attitude was to drive much of the discussion of sex underground where misinformation ran rampant. A second related reason is that for many, sexual activity, except for purposes of procreation, was a sin. Thus when sexual matters were discussed, their attendant horrors and evils were often emphasized, at least in public discussion.

These attitudes had an effect on early sex researchers who, for the most part, regarded themselves as respectable individuals. Often, when describing sexual activities, they did so in negative terms, emphasizing in the process their own respectability even if they were describing immoral or unacceptable acts. Another way they coped was to emphasize the need to protect the innocent. Thus early sex research literature is full of cases of innocent women and children contracting a sexually transmitted disease from an evil and lecherous man, usually the husband and father of those involved. Such accounts were written in general terms without actually mentioning what constituted sex. In almost all cases, whether they wrote in generalities or dealt with specifics, researchers adopted the moralizing attitudes of their contemporaries.

Yet sex itself is a subject about which almost every person considers himself or herself knowledgeable. Inevitably each generation, often shame-facedly and surreptitiously, has passed on its own erroneous ideas to the next, with additional accretions as each new generation of adolescents solidified their own ignorance with the ignorance of their peers.

The historian who begins to investigate this cycle finds that many of the erroneous assumptions about human sexuality can be traced back to the beginnings of written language, made by people and cultures who had a different worldview than our own and who obviously lacked our knowledge

7

of anatomy and physiology. Researchers, however, start with what they believe to be accepted truth, and generally they work within the system in which they find themselves. Thus when serious researchers first began to investigate sexual behavior, they tended to accept the underlying erroneous assumptions without bothering to question them, proving that scientists themselves are people of their own time and culture. Usually researchers tend to concentrate their energies in a rather narrow field, accepting as true most of the assumptions outside their own narrow specialty. This was especially the case with early sex research, where the new breakthroughs that began to occur in the last part of the nineteenth century coincided with the high tide of sexual prudishness associated with Victorianism.

A good illustration of this is the case of Denslow Lewis, a Chicago physician, who attempted to discuss the "hygiene of the sexual act" at the 1899 meeting of the American Medical Association (AMA). When the program was announced, the famous Johns Hopkins University gynecologist Howard Kelly objected to the paper on the grounds that the "discussion of the subject is attended with filth and we besmirch ourselves by discussing it in public." Though Lewis was allowed to give his paper, the AMA refused to authorize its publication in the official proceedings of the meeting.[1]

In the United States this period of sexual behavior is associated with the figure of Anthony Comstock (1844–1915), who, though today often painted as a ludicrous figure, was extremely powerful in his own lifetime. As the United States began to emerge from being a rural-agrarian country to an urban-industrialized one in the post-Civil War period, and as young people flocked to the cities, older generations of Americans were shocked at what they considered to be the evils of urban life. Restraints imposed upon individuals who lived in villages and small towns seemingly went by the wayside when these people, particularly the young of both sexes, moved to the city. Those who were upset at the changes taking place tended to look for simplistic causes. They believed they found them in what they called indecent literature, lewd art works, a growth of prostitution, and the availability of other forms of "immoral sex" in the cities. Comstock became the symbolic leader of the effort to make America pure, to give it back its "pristine innocence." Initially, he had wide enough support to be appointed a special agent by the United States Post Office with power to censor mailed materials. Comstock took his task seriously, collecting all kind of material he regarded as pornographic in order to become better acquainted with them. He prosecuted physicians who wrote on birth control, a subject he regarded as obscene. In his quest to achieve sexual purity, Comstock even went so far as to wonder why decent men and women bought and read newspapers that carried stories about "divorce or contested will cases reeking with filthy details." In his mind, it was "bad enough to have these vile details" unfold in the court, but he questioned whether they had to be admitted into the home."[2]

Women in particular had to be protected from the evils of the world. A century before Comstock's efforts in America, Thomas Bowdler (1754–1825), a well-to-do English physician, had himself become concerned over the overt sensuality present in most literary works. Dr. Bowdler enjoyed reading aloud to his family the works of the great writers, and although he was especially enamored of Shakespeare, he felt most of the works of the bard were unsuitable to be read to young women. His concern led Bowdler in 1818 to produce a ten-volume expurgated version of Shakespeare suitable for reading by "a gentleman in the company of ladies." He suggested that those works of Shakespeare which could not be "bowdlerized," such as *Othello,* had best be transferred from the parlor to the locked cabinet, to be read only by sophisticated men such as himself. Bowdler's efforts had been anticipated by others, including James Plumptre, who, in 1805, published an expurgated song book. One British writer went so far as to urge the perfect hostess to assure herself that the "works of male and female authors be properly separated on her bookshelves. Their proximity unless they happen to be married should not be tolerated."[3]

Bowdler, Comstock, Kelly, and others believed in the "sin model" of sexuality. Although it began to be supplemented in the nineteenth century by what might be called the "sickness model," it has continued to exercise an influence to the present day. The sickness model originated from an attempt by physicians to understand some of the presenting illnesses of their patients, and though it eventually developed in the twentieth century into a far more sophisticated system than the sin model, the sickness model started out by more or less accepting the sin model of sexuality. Only it defined the sinners as sick people.[4] In the twentieth century, the sickness view came to be challenged by the emerging social and behavior sciences; in the last few decades the implications of the new research have begun exploding upon the public mind. The question increasingly becomes one of how we can reconcile this research with traditionally accepted knowledge. To do this it is essential to understand our past, to examine the sources of our earlier assumptions, to sort out what is erroneous from what might be called valid.

This is important because human sexuality is a complicated mix of biological and physiological factors, psychological and sociological influences, and cultural and historical traditions. Before we can deal with the former, we have to deal with the latter. This book is an attempt to come to terms with our cultural and historical traditions. It is a subject that historians have only begun to explore.

Obviously any book requires the labor of a number of people. The authors would like to thank the copyeditor, Eugene O'Connor, who made this a much better book, and acquisitions editor, Steven L. Mitchell. The index was prepared by Michael Hayworth. He also deserves our thanks.

NOTES

1. Denslow Lewis, *The Gynecologic Consideration of the Sexual Act: and An Appendix with An Account of Denslow Lewis,* compiled and edited by Marc H. Hollender (Weston, Miss.: MTSL Press, 1970). See also "The Teaching of Sex Hygiene," *New York Medical Journal* 101 (April 24, 1915): 850. For a more complete discussion see John C. Burnham, "The Progressive Era Revolution in American Attitudes toward Sex," *Journal of American History* 59 (1973): 885–908.

2. Anthony Comstock, "How to Guard Our Youth against Bad Literature," *Chautauquan* 25 (August 1897): 520–24.

3. Quoted in Milton Rugoff, *Prudery and Passion* (New York: G. P. Putnam's Sons, 1971), p. 61.

4. Vern L. Bullough, "Sex and the Medical Model," *Journal of Sex Research* 11 (1975): 291–303. See also Vern L. Bullough, *Science in the Bedroom: A History of Sex Research* (New York: Basic Books, 1994).

1

Why the Hostility to Sex?

Western culture, at least since the advent of Christianity, has been looked upon as a sex-negative culture. Sexual activities have been regarded with suspicion if not hostility. Such attitudes did not emerge full-blown with the advent of Christianity, but rather have roots that go much further back into the past and are based upon intellectual assumptions that few would accept today. The major source of these ideas is not so much the Old and New Testaments, but rather some of the philosophical beliefs of the pagan Greeks and Romans.[1] In this respect Christianity did not make the world ascetic, but rather, in the words of the biblical scholar Morton Enslin who wrote them nearly seventy years ago, "the world in which Christianity found itself strove to make Christianity ascetic."[2]

The key to this Western hostility to sex lies in Greek dualistic thought. This divided the world into two opposing forces, described as the spiritual and the material, or the higher and lower, or the soul and the body. Put in its simplest terms, dualism held that the soul was undergoing punishment by being incarcerated in a human body. Man's purpose in life was to achieve salvation, to allow the soul to escape the domination of the flesh. Sex was bad because sexual activity represented the assertion of the bodily needs over the spiritual; moreover, the begetting of children continued the imprisonment of future souls. The origin of these dualistic ideas has been the subject of intense scholarly investigation over the past several decades. There seem to be several points of origin, all of which are shrouded in myth and legend. It is quite possible that the ideas ran deep in the consciousness of the earliest Indo-European people, since both the ancient Persians and the ancient Greeks held some of the same concepts. Though failing to agree on the starting point of this dualism, most scholars believe that the concept became fixed in the Greek-speaking world through the Orphic religion and the cult of the god Dionysus.

The Orpheus of Greek mythology is the musician who so charmed Hades, the god of the underworld, that Orpheus was allowed to bring his wife, Eurydice, back from the dead. According to the legend, however, Hades had put a condition on her return, namely, that Orpheus would not look back at Eurydice until he reached the upper world. Unfortunately, Orpheus, just before he reached his goal, glanced back, whereupon Eurydice had to return to the underworld. Later, Orpheus became the center of a cult; a singer, prophet, and teacher; and is credited with modifying or rearranging the Bacchic rites that center around the Thracian deity of vegetation, Dionysus. After investigating the surviving sources, scholars now believe that the Orphic religion taught that the soul was undergoing punishment for sin, with the body (sōma) serving as a prison or tomb (sēma) in which the soul was trapped. Release and immortality could be achieved by leading a pure life and by engaging in the secret rituals of the Orphic religion.[3]

As Orphism matured, it adopted and modified the traditional genealogy of the gods recorded by the poets Homer and Hesiod, keeping the old names but providing different explanations. According to Orphic mythology, in the beginning only night existed until a silver egg containing Eros was formed in the divine ether. When the egg burst, it separated into two elements, Heaven (the male Uranos) and Earth (the female Gaea). Eventually these elements copulated, with Gaea giving birth to Kronos and other gods known as Titans. Kronos in turn became the father of Rhea, Demeter, Hades, Poseidon, and Zeus, among others. Zeus eventually swallowed his own father, thereby encompassing all creation, after which Zeus created another world, the world we live in, over which he put Dionysus, his son by Persephone. Before Dionysus could assume his domination, he was killed, cooked, and eaten by the other Titans, who were then burned to ashes by the thunderbolts of Zeus. The goddess Athena managed to rescue the heart of Dionysus from the ashes and presented it to Zeus, who proceeded to eat it. Out of this act of cannibalism a new Dionysus was born from the seed of Zeus, though this time the mother was Semele instead of Persephone. From the ashes of the Titans, Zeus then fashioned humankind, which meant that his new creation contained something of the divine derived from the remnants of Dionysus, as well as something of the opposite, coming from the Titans.[4] It is from this legend (and similar ones) commemorating the union of the divine and the material that historians can trace the basis for many of our Western sexual attitudes.

Although the Orphic mysteries were never officially incorporated into the state religion of classical Greece, they enjoyed great popularity and exercised considerable influence on the Pythagoreans and Plato, as well as on the later Greek philosophical mystical writers, all of whom purged the Orphic dualism of some of its grosser superstitions. Pythagoras, who lived in the sixth century B.C.E., taught that the universe was ultimately divisible into two opposing principles, one of which he described as Unlimited Breath, the other as Limited. It is with the nature and operations of the latter that the famous Pythagorean teaching that all things are numbers is concerned. Limited and Unlimited are opposites, and this opposition is expressed also in light and darkness, odd and even, one and many, right and left, male and female, resting and moving, straight and curved, good and bad, square and oblong, and so on. Limit, light, odd, and male are right and good, whereas the unlimited darkness, even, and female are wrong and evil, or at least one set is superior and the other is inferior.[5]

Salvation was to be achieved through a *katharsis,* or cleansing; this required the observance of certain taboos based upon the Orphic concepts that the soul is imprisoned within the mortal body, and that the body itself is governed by evil passions which are our indwelling Furies. Pythagoras taught that individuals should not be the slaves of their bodies but should improve and save their souls by escaping from the domination of the flesh. Since sexual consummation was the primal pandering to the indwelling Furies, every symbol relating to it had to be repudiated. Though Pythagoras himself apparently did not advocate total abstinence, some of his followers did. One of them, the fifth-century philosopher and scientist Empedocles, denounced all forms of sexual intercourse. Empedocles might well have been an isolated extremist within the Pythagorean tradition, but his denunciation seems a logical step to take in light of the Pythagorean assumptions. As a result of such assumptions, E. R. Dodds has argued that sexual asceticism not only originated in Greece but was carried by a "Greek mind to its extreme theoretical limit."[6]

The most influential transmitter of these dualistic ideas was Plato (427–347 B.C.E.), who, while rejecting the cultic aspects of the Pythagoreans, elevated their philosophical ideas. Plato had only contempt for those who taught or believed that a god could be persuaded or bribed to confer blessed immortality upon initiates because they had performed special ceremonials or accepted certain doctrines or revelations. Instead, he held that the moral law was fixed and immutable, that our fate depended upon our actions during life, and that each of us had the power to rise above his or her Titanic nature. To this end, Plato postulated the existence of two universal principles, Ideas and Matter, which he equated with the intelligent and sensible worlds, respectively. Ideas were eternal and immutable, present always and everywhere, self-identical, self-existent, absolute, separate, simple without beginning or end. They were complete, with perfect existence in every respect, without taint or sense or imagery, invisible to the eye, accessible only to the mind. On the other hand, Matter, or the material world of sensible objects, existed only insofar as it caught and retained the likeness of the Idea, but in any case it was always an imperfect imitation.

Most philosophers (following Aristotle) have regarded Plato's concept of the Idea (or Form) as a universal concept that is not subject to the change that the material world undergoes. It exists in and for itself apart from the sensible world and possesses the incorporeal yet quasi-substantial sort of being commonly attributed by theologians to God. In fact, Christianity adopted so many of the Platonic concepts that Justin Martyr, an early Christian Father, never tired of reiterating that Plato must have been versed in Christian prophecy since he wrote of Christian concepts long before Jesus was born. Thus Plato, at least through his Neoplatonic interpreters, has to be regarded as a dominant force in early Christian theology.

Following the concept of Pythagoras, Plato taught that the soul, an immaterial agent, was superior in nature to the body, although it was hindered by the body in its performance of the higher psychic functions of life. Reality for Plato had two components—the *phenomena,* the changeable world of bodies, which man can know through sense perception, and the *ideas,* the timeless essence or universal realities. It was only the world of Ideas that contained the ultimate realities after which the world of sensible things had been patterned. This world could not be known through the senses but only through the *nous,* the mind or soul, which knows because it is the essence of the divine being and has an existence independent of the body. Though the soul had been born with true knowledge, the encrustation of bodily cares and interests made it difficult to recall the truth which was innately and subconsciously still present. Sense perception might aid the soul in the process of reminiscence, but only by intuitive thought, by clearing the mind of bodily concerns, by probing ever deeper by the Socratic method of questions and answers, with each answer provoking another set of questions, will truth finally be achieved.

Plato conceived of love in dualistic terms, dividing it into the sacred and profane, the former occupied with the mind and character of the beloved, the latter with the body. It was only through the higher love, the nonphysical, that true happiness could be found. To reach this highest form there was a step-by-step progression, starting with the body of the beloved, proceeding to physical love in general, then contemplation of the beauties of the mind and soul, and finally the pure form or essence of love in itself—absolute, separate, simple, and everlasting—which, without diminution or increase or change, was imparted to the continually growing and perishing beauty of all things.[7]

Plato, in the *Phaedrus,* compared the types of love to a charioteer driving two winged steeds, one of which (true love) was a thoroughbred, gentle and eager to bear its driver upward into the presence of the ideal; the other (physical love), vicious and refractory, forever bolting in pursuit of physical satisfaction. The discipline of love lay in training the unruly steed to run in harmony with its thoroughbred mate. If the charioteer was successful, the team would bear the lover and beloved away from the world of sense to the vision of absolute loveliness that alone made them truly lovely and lovable in each other's eyes. Love, in essence, implied the mutual attainment of self-mastery that cured the disease of physical craving.[8] Copulation, or physical love, lowered a man to the frenzied passions characteristic of animals, and for this reason Plato relegated sexual desire to the lowest element of the psyche (i.e., soul).[9]

Many other Greek writers of philosophy, including those who started with assumptions different form Plato's, seemed to assume that the true state of goodness was one devoid of physical, sexual activity. Even Democritus, the fifth-century proponent of the atomistic nature of the universe, who taught that enjoyment of pleasure was the end naturally sought by man, held that all pleasures were not equally good. He proclaimed that the pleasures of the senses were short-lived, agitating, and in the long run led only to pain, while the pleasures of the mind were painless, calm, and enduring. This led him to define virtue as a matter of the exercise of intelligence, and since sexual activity tended to interfere with the pleasures of the mind, Democritus ended by disapproving of such activity. One of the more famous statements attributed to him was the definition of a brave man as one "who overcomes not only his enemies but his pleasures." He then added that there were men who were masters of cities but slaves to women, and to be a slave to a woman was the ultimate disgrace for a man. Thus the man who selected the true pleasures, those which were good for the soul, made a "divine choice," while the one who chose the good of the body made simply a "mortal choice."[10] Epicurus, the fourth-century B.C.E. disciple of Democritus and the founder of the Epicurean school, became even more specific in his condemnation of sex. Sexual intercourse, he held, "never benefitted any man," and he believed that the good life could not result from "sexual intercourse with women."[11] The Epicurean school continued to exercise its influence on Rome. The Romans' best known Epicurean adherent was Lucretius (98–54 B.C.E.), who held that sexual desire was a sickness and advised the wise man to avoid the "madness" of love altogether.[12]

The Cynics, a somewhat less influential group than the Epicureans, but also dating from the fourth century B.C.E., expressed similar ideas. Diogenes, considered the founder of the school and known to most of us for his search for an honest person, sought to reduce human desires and appetites to only those that were absolutely indispensable to life. All others he tried to renounce. Diogenes praised those who were about to marry but refrained from doing so,[13] although his condemnation of marriage was not so much because it implied sexuality but because it imposed such a burden on a husband. Interestingly, most of these Greek philosophers wrote in terms of men, and not of women, giving the strong implication that women were essentially not that important in making the basic decisions about life.

Zeno (340–265 B.C.E.), the founder of Stoicism, patterned his personal life after that advocated by the Cynics,[14] but considerably modified their teachings. Later Stoics continued to admire the ascetic values advocated by individuals such as Diogenes, although they recognized that men and women were human beings living in a material environment. Thus instincts and emotions were not necessarily antagonistic to right living, provided they were kept in submission to the ruling principle. Sex was not bad in itself (in fact it was necessary for reproduction), but immoderation in sex as well as in other bodily activities was bad because it made individuals dependent upon their own body.[15] The Stoic watchwords became nature, virtue, decorum, and freedom from excess. Marriage was recognized and accepted, but passion in marriage was suspect. The only real justification for marriage was the necessity to propagate the race.

Some Stoics, such as the first century C.E. philosopher Musonius Rufus, went so far as to claim that marital intercourse was only permissible when the purpose was procreative; sexual intercourse for pleasure, even within marriage, was reprehensible.[16] His Stoic contemporary Seneca urged the wise man to love his wife with judgment, not with affection. "Let him control his impulses and not be born headlong into copulation." Seneca cautioned husbands to imitate the beasts and not copulate when their wives were pregnant, to avoid loving a wife as if she were an adultress.[17] Stoic concepts also influenced medical writers such as Celsus, who wrote in his *De medicina* that sexual intercourse should be neither avidly desired nor overly feared.

He added that if intercourse was performed infrequently it tended to revive people, but if performed frequently it weakened them.[18] In short, the Graeco-Roman medical, scientific, and philosophic teachings increasingly emphasized that sex was to be confined within the marriage relationship, where its purpose was to be procreative rather than pleasurable.

How much influence did these philosophic ideas have on ordinary Greeks and Romans? Probably very little since for the most part sexual practices were a matter not of civil law but of tradition. But tradition is influenced by a culture, and the major cultural determinant in earlier civilizations was religion. By the first century B.C.E., when the center of philosophical speculation in the Graeco-Roman world had shifted from Greece to Alexandria in Egypt, it is possible to see such speculations becoming strongly entrenched in religious teaching. Particularly influential on later Christian writers was Philo, an Alexandrian Jew born in the last quarter of the first century B.C.E. Though Philo accepted Jewish teaching on the necessity to procreate and replenish the earth, he followed the Graeco-Roman philosophic tradition that sexual intercourse could only be justified when there was hope of legitimate offspring. He described those who mated with their wives with no intent of begetting children as being "like pigs or goats."[19] Such an attitude led him to hold that those men who mated with barren women deserved condemnation, because in their pleasure-seeking they destroyed the "procreative germs" with deliberative purpose.[20]

Following Plato, Philo (ca. 30 B.C.E.–45 C.E.) conceived of sex in dualistic terms. The highest nature of man was asexual, in imitation of God, and it was only the irrational part of the soul that contained the categories of male and female and existed in the realm of the sexual. For Philo the original sin of Adam and Eve was sexual desire, and sexual pleasures were the "beginnings of wrongs and violation of the law."[21] He justified the Jewish custom of circumcision as necessary to curb man's sexual desires by making the penis less sensitive.[22]

Philo was just one of many writers active in Alexandria, but because he was Jewish he had particular influence on Judeo-Christian thought. Alexandria itself became a center of Neo-Pythagorean and Neoplatonist thinking. Although the Alexandrian writers did not necessarily advocate complete celibacy, they usually insisted that sexual relations be motivated only by the necessity of propagating the species and not by the "promptings of nature."[23]

The dominant figure in terms of Christian thought, however, was not Philo but Plotinus, who lived and wrote during the third century of the modern era. Plotinus was a religious mystic whose mysticism and piety were so dependent upon reason and intellectual balance that he refused to affiliate himself with any organized worship on the grounds that the gods must come to him and not vice versa. Plotinus differed from Plato in his great emphasis on religious and mystical orientation, insisting that the nature of the Real was obtainable only in a state of mystical ecstasy from which the last trace of sensible as well as intelligible experience had been erased. Immortality for him was not a personal matter, but rather a merger with the universal spirit. The path to redemption was long and gradual, taking eons of reincarnation to traverse, but in the end the soul could be united with the divine in indescribable ecstasy.[24]

The first step in achieving this union was to gain perfection in the practice of ordinary and practical virtues. This entailed living an upright life; participating nobly in worldly affairs; and being honest, generous, and friendly with others, all of whom were to be regarded as brothers and sisters.[25] The body and its needs were not to be despised and suppressed, but instead disciplined so that they did not distract the soul from its contemplation of higher things.[26] The key to human virtue lay in detachment from worldly (i.e., evil) desire; only this kind of indifference could put an individual out of reach of the caresses and ties of material life. Having achieved this kind of "apathy" from the material world, the soul was free to turn its attention upon the intelligible world, to identify with the path toward divine reason, on which truth lay.[27] By implication it was necessary to become indifferent to sex. The necessity of this indifference was clearly spelled out by Plotinus' pupil Porphyry (ca. 234–ca. 305 C.E.), who edited and expanded on his master's teachings. Porphyry condemned any kind of pleasure as sinful, including not only sexual intercourse under any condition, but theater-going, horse-racing, dancing, and eating meat.[28]

It was in this intellectual setting that Christianity appeared, and while these ascetic ideas are not particularly influential on the minds of the writers of the New Testament who, as a group, looked more to the Jewish than the Graeco-Roman tradition, the later disseminators of the Christian message, the so-called Fathers of the Church, drew heavily from these pagan writers. So, for that matter, did the rivals of Christianity, particularly the Gnostics, and since Christianity was competing with Gnosticism and other redemptive cults, it both was influenced by and exercised influence upon its rivals. In fact, it is not too far-fetched to suggest that within the various Christian communities, as the movement spread across the Mediterranean world, the degree of sexual repression among its members depended upon the practices of Christianity's leading rivals. This helps explain why, within Christianity, there was a narrow range of conflicting opinions from permitting copulation if motivated by a desire for children to an outright demand for celibacy for all church members. At times it seems that the Christian communities tried to gain status and adherents by outdoing their pagan rivals at ascetic practices. Such a hypothesis might also serve as a possible explanation for the statement by the physician Galen (ca. 129–190 C.E.) that the Christian community in Rome included men and women who, like the philosophers, refrained from "cohabitating all through their lives."[29]

Central to Gnostic speculation were the dualistic beliefs so much a part of Greek thought. Men and women had within them elements of both evil and good, the material and the spiritual, and their purpose on earth was to seek redemption through the secret knowledge, or *gnosis,* which the Gnostics claimed had been revealed only to them. This knowledge, as we can reconstruct it, concerned the supreme God, superior to God the Creator of this world. Recognition of this supreme God and living the life demanded by such a god ultimately allowed the individual to escape this alien world. Since on earth the spiritual souls were imprisoned in physical bodies, the key to salvation lay in freeing the spirit from corporeal bondage. Escape entailed abstaining from sex and adopting an ascetic life.[30] John T. Noonan, one of the leading Catholic experts on canon law and Christian sexuality, labeled Gnosticism a special mixture of "Christian theology and sexual morality."[31]

Gnosticism, however, apparently embraced conflicting prophets, and some Gnostics went to the opposite extreme, arguing that since human actions were not subject to moral law, every kind of sexual activity was to be considered permissible. At any rate, the early Church Fathers spent a good deal of their time trying to deal with the teachings of the Gnostics. While recent discoveries have given us new information about the Gnostics, most of what we know about them comes from antagonistic Christian writings of the early Church. It matters little whether these sources are a true reflection of what the various Gnostics taught, because in the long run it was the Christian interpretation of and reaction to them that was important in forming Christian ideas.

Clement of Alexandria, a second-century Church Father, said that one group of Gnostics, called the Marcionites, regarded nature as evil because it was created out of evil matter. They therefore refused to propagate in any world made under such conditions and abstained from all marriage.[32] Marcion (d. ca. 160 C.E.) himself was said to have denied that Jesus had been born of Mary in order that he would not have to admit the material flesh of Jesus.[33] Rather, he claimed, Jesus had descended from heaven as a fully formed adult without undergoing birth, boyhood, or temptation.[34] Marcion not only refrained from sexual relations, but prohibited marriage for all his followers,[35] limiting the sacraments of baptism and the Eucharist to virgins, widows, and those married couples who agreed together to "repudiate the fruit of their marriage."[36]

Sharing the ascetic antisexual outlook of Marcion was another second-century Gnostic leader, Julius Cassianus, who taught that men and women were most beastlike when they engaged in sexual intercourse.[37] He believed that the mission of Jesus in the world had been to save man from copulating:

> Let no one say that because we have these parts, that the female is shaped this way and the male that way, the one to receive, the other to give seed, sexual intercourse is allowed by God. For if this arrangement had been made by God, to whom we seek to attain, he would not have pronounced the eunuchs blessed [Matt. 19:12]; nor would the prophet have said that they are "not a fruitless tree" [Isa. 56:3–4], using the tree as an illustration of the man who chooses to emasculate himself of any such notion.[38]

Gnostic interpreters of Christianity based much of their antagonism to sex upon the Gospel According to the Egyptians, only fragments of which have survived.[39] According to the fragments, men were going to suffer and die as long as women bore children, and this was interpreted by the Gnostic Christians as an implicit injunction to defeat death by ceasing from procreation.[40]

In spite of the denunciation of such Gnostic interpretations by more orthodox Christians, Gnosticism continued to exercise great influence upon Christian belief, most notably through the influence of Justin Martyr (ca. 100–ca. 165 C.E.). A convert to Christianity after studying under Neo-Pythagorean teachers, Justin insisted that Christianity was the one supreme and true religion. Still, it is evident that he carried over into Christianity many of his own philosophical beliefs. Justin's concepts of the workings of Christianity were deeply influenced by his Neo-Pythagorean background.[41] For example, he contrasted the virtuous lives of Christians with their heathen contemporaries, describing in favorable terms a Christian youth who asked surgeons to emasculate him in order to better protect his bodily purity. Justin also pointed with pride to those Christians who renounced marriage in order to live in perfect continence.[42]

Almost equally influential was Justin Martyr's disciple, Tatian (ca. 120–173 C.E.), the leader of a group known as the Encratites, i.e., the "self-controlled," who taught that marriage was corruption, and who prohibited sexual intercourse, intoxicants, and meats.[43] Tatian preached that since sexual intercourse had been invented by the Devil, anyone who attempted to be married and remain Christian was attempting to serve two masters.[44] Individuals had to choose between sex and the Devil on the one hand and celibacy and Jesus on the other. Tatian's followers believed wedlock to be so polluted and foul that they made special efforts to encourage all Christians about to wed to promise to abandon filthy intercourse.[45] Tatian's greatest influence was on the Syrian Christian Church, which for a time in the third century held that the Christian life was unthinkable outside the bounds of virginity.[46]

By the end of the second century of the modern era, the organizational ability of the more orthodox Christians had begun to win the battle for control of Christianity over the groups we now associate with Gnosticism. By insisting upon the importance of the community as opposed to individuals, by emphasizing the teaching of the Hebrew Scriptures, yet incorporating pagan philosophy, orthodox Christianity eventually succeeded in overcoming the extremes of Gnosticism. Still, the Christian Church retained a strong undercurrent of hostility to sex, and in this respect was more like the ascetic Gnostic than the earthy Jews who were willing to accept the joys of intercourse. The extent of the Gnostic influence is indicated by the fact that one of the most avid opponents of Gnosticism, Tertullian (ca. 155–220 C.E.), seemingly adopted many of the Gnostic ideas. Tertullian stopped just short of condemning intercourse in marriage and actually seemed uncertain why God ever permitted it.[47] The Gnostic appeal rested in part on the similarity of the Gnostic attitude to the Christian stress on virginity, with the Gnostics only carrying to logical conclusion what many orthodox Christians seemed to want to believe. The latter, however, hesitated to go quite so far, if only because of the biblical sanction given to marriage, something which they felt they could not deny.

With the decline of Gnosticism, it would seem that Christianity should have been able to reassess its position and tone down some of its extreme antisexuality. That this did not happen was mainly due to the influence of St. Augustine (354–430 C.E.), who, in responding to a new religion, Manichaeism, a sort of Gnostic synthesis which for a time presented a renewed threat to Christian dominance, refortified the negative sexual attitudes of the second century. Manichaeism was based upon the teachings of the prophet

Mani (216–277 C.E.) who lived and was crucified in southern Babylonia. Mani incoporated into his teachings elements of Gnosticism, Christianity, and Zoroastrianism, as well as the philosophical ideas of the Neo-Pythagoreans and Neoplatonists. By the time of Mani's death his religion had spread to Egypt, Palestine, Rome, and soon afterward it appeared in Asia Minor, Greece, Illyria, Italy, and North Africa. Manichaeism was similar to Christianity in that it had a savior (Mani) and a canonical scripture (the seven books of Mani), claimed to be a universal religion, and had a hierarchy and apostles. Similarly, Manichaeism was a missionary faith and one of its converts, Augustine, was, for better or worse, later to become the most influential teacher in the Western Christian Church about sexuality and marriage.

Manichaeism was a dualistic religion combining science, philosophy, and religion in a new synthesis. Although claiming the authority of revelation, the Manichaeans also paid the highest deference to reason. Following the cosmology of Zoroastrianism and its offshoot Mithraism, the universe was divided into two portions, the Kingdom of Light and the Kingdom of Darkness, which were in juxtaposition, each reaching out into infinity. Light and darkness were both eternal and uncreated powers in everlasting opposition and conflict, although the God of Light alone was prescient, i.e., able to know the future. Eventually Light would overcome Darkness, and the purpose of man's life on earth was to release the light imprisoned in his material body. Light could be released by eating bread, vegetables, or fruit containing seeds, but could be more deeply imprisoned by eating meat or animal products. The release of light could also be effected or impeded by sexual actions since the seed of man contained light. Procreation to the Manicheans was an act of evil since it kept the light imprisoned within the material man. The true Manichean adherents were the Adepts, those who had been able to tame concupiscence and covetousness, to refrain from eating flesh, and to refuse to have sexual intercourse. Those who believed in the teaching of Mani but were not yet Adepts were regarded as Auditors, men and women of goodwill who could not yet contain themselves, but were trying to do so. In the meantime they supported the Adepts. The rest of humankind were classed as the sensual members of society; since they had rejected the gospel of Mani, they were totally lost in their wickedness.

The soul of God was constantly being freed from its physical fetters in the natural process of growth and death, but it was also continually being reencumbered by the act of procreation. Sexual intercourse chained the soul to Satan, denying it progress into the Kingdom of Light. Marriage was a sin; procreation was defined as defiling the divine substance. For the Manicheans sexual sins consisted not only in the overt acts of sex but in the impulse; thus marriage was not a greater offense than the desire to marry or to beget children. Within the hierarchy of membership, however, marriage was only a sin for the Adept. Auditors were permitted to follow their natural inclinations since Mani was the truth, the light, and the way, and no man was to be forced to do what he could not do. Eventually, it was believed, the Auditor would find his or her way to becoming an Adept.[48]

Augustine was an adherent of the Manichean faith for some eleven years but never reached the Adept stage, in part because of his difficulties with sex. He remained an Auditor, living with a mistress, and feeling uncomfortable about his inability to control his lustful desires. In fact Augustine's lack of restraint ultimately led to a crisis in his life which induced him to renounce Manichaeism and accept Christianity. Though he then rose rapidly in the Christian hierarchy, Augustine carried with him many of his Manichean ideas about sex. Perhaps inevitably, sexual intercourse for Augustine came to be regarded as the greatest threat to spiritual freedom. He wrote:

> I know nothing which brings the manly mind down from the heights more than a woman's caresses and that joining of bodies without which one cannot have a wife.[49]

With such attitudes Augustine had difficulty in accepting any kind of sex, even though he recognized that it had biblical justification. Finally he concluded that sexual intercourse could be justified only in terms of procreation.[50] Celibacy for him was the highest good, while intercourse remained in essence only animal lust; in marriage, however, and only in marriage, was intercourse justified because of the need for procreation. Marital intercourse itself could be both good and evil; it was only through procreation that the evil act became good. After examining various forms of intercourse as well as various positions, Augustine concluded that the proper position was the woman on the bottom with her face up and the man on top. He was opposed to any foreplay and insisted that only the proper orifice, the vagina, be used with the proper instrument, the penis. All other forms of sexual activity were evil.

With Augustine the basic sexual attitudes of the Christian Church were set. Virginity was the preferred state of existence, but for those unable to adapt to this state, marriage was permitted. Within marriage, intercourse was tolerated, but only for the purpose of procreation. Although the Christian Church never quite rejected sex altogether, its leaders felt uncomfortable in accepting it, and probably did so only because of the biblical sanctions. Beyond this, Christian ideas on sex were not primarily derived from any biblical teaching. Rather, they were based upon the intellectual and philosophical assumptions of the Graeco-Roman world, assumptions that must be regarded as the value system of a people lacking any real scientific knowledge. Inevitably Christians became—in spirit if not always in practice—ascetics, justifying sexual activity only in terms of progeny. Inevitably any kind of sexual activity not resulting in procreation had to be condemned. Moreover, even when children resulted from an act of intercourse, sex itself was not necessary something to be enjoyed but rather engaged in because it was God's will. The Church Fathers regarded sex as, at best, something to be tolerated, a necessary evil out of which procreation resulted. The dominant Western attitudes have been conditioned by these beliefs ever since. Americans, whether or not they are Christians, are heirs to this tradition, and understanding this background might help us to come to terms with our own ambiguous feelings about sex.

NOTES

1. Several pioneering studies were made in the nineteenth century of these Greek influences upon Christianity, although the sexual aspects were not so much emphasized. The most influential was Adolf Harnack's *Lehrbuch der Dogmengeschichte,* first published in 1886 and translated into English by Neil Buchanan under the title *The History of Dogma* (Boston: Roberts Brothers, 1895-1903). There was a one-volume summary of the work made by Harnack himself titled *Outlines of the History of Dogma,* first published in English in 1893 and since then often republished (Boston: Beacon Press, 1957). Also important was Edwin Hatch, *The Influence of Greek Ideas on Christianity,* first delivered as the Hibbert Lectures in England in 1888. It has been periodically republished since, including an edition with an introduction by Frederick C. Grant (New York: Harper and Company, 1957).

2. Morton S. Enslin, *The Ethics of Paul* (New York: Harper, 1930), p. 180.

3. See Jane Harrison, *Prolegomena to the Study of Greek Religion* (reprint New York: Meridian Books, 1955), chaps. IX, X, XI. There has been considerable scholarly work since Professor Harrison first wrote, but her work serves as a good starting point. For a classical reference see Plato, *Cratylus,* translated by H. N. Fowler (London: William Heinemann, 1953), 400C.

4. See Martin F. Nillson, *A History of Greek Religion* (New York: W. W. Norton, 1964), pp. 214–17, and W. K. C. Guthrie, *The Greeks and Their Gods* (Boston; Beacon Press, 1950), pp. 318–20. Joseph Campbell, *The Masks of God: Occidental Mythology* (New York: Viking Press, 1964), includes many of the stories.

5. See Aristotle, *Metaphysics* 1.5. 3–7 (1986A), edited and translated by Hugh Tredennick (London: William Heinemann, 1936).

6. E. R. Dodds, *The Greeks and the Irrational* (Boston: Beacon Press, 1957), p. 155. See Diogenes Laertius, *Lives of the Eminent Philosophers* 8. 1, edited and translated by R. D. Hicks (London: William Heinemann, 1950), for some of the statements about sex attributed to Pythagoras.

7. Plato, *Symposium* 211B, edited and translated by W. R. M. Lamb (London: William Heinemann, 1953).

8. Plato, *Phaedrus* 246–47, edited and translated by Harold North Fowler (London: William Heinemann, 1953).

9. Ibid., 250–53.

10. For some surviving fragments from Democritus see J. M. Robinson, *An Introduction to Early Greek Philosophy* (Boston: Houghton Mifflin, 1968), pp. 227–30.

11. Diogenes Laertius, *Lives of the Eminent Philosophers* 10. 1; 118, 132.

12. Lucretius, *De rerum natura* 4.1052–1120, edited and translated by W. H. D. Rouse (London: William Heinemann, 1959).

13. Diogenes Laertus, 6. 2. 29. See also M. I. Finley, *Aspects of Antiquity* (New York: The Viking Press, 1968), p. 94.

14. Diogenes Laertius, *Lives of the Eminent Philosophers* 6. 6.

15. A good discussion of this appears in Epictetus, *Discourses,* edited and translated by W. A. Oldfather, 2 vols. (London: William Heinemann, 1956, 1959), although no particular passage can be cited.

16. A. C. Van Geytenbeck, *Musonius Rufus and Greek Diatribe,* translated by B. L. Hijamans, Jr. (Assen, The Netherlands: Van Gorcum & Company, 1963), pp. 71–77.

17. Seneca, *Fragments,* in vol. III of *Opera,* no. 85, edited by Frederich G. Haase (Leipzig: Teubner, 1853). The passage is found in Jerome, *Against Jovinian* (1–30), and has not survived in any other form. Haase claims the passage came from a lost Senecan treatise, *De matrimonio* (*On Marriage*).

18. Celsus, *De medicina* 2.1.4, edited and translated by W. G. Spencer, 3 vols. (London: William Heinemann, 1935–38).

19. Philo, *On the Special Laws* (*De specialibus legibus*) 3. 113, edited and translated by F. H. Colson (London: William Heinemann, 1958).

20. Ibid., 3.34–36.

21. Philo, *On the Creation,* 69–70, 151, 162, edited and translated by F. H. Colson and G. H. Whittaker (London: William Heinemann, 1963).

22. Philo, *On the Special Laws* 3.6 (37–42), and Richard A. Baer, Jr., *Philo's Use of the Categories Male and Female* (Leiden: E. J. Brill, 1970), p. 58.

23. See, for example, Ocellus Lucanus, *De universi natura,* sec. 44, text and commentary by Richard Harder (Berlin: Weidmannsche, 1926), pp. 121–26, and K. S. Guthrie, *Numenius of Apamea* (London: George Bell and Sons, 1917), p. 133.

24. Plotinus, *The Enneads* 5.3: par. 1–9; 1.6: par. 9, edited and translated by Stephen MacKenna, revised by B. S. Page (London: Faber and Faber, 1956).

25. Ibid., 1.3: par. 6, 4: par. 1.

26. Ibid., 1.4: par. 1.

27. Ibid., 1.3: par. 1; 5.9: par. 1.

28. Porphyry, *Abstinence from Animal Foods* 1.45; 4.1, 20, translated from the Greek by Thomas Taylor (London: Thomas Rodd, 1823). There are many other references.

29. R. Walzer, *Galen on Jews and Christians* (London; Oxford University Press, 1949), p. 65.

30. An early pioneer in the study of Gnosticism was G. R. S. Mead, *Fragments of a Faith Forgotten: The Gnostics* (1900; reprint New York: University Books, n.d.). The discovery of Coptic manuscripts at Nag Hammadi in Egypt in 1945 as well as subsequent discoveries in the area revolutionized the study and gave renewed emphasis to the influence of Gnosticism on Christianity. Particularly important is the Gospel of Thomas, which some now regard as important as the canonical gospels of the Christian New Testament. See, for example Jean Doresse, *The Secret Books of the Egyptian Gnostics* (London: Hollis & Carter, 1958), and Kurt Rudolph, *Gnosis: The Nature & History of Gnosticism* (New York: Harper and Row, 1984). Most helpful is *The Nag Hammadi Library: In English,* edited by James M. Robinson and translated by a number of scholars (New York: Harper and Row, 1977).

31. John T. Noonan, *Contraception: A History of Its Treatment by Catholic Theologians and Canonists* (Cambridge, Mass.: Belknap Press of Harvard University, 1966) p. 58.

32. Clements, *Stromata* 3. 3 (12), in vol. II of *The Ante-Nicene Fathers,* edited and translated by Alexander Roberts and James Donaldson (Grand Rapids, Mich.: Eerdmans Publishing Company, 1961). It is worth a comment that the nineteenth-century editors refused to translate this section into English but instead put it in Latin. There is a more recent translation of the third book in John F. L. Oulton and Henry Chaduck, *Alexandrian Christianity* (Philadelphia: Westminster Press, 1954).

33. Tertullian, *On the Flesh of Christ,* cap. 1, in vol. III of *The Ante-Nicene Fathers,* edited by Alexander Roberts and James Donaldson. American ed. editor A. Cleveland Coke (reprint Grand Rapids, Mich.: W. B. Erdemans Publishing Company, 1966).

34. Tertullian, *Against Marcion* 4.7, in vol. III of *The Ante-Nicene Fathers.*

35. Ibid., 5.7.

36. Ibid., 4.34.

37. Clement, *Stromata* 3.17 (102).

38. Ibid., 3.9 (64).

39. There is a Gospel of the Egyptians in the Nag Hammadi collection, but though similar in content it does not correspond to the surviving fragments mentioned here. See Doresse, *The Secret Books,* p. 181. See also Robinson, *Nag Hammadi Library,* pp. 195–205.

40. Ibid., 3.9 (64).

41. Arthur O. McGiffert, *A History of Christian Thought,* 2 vols. (New York: Charles Scribner's Sons, 1932), 1:100. See also Justin Martyr, *Dialogue with Trypho,* 1.2, in vol. I of *The Ante-Nicene Fathers.*

42. Justin Martyr, *Apology* 1.29, in vol. I of *the Ante-Nicene Fathers;* see also *Dialogue with Trypho* 100, and Erwin R. Goodenough, *The Theology of Justin Martyr* (Amsterdam: Philo Press, 1923), pp. 181–82, 235–39.

43. Eusebius, *Ecclesiastical History* 4.29, edited and translated by Kirsopp Lake (London: William Heinemann, 1959); Irenaeus, *Against Heresies* 1.28, in vol. I of *The Ante-Nicene Fathers.*

44. Clement, *Stromata* 3.12 (8).

45. *Acts and Martyrdom of Andrew,* in vol. VIII of *The Ante-Nicene Fathers,* p. 512, and *Acts of Thomas* in vol. VIII of *The Ante-Nicene Fathers,* p. 537. See also William E. Phipps, *Was Jesus Married?* (New York: Harper & Row, 1970), p. 133.

46. Arthur Vööbus. *History of Asceticism in the Syrian Orient* (Louvain: Corpus Scriptorum Christianorum Orientalium, 1958), I: 69.

47. Tertullian, *On Monogamy,* cap. 3, in vol. IV of *The Ante-Nicene Fathers.*

48. See Henri-Charles Puech, *Le Manichéisme* (Paris: Civilisations du Sud [S.A.E.P.], 1949). The best sources are the various writings of Augustine, particularly *The Way of Life of the Manichaeans* 18 (65–66), translated by Donald A. Gallagher and Idella J. Gallagher in vol. 56 of the *Fathers of the Church* (Washington, D.C.: Catholic University Press, 1966). Also invaluable is the *Fihrist of al-Nadim,* 2 vols. (New York: Columbia University Press, 1970). See also Noonan, *Contraception,* pp. 107–30.

49. Augustine, *Concerning the Nature of God,* cap. xvii, in *Basic Writings of St. Augustine,* translated by A. H. Newman and edited by Whitney J. Oates (New York; Random House, 1948), p. 455.

50. Augustine, *Soliloquies* 1.20 (17) in vol. 1 of *Fathers of the Church,* translated by Thomas F. Gilligan (New York: Cima Publishing Company, 1948ff).

2

Alternative Views of Sexual Activity

The deeper one delves into Western attitudes, the more apparent it becomes that the dual nature of the human being, with the sexual aspect being set apart as evil, keeps reappearing in different forms. This Greek dualistic view, as adopted by Christianity, however, is not the only possible approach; even among the ancients there were alternative views which ultimately led other cultures to develop different attitudes toward sex than ours. Even those cultures that saw male and female as opposites, as the ancient Chinese did, never emphasized that conflict between the spiritual and the material so prominent the Greek-oriented West. Instead the Chinese accentuated the inherent unity of the opposing forces. This is especially evident in Taoism, the ancient indigenous religion of China, which continued to exercise considerable influence upon Chinese thought even after Buddhism and Confucianism had become more prominent.

CHINA

In the Chinese view, men and women composed a miniature worldview (microcosm) functioning in the same way as the world at large (macrocosm). The sexual union of the male and female was a repetition of the larger interaction of heaven and earth. The *I Ching* (*Book of Changes*), one of the oldest of Confucian classics, states:

> There is an intermingling of the genial influence of heaven and earth, and transformation in its various forms abundantly proceeds. There is an intercommunication of seeds between male and female, and transformation in its living types proceeds.[1]

29

As in Western thought, heaven was regarded as male and the earth female, but the simile was carried further. Clouds were the vaginal secretion of the lining of the womb, essential for allowing the heavenly sperm, the rain, into the womb of the earth. It was from the union of these two forces, heaven and earth, male and female, that all life originated.

Ultimately the Chinese used the terms *yin* and *yang* to describe these dual cosmic forces. Yang was heaven, yin was earth, yang the sun, yin the moon, yang male, yin female. The two forces came together through intercourse, the principle of universal life. In the *I Ching,* one of the earliest and most important of ancient Chinese classics, we find the core of Chinese philosophical thinking. This book deals with the interpretation of eight trigrams and sixty-four hexagrams of which the hexagram symbolizing sexual union is a key. A combination of the trigram *k'an* (water, clouds, or woman) on top and the trigram *li* (fire, light, or man) on the bottom, it is written thus:

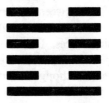

This hexagram was believed by the Chinese to indicate that everything was in its proper place, with the strong lines in the strong places, and the weak lines in the weak places, thus emphasizing the combination of perfect harmony of man and woman complementing and completing each other.[2]

Sexual union was pictured as the intermingling of heaven and earth—absolutely essential to achieve harmony as well as a happy and healthy sex life. It was the operation of the two opposing forces which produced universal phenomena and determined human conduct. Though male and female were dominated by different essences, within the human body there was both yin and yang, the yin essence being more important in women, the yang in men. The body surfaces of both sexes were regarded as yang, the interior yin; yang was the back part, yin the front. Yin was in the liver, heart, spleen, lungs, and kidneys, while yang was in the gallbladder, stomach, large and small intestines, and the "warmer," a term interpreted by some modern scholars to mean the lymphatic system.

Medically it was important for yin and yang to be kept in balance.

The aura of the yang nourished the mind and influenced the muscles; if there was an insufficient amount or if it was overpowered by the yin, coldness would set in, swelling would occur, ulcers would penetrate the flesh, the blood vessels would be weakened, and the patient would become full of anxiety and fears. Eventually the body would waste away until the person died. On the other hand, if the yin essence became too strong, the patient would become hotter, perspire incessantly, grow increasingly nervous and apprehensive, and eventually these reactions would also result in death. The key to keeping the yin and yang in balance was sexual intercourse, an essential part of human activity.[3]

The ancient Chinese believed that at birth an individual was filled with the principles of primordial yang and yin. Both would grow as the body grew until maturity, when the yang ceased to grow and began to wane. The yin, however, continued to increase even when the yang had ceased to grow; this imbalance between the yin and yang was the ultimate cause of death from old age. If a man could slow down the waning of his yang, he would be able to live much longer than average; to do this, he needed to continually replenish his yang, which was possible through sexual intercourse. From the male point of view the highest achievement possible in intercourse involved the conservation of as much of the seminal essence (*ching*), or the divine element, as possible by causing the *ching* to return (*huang ching*). This was because yang was produced in the semen, and the loss of undue amounts of semen in intercourse could prove draining upon the male unless he learned to use it to his advantage. Correct methods of intercourse were thus essential to strengthen the male's vitality and prolong his life. This entailed absorption of some of the woman's yin essence, of which she had an abundant supply, while in the process conserving his own yang. Moreover, the yin force gained from women fed the yang force in man, thus allowing the male to remain in good health, live a long life, and beget male children. Women, for their part, probably tried to obtain the yang element from the male, but the sex books that have survived were all written from a male point of view.

The secrets of sexual intercourse set forth by Taoist teachers were intended to increase the amount of life-giving *ching* through sexual stimulus, while at the same time avoiding as much as possible any loss of the precious seminal essence. This meant that except at those times on the calendar considered to be right for conception, the male was to avoid depositing semen in the female's vagina. Instead he was to practice *coitus reservatus,* keeping his penis inserted but avoiding ejaculation. This entailed practicing *huan ching pu nao,* literally, "the method of making the semen return to restore the brain." Men were taught to put pressure on the urethra at the base of the scrotum and anus at the moment of ejaculation, an action which we know diverts the seminal secretion into the bladder where it is later excreted with the urine. The Taoists, however, did not understand modern physiology. Since by observation the semen was no longer present, they held that this method, when combined with positive thinking, could encourage the seminal essence to ascend to the brain where it rejuvenated or revived the upper parts of the body.[4] If at the same time the male could arouse the woman to orgasm, his yang would be further strengthened by her yin infusion.

To explain the secrets of intercourse, a number of manuals were written, known collectively as the *fang chung,* literally "inside the bedchamber." The oldest yet discovered date from the second century B.C.E., but we know the tradition is older than that. Three of these were found in 1973 at the Ma-wang-tui Hans Tomb, No. 3. Their titles are *Ten Questions and Answers (Shi-wan), Methods of Intercourse between Yin and Yang (He-yin-yang-fang),* and *Lectures on the Super Tao in the Universe (Tian-xia-zhi-tao-tan).*[5] Prior to this discovery, we possessed only fragments of these ancient texts. Even later manuals are preserved mostly in Japanese versions because in the twelfth and thirteenth centuries China entered a period of prudishness under Neo-Confucian rulers. The result was that sexual teaching became the cult secret of a few, taught only to adepts, and this information was kept hidden from the general public. Fortunately, several works had been translated into Japanese, and it is from these versions that Taoist teachings could be reconstructed.

The most valuable treatise in the Japanese collections is that by Tamba Yasuyori, dating from the late tenth century, titled *Ishimpo (Essence of the Medical Prescriptions).*[6] Some thirty coital positions are described in the *Ishimpo,* most named after animals that metamorphically seem the most suitable. Positions are described, for example, as the Shifting Turning Dragon, the Galloping Steed, the Paired Dance of the Female Phoenix, and the Dog of Early Autumn.[7] The leading character in most of the sex manuals is the Yellow Emperor, Huang-ti, a mythological character believed by the Chinese to have taught humans the various earthly skills. In addition to the Yellow Emperor several female participants are usually involved, identified by such names as Woman Plain, Woman Selective, or Woman Profound. These women belong to the immortals, since they reversed the process prescribed for males by engaging in coitus with innumerable virgin boys when their youthful yang was at its height and before they had learned the secret of *coitus reservatus*. The importance of sexual intercourse was explained by the Woman Profound:

> Between Heaven and Earth, movements must [accord with] the female and male elements. The male element gets the female one and is converted; the female element gets the male one and is moved. The female element and the male element must operate in mutuality. Therefore, if the male [penis] feels, firm and strong, and the female [vagina] moves, open and extended, two life forces exchange emissions and flowing penetrates mutuality.[8]

Though China, like the West, went through periods of greater or lesser public prudery, it now seems clear that individually the Chinese always enjoyed sex and were never plagued with the guilt that seemingly afflicted the West. There were few limitations on the kind of sex in which a person could engage. Oral-genital contacts were allowed, although fellatio was not to result in a complete emission because then there would be no compensating yin essence from the woman. Cunnilingus, however, met with approval at all times by the male writers of the sex manuals since it not only prepared the woman for the act of sex but also procured yin essence from the woman. Anal intercourse with a woman was permitted since a man could obtain yin essence in this way as well as through the vagina. Male masturbation was frowned upon because of the possible loss of yang essence, but female masturbation was more or less ignored if not encouraged. Homosexuality was tolerated.[9] In fact, the only people viewed with contempt and profound suspicion were those who professed celibacy or voluntarily abstained from sexual intercourse.[10] In sum, the ancient Chinese, in spite of their recognition of opposing male and female elements, developed quite different views of sexuality than those that became dominant in the West.

INDIA

Taking still another viewpoint were the people of the Indian subcontinent, where Hindu influence has been dominant. Hindu mythology, in fact, taught that the literature of sex was of divine origin, derived from a collection of all knowledge compiled by Prājapati, the supreme god, creator of heaven and earth.[11] The history of this transmission of sexual information was recorded in the fifth century C.E. by Vātsyāyana, whose *Kāmasutra* is the oldest surviving sex manual we possess. According to tradition, Vātsyāyana was an ascetic celibate who wrote an encyclopedic survey of the ways of women in order that men might obtain the maximum pleasure from sexual activity. Though he admittedly lacked personal experience in the matter of sexual intercourse, Vātsyāyana was able to write about it so expertly because he had been instructed in such matters by the gods. His writing set a pattern for sex manuals and a number of others have survived, although for the most part they are based on more worldly experience. The more prominent titles include *Kuttani-mata* (*Lessons of a Prostitute*), *Samaya-mātrika* (*Prostitute's Breviary*), *Rati-rahasya* (*The Mysteries of Passion*), *Pānchasāyaka* (*Five Arrows [of the Love God]*), *Ananga Ranga* (*Theater of the Love God*), *Nagara-sarasva* (*Complete Citizen*), *Rati Mānjarī* (*Blossoms of Love*), and *Rati-ratna-pradīpakā* (*Love Jewel Lamp*). There are literally hundreds of lesser known manuals.[12]

If only because of the number of erotic classics available and the belief that they were associated with gods, it is evident that the peoples of the Indian subcontinent had a much more positive view of sex than the Christians of the West. Further evidence for this more positive attitude comes from the *Vedas,* the primary scriptures of Hinduism which, according to Hindu tradition, have existed since time itself began. Sexual arousal was in fact responsible for creation, since in the beginning there was neither existence nor nonexistence. Then the One breathed airless by self-impulse, and sexual desire made its appearance:

> In the beginning there was desire,
>   which was the primal germ of the mind;
> the sages searching in their hearts with wisdom
>   found in nonexistence the king of existence.[13]

The *Atharva Veda,* the fourth of the Hindu Vedas, includes a number of spells, incantations, and charms designed to help or hinder lovemaking. There are charms for being successful in love, spells for the recovery of virility, and incantations to put a household to sleep in order that a lover might steal into the house of his beloved unobserved. Conversely, there are spells to make a man impotent, to keep a rival a spinster, and so forth. The explicitness of some of these can be illustrated by the spell devised to deprive a man of his virility:

. . . turn this man for me today into a eunuch
that wears his hair dressed!
. . . Turn him into a eunuch that wears his
hair dressed, and into one that wears a hood!
Then Indra with a pair of stones shall break
his testicles both. . . . O eunuch, into a eunuch
thee I have turned; O castrate, into a castrate
thee I have turned; O weakling, into a weakling
thee I have turned! . . . As women break reeds
for a mattress with a stone, thus do I break thy
member.[14]

Hinduism, however, was not without sex prohibitions, including those against intercourse with sisters by the same mother and with the wives of a son or a friend, as well as against rape and against intercourse with a menstruating woman.[15] The reason for most of these prohibitions, however, is that the acts enjoined resulted in ceremonial impurity; however, those who violated the prohibitions could purify themselves by performing the prescribed ablutions.

Sex in Hinduism, in addition to being the means of procreation, was also regarded as a source of pleasure, of power, and even of magic. The various sex manuals usually pay little attention to the procreative aspects of sex but devote considerable attention to the others, particularly to ways of gaining pleasure.[16] Pleasure, however, is defined primarily from a male point of view. Women were regarded as voluptuous creatures who were fair game for the more predatory male. This appears most obviously in the handbooks devoted to *stritantra,* literally the female lore; these list the different kinds of females, outline the proper behavior for women in the sex act, and examine various female functions and duties.

The *stritantra* explain that sexual desire in a woman is dependent upon several things, including her education, life experience, physical type, and the stimuli necessary to arouse her. This last is regarded as the function of the male who is supposed to acquire a thorough knowledge of the female's erogenous zones—the breasts, nipples, nape of the neck, folds of the buttocks, the labia, and the clitoris. In some women, there are special sensitive areas such as the earlobe, the middle of the palm, the navel, the anus, or the arch of the foot. Stimulation of these "passion pulse areas" not only helps to bring about orgasm but ensures the birth of a son, an act as much desired in India as it is in China.[17]

In the sexual handbooks lovemaking is often referred to as a refined form of combat, with the man attacking, the woman resisting. Through this subtle interplay of advance and retreat, assault and defense, desires were mutually built up. Unlike war, however, the final result was a "delightful victory" for both parties. At the height of passion, consciousness was enhanced by intensive stimulation, often through sadistic acts, since the senses were believed to have become so dulled to the unpleasantness of pain that the subject found sharp delight in it. The handbooks term this combat *prahanana*: during this phase it was possible to bite, scratch, pull the partner's hair, and beat or slap with the palm of the hand, the back of the hand, the side of the hand, a half-open or closed fist, on the shoulders, back, chest, and buttocks, although partners were cautioned against becoming too violent.[18] As in China, postures are often named after animals, but the positions are more numerous. Vātsyāyana is said to have described eighty-four different postures, while another commentator listed 729 different variations, although not all could be performed by a single couple. When so many positions are named, the differences between them become almost infinitesimal. For example, when a woman engages in coitus standing on her feet but with her hands on the floor like a four-footed animal and her lover mounts her like a bull, it is called the congress of a cow. With only slight variations it becomes the congress of the goat, deer, ass, cat, tiger, elephant, and so forth. In general, the positions are divided into categories according to the postures involved, that is standing, leaning against a pillar, sitting, half reclining, reclining, flexed, extended, face to face, front to back, lateral or sideways, astride, upside down, and reverse. Movements accompanying the postures are described as being like a pair of tongs, spinning the top, biting the board, churning the milk, swinging, squeezing, and so on.[19]

Sex also had mystical or magical powers. In its profound esoteric sense, the *yoni* (female genitalia) was the sacred field in which the seed of all creatures was planted and nourished. It was the emblem of the ultimate and the keeper of the great mysteries, so much so that portions of the female anatomy were compared to the parts of the sacrificial altar. The hips and the haunches were like the sacrificial grounds, the genitalia the altar, the pubic hair the grass, and sexual intercourse itself a higher form of worship.[20]

The sex act was also a psychospiritual communion. The rich, deep fulfillment of love between a man and a woman created a condition of happiness so natural, so simple, yet so real, that it was the best of all earthly states. Inevitably it was also employed by the mystics as a symbol of divine communion. Sex in its transcendent and esoteric aspects was believed to be a way to discover the hidden truths of the universe, thus making redemption possible through pleasure, although to achieve this it was necessary to transcend the carnal state of sexual activity and rise above passion. To realize such a state of absoluteness, the male had to conceive of himself as the male deity, then by worship he transfigured his partner into his divine female counterpart, and ultimately they united physically, mentally, and spiritually.

Within Hinduism there were so many varying interpreters of the esoteric meaning of sex that numerous sects arose advocating different interpretations. Some sects taught that promiscuous intercourse was an act of devotion. The highest union was that resulting in the total breakdown of distinctions between one woman and another, so that one's sister, daughter, or even mother was the same as any other woman. There was no evil or good in sex, just as there was no deed that could not be done, and no woman who was not available for enjoyment.[21] Other Hindu sects, including the more orthodox, advocated asceticism and abstinence, although not total celibacy since human beings were meant to reproduce. The great twentieth-century Hindu leader, Mohandas Gandhi, however, came to advocate *bramacharya* (continence) for his devoted disciples. Traditionally then, within orthodox Hinduism, there has been a double standard.

Since it was widely believed that an unmarried woman posed enormous dangers, the Hindus emphasized that all adult women should be married. Moreover, a woman with her hymen still intact at marriage would, it was thought, damage the penis of her husband, perhaps so severely that he could never again engage in intercourse. Thus defloration was widely practiced and it began early in the life of a girl. Mothers, through a process known as deep cleaning, would penetrate deep into the vagina of their female children, tearing the hymen and enlarging the vaginal opening. Menstruating virgins were regarded as particularly dangerous, but even married women during their menses were regarded as unclean, and a man who touched such a woman became as impure as if he had touched a corpse.[22]

Though masturbation generally was frowned upon as wasting seed, some cults encouraged it; in fact, within the Indian subcontinent almost all forms of sexual behavior were practiced or encouraged by one sect or another. Since there was a general belief that all desire was holy if the mind was pure, some adepts tried to demonstrate their purity by engaging in activities that revolted them personally. For example, some tantric rituals involved acts of necrophilia during which the adept meditated upon death, corpses, decay, and putrefaction by sitting in a graveyard or cremation ground with a skull pressed against his genitals. In another ritual he lay prostate or squatted upon the cadaver and then ate the flesh. In the so-called black ritual the adept sat astride the body of a newly dead male and animated the body by occult means until the penis became erect and ejaculated.[23] In short, the peoples of the Indian subcontinent embraced sex, gave it a mystical connotation, and although attitudes varied from sect to sect, almost anything in the sexual field received approval from some segments of Hindu society. It is as if Hinduism had turned the ideas of the West almost totally on their head until what was desirable in the West became undesirable in India, and vice versa.

ISLAM

Even within the Jewish or Graeco-Roman cultures, there were alternative views that Christianity could have taken toward sex. This is most evident from what happened in Islam which has much more in common with Christianity and Judaism than with the religions of India or China. Islam, in fact, looks to the Jewish Scriptures in much the same way that Christianity does, and while it includes references to Jesus, John the Baptist, and other Christian figures, it is far more sex-positive than Christianity. Intercourse in Islam, in fact, is regarded as a good religious deed. As the Koran states:

> Your women are a tilth [field] to you (to cultivate) so go to your tilth
> as ye will, and send (good deeds) before you for your souls, and fear
> Allah and know that ye will (one day) meet him. Give glad tidings to
> believers (O Muhammad).[24]

As far as morals are concerned, Islam in general emphasizes that avoidance of excess is a virtue,[25] and this applies to sexual matters as well. What constitutes moderation, however, is culturally defined: according to the Koran, moderation for a male meant that he should limit his activities to his legal wives and concubines. Nonetheless, Allah was merciful and forgiving, and would put away the guilt of the worst actions, rewarding the best actions of those who believed. Most commentators on Islam seem to hold that a single punishment for a sex act would answer for all previous repetitions of the act, since punishment was visualized as a way of deterring people from the perpetuation of things that God had forbidden. If such action could not be prevented by a single punishment, there was little hope that multiple punishments would be any more successful. The matter then became something between Allah and the individual, not one for the state to continually punish.[26]

In some ways, however, Islamic sexual mores are similar to those of Christianity. Intercourse between persons who are not in a state of legal matrimony or concubinage is a sin; chastity is the mark of a believer.[27] Adultery is a sin, particularly for women, and the punishments are harsh, although the Koran makes such activities difficult to prove since it requires four witnesses to the act. Women found guilty of adultery and fornication are to be locked up in their houses until they die.[28] Later, death by stoning becomes the normative punishment for an adulterous woman. A husband who catches his wife in adulterous relations, however, is allowed to testify four times in lieu of four witnesses,[29] and if the husband, finding his wife and her paramour *in flagrante delicto,* kills them, he is not liable for punishment. Adultery by the husband, on the other hand, is not regarded as particularly evil conduct. The hostility to female adultery seems to derive more from a concept of wives as property belonging to their husbands than from any hostility to the sex act. Obviously Islam, like most religions, tolerated a double standard.

Divorce was and still is easy in Islam, at least for the husband, thus allowing the male to divorce an unattractive woman and marry a more attractive one. Moreover, some of the prohibitions against intercourse outside of legal matrimony could be avoided through the practice of *mut'a,* a short-term marriage. Often prostitutes entered into such relationships, and this had the advantage of making the offspring of irregular sexual liaisons legitimate.[30] Some Islamic states no longer permit *mut'a,* and some have made divorce easier for the woman as well.

Masturbation was not particularly condemned in Islamic countries. In fact, some commentators on the Koran have gone so far as to justify it as necessary to alleviate excessive lust:

> Who practices it to alleviate his overexcessive lust which occupies totally his heart and he is single and has no woman I hope that he would be excused and no punishment would be inflicted upon him, but he who practices it to arouse himself sexually is deemed a sinner.[31]

No specific punishment is mentioned for homosexual conduct in the Koran, although in the Koran the story of Lot and the Sins of Sodom and Gomorrah are clearly equated with men lusting after men instead of women.[32] The destruction of the cities, however, was never utilized by Islamic commentators as it was by the Christians as an absolute condemnation of such sexual activity. In fact, most commentators tended to be fairly specific, with the result that, if the Koran did not specifically condemn an action, it was regarded as permissible. Among the specific prohibitions, usury, adultery, homicide, theft, and the drinking of wine, the only "sex crime" is adultery and, as indicated, it is more of a violation of property than a sex crime.[33]

In practice, homosexuality was not punished with any great severity and its prevalence among Islamic peoples has often been noted.[34] Part of the difficulty was that Islam had created a dilemma for itself. By allowing polygamy and concubinage it decreased the supply of available women, and by strictly segregating men and women it also made it difficult to establish normal relations between the two sexes. Marriage was not for love but to establish a family and to produce children. Since fornication and adultery were frowned upon, prostitution, homosexuality, and masturbation were tolerated as alternate means of sexual relief, and since Islam regarded sex as good and not evil, both prostitution and homosexuality prospered.

Some indication of the general sexual attitude appears in the *Qābūs-nāma* (*Mirror for Princes*), written in the eleventh century by Kai Kā'ūs ibn Iskander as a guide for his son. In a chapter titled "On Taking One's Pleasure," he cautioned his son not to indulge in sexual intercourse indiscriminately since it was only the beast who indulged every time the thought occurred. Man, on the other hand, had to select the proper season, if only to preserve a distinction between himself and a beast. But if the season was proper, the boy was advised not to "confine" his inclinations to one particular sex since both women and youths offer enjoyment. While excessive copulation was harmful, complete abstention also posed dangers, and so Iskander ended up advising the young men to engage in intercourse in "accordance with appetite and not as a matter of course."[35]

Once one engaged in intercourse there was no prescribed position, although the male superior, or "man on top," was preferred. Unlike Christianity, which attempted to limit sexual activity to vagina and penis, Islamic writers regarded any orifice as suitable for sex. There is an old Arabic saying that a woman is "apt for two tricks" which is usually taken to mean that both vaginal and anal intercourse were possible. Oral-genital contacts were also permissible, as was mutual masturbation; in fact, as long as the couple eventually had children, there were almost no restrictions except on bestiality. Even this act might be condoned if done in order to prevent a greater crime.[37]

Islam did not escape entirely from the Greek Neoplatonic and Neo-Pythagorean traditions that were so influential in forming Christian thought. Generally, however, this tradition was confined within the movement known as Sufism, and even here, it never went to quite the extremes of Christianity. Though the Sufis, like the Gnostics and the Manicheans, believed that the soul was confined to a material cage (the body), they never made a distinction between good and evil. In their mind there could be no difference, since both were reduced to Unity, with God being the real author of the acts of mankind. One Sufi mystic, when questioned as to what was evil, answered, "Evil art thou," and when further questioned as to the worst evil, replied, "Thou when thou knowest it not."[38]

Sufism followed not just one path to salvation, but many, with competing sects of Sufis advocating different ways. One group known as the Malamatis deliberately acted in ways to incur blame, thus compounding virtue with vice, or vice versa. Another sect, the Mūhābīyāh, maintained a community of property and women. Other groups refused to hold themselves responsible for sins committed by the body, since this was only a miserable robe of humanity encircling the pure in spirit.[39]

Generally, however, Islam accepted sex as a positive good. Even when certain forms of conduct were prohibited, the prohibition was not necessarily strictly observed since there might be extenuating circumstances. In general Islam emphasized tolerance; believers who strayed were never entirely regarded as lost souls provided they eventually repented. Sufism encompassed many concepts found in Gnosticism and Manichaeism, but Islam never felt called upon to modify its own version of sexuality to meet these challenges as Christianity did; rather it was content to allow Sufism to exist as a viable alternative.

This chapter is simply an introduction to what might be called comparative sexology. There is a tremendous variety out there. The ancient Greeks, for example, not only tolerated but encouraged the love of adolescent boys by older men. In parts of New Guinea, males are initiated into manhood by sucking the penis of an older man. In parts of Africa, women undergo circumcision involving removal of the clitoris (clitorectomy), the labia minora, and the labia majora, and sewing up the entrance to the vagina. In India, male members of a cult that worships Rādhā, the favorite consort of the god Krishna, dress like women and affect the behavior, movements, and habits of women, including menstruation. Many of them in the past emasculated themselves, and all were supposed to play the part of women during intercourse, allowing themselves to be penetrated as an act of devotion.[40] Obviously there were and are many different approaches to sex that the Western world could have adopted; but the fact that it opted for one emphasizing a distrust of sexual activity has afflicted Western culture with an underlying hostility toward sex that has been challenged only in the twentieth century—a challenge we shall examine in later chapters. We shall also review some of the effects these sex-negative attitudes have had on law, literature, science, and research on sex in general.

NOTES

1. *I Ching*, translated by James Legge, in *The Sacred Books of the East*, edited by F. Max Müller, 2d ed., vol. 16 (Oxford: Claredon Press, 1899), *The Great Appendix*, section II, chap 5, par. 43, p. 393. The Chinese name for this section is *To Chuan* or the *Hsi Tz'us-Chuan*, literally the "Commentary on the Appended Judgments." There is a slightly different version in Cary F. Bayne's English translation of Richard Wilhelm's German edition in the Bollingen Series, 3d ed., XIX (Princeton: Princeton University Press, 1967), Section II, chap 5, 13, pp. 342-43. Numerous other translations are available.

2. *I Ching*, LXIII

3. See Heinrich Wallnöfer and Ana Rottasucher, *Chinese Folk Medicine*, translated by Marion Palmedo (New York: Crown, 1965), pp. 10-12, 93-94.

4. See Joseph Needham, assisted by Wang Ling, *Science and Civilization in China*, vol. 2 (Cambridge: Cambridge University Press, 1956), pp. 147-50, and R. H. Van Gulik, *Sexual Life in Ancient China* (Leiden: E. J. Brill, 1961), *passim*, but especially pp. 70-71.

5. For a discussion of these see Fang Fu Ruan, *Sex in China: Studies in Sexology in Chinese Culture* (New York: Plenum Press, 1991), pp. 2-3, 29-46.

6. This has been translated into English by Akira Ishihara and Howard S. Levy under the title of *The Tao of Sex* (Yokahoma: Shibundö, 1968).

7. Ibid., and Van Gulik, *Sexual Life in Ancient China*, pp. 125-34.

8. Ishihara and Levy, *Tao of Sex*, chap. 1, pp. 19-20.

9. See Vern L. Bullough and Fang Fu Ruan, "Lesbianism in China," *Archives of Sex Research* 21, no. 3 (1992): 217-26; Vern L. Bullough and Fang Fu Ruan, "Same-Sex Love in Contemporary China," *The Third Pink Book*, edited by Aart Hendriks, Rob Tielman, and Evert van der Veen (Amherst, N.Y.: Prometheus Books, 1993), pp. 46-55; Bret Hinsche, *The Male Homosexual Tradition in China* (Berkeley and Los Angeles: University of California Press, 1990); Fang Fu Ruan and Y. M. Tsai, "Male Homosexuality in the Traditional Chinese Literature," *Journal of Homosexuality* 14 (1987): 21-33; Fang Fu Ruan and Y. M. Tsai, "Male Homo-

sexuality in Contemporary Mainland China," *Archives of Sexual Behavior* 17 (1988): 189–99.

10. Needham, *Science and Civilization in China,* pp. 49–50.

11. Vātsyāyana recounts the history of this transmission in the introduction to his *Kāmasutra.* I have used the translation by Richard Burton (reprint New York: E. P. Dutton, 1962), p. 55.

12. A valuable summary can be found in Benjamin Walker, *The Hindu World,* 2 vols. (New York: Praeger, 1968), 1: 517–19. See also the introduction to Kaly-anamalla, *Ananga Ranga,* translated with an introduction and comments by Tridib-nath Ray (New York: Citadel Press, 1964); S. K. De, *Ancient Indian Erotics* (Calcutta: Mukhopadhyayi, 1959), and Edward Powys Mathers, *Eastern Anthology,* 12 vols., reprinted in four (London: J. Rodker, 1927–1930).

13. *Rig Veda,* X, 129, the "Hymn of Creation," translated by Abinash Chandra Bose, in *Hymns from the Vedas* (Bombay: Asia Publishing House, 1966), p. 305. Each translator renders the verses in a slightly different way.

14. *Hymns of the Atharva Veda,* VI, 138, translated by Maurice Bloomfeld in vol. 42 of *The Sacred Books of the East,* edited by Max Müller (reprint Delhi: Motilala Banarsidass, 1964), pp. 108–109, and also pp. 94–110 for a list of other charms.

15. *The Laws of Manu,* IV, 131, VIII, 364–65, 369–70; XI, 171, 172, 175, 213, translated by G. Buhler, in vol. 25 of *The Sacred Books of the East,* pp. 150, 317, 318, 465, 466, 474.

16. Vātsyāyana, *Kāmasutra,* I, chap. 5, pp. 81–84.

17. Walker, *The Hindu World,* 1: 433–37, and Kalyanamalla, *Ananga Ranga.* chap. 2, pp. 55–56.

18. Kalyanamalla, *Ananga Ranga,* chap. 10, pp. 243–47.

19. Ibid., chap. 10, secs. 1, 2, 3, 4, 5, pp. 217–42; Vātsyāyana, *Kāmasutra,* II, 6, 7, 8, 9, 10, pp. 112–32, and Walker, *The Hindu World,* 1: 334–40.

20. See, for example, *Chandogya Upanishad,* V, 8, 1–2, in the *Principal Upanishads,* edited with an introduction by S. Radhakrishana (London: George Allen & Unwin, 1953), p. 43; the *Bridhadaranyake Upanishad* in the same collection, II, 7.23, VI, 4.3, pp. 230, 313, 321, and the *Bhagavadgītā,* XIV, translated by Kashinath Trimak Telan in vol. 7 of *The Sacred Books of the East,* p. 196.

21. Walker, *The Hindu World,* 1:51–54. See Also John Woodroof, *Sakti and Sākta;* 7th ed. (Madras: Ganesh and Company, 1969), pp. 476–512; David N. Lorenzen, *The Kāpālikas and Kālāmukhas* (Berkeley and Los Angeles: University of California Press, 1972), and Shashi Bhusan Dasgupta, *Obscure Religious Cults,* 2nd ed. (Calcutta, Firma, K. L. Mukhodpadhay, 1962).

22. *Laws of Manu,* IV, 41, p. 135.

23. Walker, *Hindu World,* I, 132–33.

24. Koran, II (The Cow), 223. There are various English translations of the Koran, none of them official, since Allah has forbidden anyone to change his Arabic,

the language that Muslims believe God spoke. Most of the translations in this section have been taken from the English version of Muhammed Marmaduke Pickthall which is widely distributed. It was published by New American Library in 1953 and has been reprinted by a number of publishers. Occasionally other versions are used because they seem better able to express the original Arabic.

25. Dwight Donaldson, *Studies in Muslim Ethics* (London: SPCK, 1963), p. 122.

26. Ali ibn Abī Bakr, Burhan al-Din, al Marghīnanī, *The Hedaya or Guide: A Commentary on the Mussulman Laws,* Book VIII, chap. 5, translated by Charles Hamilton, and edited with a preface by Standish Grove Grady, 4 vols. in one (reprint Lahore: Premier Books, 1957), pp. 202.

27. Koran, XVII (Children of Israel), 32; XXV (The Criterion), 68, and XXXIII (The Clans), 30.

28. Koran, IV (Women), 19.

29. Koran, XXIV (Light), 4–9.

30. Koran, XXIV (Women), 24. For more information see Vern L. Bullough and Bonnie Bullough, *Women and Prostitution* (Amherst, N.Y.: Prometheus Books, 1987), pp. 71–79, and W. Heffening, "Mut'a," in *Shorter Encyclopedia of Islam,* ed. H. A. R. Gibb and J. H. Kramers (Ithaca, N.Y.: Cornell University Press, 1953), pp. 418–20.

31. Makhluf, *Fatawa Shareia (Legal Decisions)* (Cairo, 1965), p. 117, in Arabic.

32. Koran, VII (The Heights), 80–81, XXVI (The Poets), 165–80.

33. Joseph Schact, *An Introduction to Islamic Law* (Oxford: Clarendon Press, 1964), p. 178.

34. This was particularly true in the nineteenth century. See Thomas Patrick Hughes, *A Dictionary of Islam* (1895; reprint Clifton, N.J.: Reference Book Publishers, 1965), p. 601, where he makes a reference to the widespread existence of sodomy among the Muslims. See also the essay titled "Pederasty" by Richard F. Burton in his edition of *The Books of the Thousand Nights and a Night,* translated and annotated by Richard F. Burton (reprint 6 vols. in three, New York: Heritage Press, 1934), section D, pp. 3748–4782; T. E. Lawrence, *Seven Pillars of Wisdom* (reprint Garden City, N.Y.: Doubleday, Doran and Company, 1937), pp. 508–509. There are many more.

35. Kai Kā'ūs ibn Iskander, *A Mirror for Princes (The Qābus-nāma),* translated from the Persian by Reuben Levy (London: The Cresset Press, 1951), chap. 15, pp. 77–78.

36. Burton, *Thousand Nights,* "The Man's Dispute with the Learned Woman," 423rd Night, III, p. 1727.

37. There is considerable discussion of sexual positions in Sheik Nefzawi, *The Perfumed Garden,* translated by Richard Burton (reprint New York: Castle Books, 1964). See also Marghīhānī, *Heydaya,* Book VII, chap 2, and Raphael Patai, *Sex and Family in the Bible* (Garden City, N.Y.: Doubleday & Company, 1959), pp. 176–78.

38. Reynold Alleyne Nicholson, *Studies in Islamic Mystcism* (Cambridge: Cambridge University Press, 1921), p. 53.

39. Probably the best known of the Sufi orders is that of the Mevlevis, or whirling dervishes. See Ira Friedlander, *The Whirling Dervishes* (New York: Collier Books, 1975).

40. We have explored these and other forms of sexual activity in a number of different books. See Vern L. Bullough, *Sexual Variance in Society and History* (Chicago: University of Chicago Press, 1976); Vern L. Bullough and Bonnie Bullough, *Cross Dressing, Sex, and Gender* (Philadelphia: University of Pennsylvania, 1993); Vern L. Bullough and Bonnie Bullough, *Human Sexuality: An Encyclopedia* (New York: Garland, 1994).

3

"Unnatural" Sex

While it was the early Christian theologians who gave Christianity a mindset hostile to sexuality, it was the institutional church that translated these ideas into regulations about everday conduct. Ultimately church officials also tended to distinguish between the various sexual activities, making some greater sins than others. To examine how this happened we have to turn to other sources. Some of these are religious, such as penitentials (which prescribed penalties for various sins) and church (or canon) law; but since religious attitudes also carried over into secular law, it is necessary to examine these along with court cases and various legal commentaries.

One standard used by various authorities, theological as well as secular, to differentiate sexual activities was the belief that certain sexual activities were "unnatural." In fact, until well into the twentieth century, Anglo-American law classified many sexual acts as "against nature." Because they were against nature, they early moved from the category of sin to that of crime, and in order to avoid mentioning them they were often described as "crimes not fit to be named."

The biblical source of much of the Christian tradition for the use of this concept derives from the Pauline Epistle to the Romans, where it is stated that God had given up on some idolatrous pagans because they had dishonored their own bodies:

> Who changed the truth of God into a lie, and worshipped and served the creature more than the Creator, who is blessed forever, Amen. For this cause God gave them up into vile affections, for even their women did change the natural use into that which is *against nature*; and likewise also the man, leaving the natural use of the woman; burned in their lust toward one another; men with men working that which is unseemly, and receiving in themselves that recompense of their error which was then meet.[1] (Italics ours)

Biblical and other scholars are still not in agreement which sexual acts were meant to be included in the category of unnatural.[2] The purpose in citing the passage, however, is not to determine exactly which acts were against nature, but rather to establish the biblical use of nature as a criterion for determining the seriousness of sexual sins. Key to such usage is the belief that humans, by observation of the world around them, could discover the basis for right conduct. Put in these terms the idea is not particularly Christian, and in fact would seem to be opposed to those Christian teachings which attempt to distinguish humans from animals and to separate them somewhat from the material world.

Like so many other ideas about sex, the concept of natural versus unnatural can be traced to pre-Christian teachings of the Greeks and Romans. Inevitably many of the early Church Fathers turned to the philosophers for an understanding of what could be deemed contrary to nature. Aristotle (384–322 B.C.E), for example, used observations based upon nature to prove the inferiority of the female. Later the Stoics turned to nature to determine a basis for right conduct, assuming that natural law could be discovered through the reasoning process.[3] Some of the same concepts used to demonstrate that celibacy was the most desirable form of sexual activity were also utilized by the promoters of abstinence to bolster the idea that most forms of sexual activity were unnatural. Philo of Alexandria (ca. 13 B.C.E.–ca. 50 C.E.), for example, felt that all sexual activity not leading to procreation debased the "sterling coinage of nature": he compared those who engaged in such practices to bad farmers in that they let the

> deep-soiled and fruitful fields lie sterile, by taking steps to keep them from bearing while . . . [they spend their labor] night and day on soil from which no growth at all can be expected.[4]

Tied in with these pre-Christian ideas was the biblical story of Sodom and Gomorrah, which also deeply influenced Western ideas about "unnatural sex." In the Genesis account of the visit of two angels to Lot at his home in Sodom, the men of Sodom are reported as having called to Lot asking him to bring the two visitors out so that they might "know them."[5] The Hebrew word *yadha* (to know) here is a double entendre since it can imply "knowing" in terms of sexual intercourse as well as in the sense of becoming acquainted.[6]

Traditionally the passage has been interpreted as referring to "unnatural intercourse." This interpretation is in part derived from Lot's reply volunteering to send forth to the crowd two daughters who had not yet "known" men, in effect offering them as sexual partners. The crowd, however, persisted in their demands to know the two strangers, and the people were thwarted in their demands only when they were struck blind. In spite of Lot's willingness to prostitute his daughters, the next morning the heavenly visitors took Lot and his family out of the city, after which Yahweh destroyed it and four other cities with brimstone and fire from heaven. In an exhaustive study of the story Derrick Sherwin Bailey concluded that the association of Sodom and Gomorrah with unnatural intercourse was not an original part of Jewish Scripture but a later interpolation, inserted to emphasize the hostility felt in Palestine toward the Greeks and other outsiders who were believed to be undermining traditional religion.[7] Bailey argues that the original reference to the destruction of Sodom portrayed it as being destroyed for inhospitable treatment of the visitors sent from the Lord. Interestingly, although Sodom is used as a symbol of evil in numerous other places in the Bible, in no other case is the sin of Sodom specified as due to unnatural sexual activities. The Book of Ezekiel, for example, summarizes four charges against the residents of Sodom: (1) pride, (2) unwillingness to aid the poor and needy even though the city had an excess of food and was prosperous to the extent of idleness, (3) haughtiness, and (4) abom-inations.[8] It is not until the appearance of the Palestinian Pseudepigrapha, the noncanonical books of the Bible written between 200 B.C.E. and 200 C.E., that the sexual aspects clearly appear.[9] In short, what had started out as a sin of pride and arrogance became, with the changing times, a sexual sin.

It was this later definition of the sin of Sodom that found its way into Western literature. The pagan concern over "unnatural" had been extended to include a punishment by God to those who engaged in unnatural sex. But what constituted unnatural sex? The Christian writers seemingly used three criteria to determine this. In the first instance, the sexual process was compared to the sowing of a field, and was therefore natural, so that only those sexual activities aimed at seeding or procreation could by definition be natural. Second, sexual behavior in man was compared to that in animals; what animals did was natural and what they did not do was unnatural. Humans were therefore natural only when they followed specified animal models. But not all animal acts were acceptable, since the third criterion stipulated that the different body structures of man and animals had to be taken into consideration. In all cases, the obvious function of the organ was the natural and self-evident one: just as eyes were for seeing and ears for hearing, so the genital organs were for procreation. Unfortunately, not all functions are self-evident, and when this was the case, the Christian writers proved to be very selective in what they regarded as natural. Even when using agricultural models, they refused to accept practices contrary to their essentially ascetic notions. For example, it was common practice to dam a river or stream in order to divert the water, but if a male diverted his semen this was regarded as human intervention in nature. Thus *coitus interruptus* was prohibited. When human conduct was compared with that of animals, certain animals were excluded, such as the hyena, because it was believed to have sexual organs of both sexes, and thus sex was for pleasure and not for generative purposes. The same selectivity was evident when Christian writers determined the functional purposes of various parts of the body. In effect, when the Christian writers used nature in reinforcing theoretical positions they had already adopted, they tossed out any contrary observations.[10]

Instead, they increasingly turned to procreation as a criterion for judging, holding that a sexual activity could only be natural if it was capable of leading to procreation. Some went so far as to state that engaging in sexual intercourse for any purpose other than the procreation of children was to do injury to nature.[11] Those who so succumbed to the passions of the material body that they went beyond the laws of nature (i.e., engaged in nonprocreative intercourse) were to be banished not only from the shelter of the Church but the Christian community as well, since they had committed not just sins but "monstrosities."[12] The *Didascalia* (also known as *Apostolic Constitutions*), dating from the third century, emphasized that Christians were to abhor "all unlawful mixtures" and that those individuals who engaged in activities "contrary to nature" were to be regarded as "wicked and impious."[13] Though not all the early Church Fathers agreed on the criteria for determining what was natural, particularly in the Eastern portion of the Roman Empire, the pattern for the Western Christian Church was set by St. Augustine (354–430). Augustine saw nothing rational, spiritual, or sacramental in the act of intercourse, although he recognized that there was biblical sanction for marriage. In fact, it was only because there were such specific sanctions for marriage and childbearing that Augustine accepted sexual intercourse as a good, but only if it was intended to lead to offspring.[14] His beliefs on the subject need to be quoted at length because there is a kind of inherent contradiction in Augustine that has continued to trouble Western thinking about sex. The contradiction results because Augustine recognized the right of one partner (usually the husband) within the marriage relationship to demand intercourse with the other, even when procreation, because of age or other factors, could not be involved.

For what food is to the health of man, intercourse is for the health of the race, and both are not without carnal pleasures, which, however, when modified and put to its natural use with a controlling temperance, cannot be passion. However, what unlawful food is in sustaining life, this is the fornication or adultery in seeking a child [i.e., it is prohibited even if it produces offspring], and what unlawful food is in the excessive indulgence of stomach and palate, this is unlawful intercourse in a passion seeking no offspring; and what is immoderate appetite for some as regards lawful foods, this is that pardonable intercourse in spouses.[15]

Augustine himself was not pleased about the fact that carnal pleasure existed within marriage, and he tried to put rigid restrictions upon marital intercourse by adopting the concept of "natural use":

For although the natural use, when it goes beyond the marriage rights, that is beyond the need for procreation, is pardonable in a wife but damnable in a prostitute, that use which is against nature is abominable in a prostitute but more abominable in a wife. For, the decree of the Creator and the right order of the creature are of such force that, even though there is an excess in the things that have been granted to be used, this is much more tolerable than a single or rare deviation in those things which had not been granted . . . when a husband wishes to use the member of his wife which has not been given for this purpose, the wife is more shameful if she permits this to take place with herself rather than with another woman.[16]

Since Augustine felt called upon to classify many of the sexual activities engaged in by a husband and wife as against nature, inevitably all sexual activity outside marriage was against nature, but in his hierarchy of sins Augustine condemned especially those said to have been committed in Sodom and Gomorrah. These acts

ought everywhere and always to be detested and punished. If all nations were to do such things they would (equally) be held guilty of the same crime by the law of God which has not so made men that they should use one another in this way.[17]

Inevitably Christian concepts about sex began to appear in Roman legal writing. The earliest Roman legislation against sexual activity other than rape or adultery came under the Christian co-emperors Constantius and Constans in 342, and this quite clearly is aimed at homosexuality.[18]

The term "unnatural," however, was not used until the time of the Christian emperor Justinian in the sixth century. One of Justinian's laws referred to certain types of men who,

> seized by diabolical incitement, practice among themselves the most disgraceful lusts, and act *contrary to nature*. We enjoin them to take to heart the fear of God and the judgment to come and to abstain from such like diabolical and unlawful lusts, so that they may not be visited by the just wrath of God on account of these impious acts, with the result that cities perish with all their inhabitants. For we are taught by the Holy Scriptures that because of the impious conduct cities have indeed perished, together with men in them. . . .[19] (Italics ours)

Subsequent religious legislation on sexual matters also adopted the catchall category of activity against nature, defining it so broadly that all sexual activities not leading directly to procreation could be included.[20] The religious concepts behind such legislation reached the ordinary Christian communicant through the penitential literature, a listing of the sins the devout were supposed to avoid along with their accompanying punishments. Before undergoing punishment, however, communicants were supposed to confess and do penance.

The earliest penitential literature was fairly specific about sexual acts since the writers argued that the physicians of the soul had to know the hidden recesses of the mind as much as the physicians of the body knew all parts of the body as well as its excrements.

> For no one can raise up one who is falling beneath a weight unless he bends himself that he may reach out to him his hand; and no physician can treat the wounds of the sick, unless he comes in contact with their foulness. So also no priest or pontiff can treat the words of sinners or take away the sins from their souls, except by intense solicitude and the prayer of tears. There it is needful for us, beloved brethren, to be solicitous on behalf of sinners, since we are "members one of another" and "if one member suffers anything all the members suffer with it."[21]

An early Welsh penitential, *The Preface of St. Gildas on Penance* (495–570), starts out rather bluntly by proscribing sexual activities for deacons or priests: "A presbyter or a deacon committing natural fornication or sodomy who has previously taken the monastic vow shall do penance for three years."[22] Though the general meaning seems clear, there are still doubts about what specifically is meant since sodomy is undefined, and confusion is encouraged by the fact that the writer regarded sodomy as no worse a crime than fornication. As the penitential literature blossomed, however, the various sexual acts were spelled out in detail with a distinction made between coitus *in ano* (the anus), coitus *in femoribus* (the groin), coitus *in manu* (the hand, i.e., masturbation), *coitus interruptus,* bestiality, nocturnal emissions, heterosexual fornication, and so forth, although different penitential writers differed from one another on the stipulated punishments. Some held that simply thinking about forbidden activities was a sin although the penalties they prescribed varied, with lighter penances when just intent was involved and more serious ones if actual sexual activity took place.[23]

Because each penitential writer seemingly prescribed a somewhat different penance from the others, and many of them did not punish "unnatural" sex more severely than "natural," there was a growing criticism about the imposition of penalties. One of the leading critics of the lack of common standards was the eleventh-century theologian Peter Damian, who felt that every kind of sin against nature deserved the maximum penalty without even taking into consideration whether there were mitigating circumstances.[24] Peter, however, also worried that the mere mention of various kinds of sexual activity might encourage individuals to practice them. Even Pope Leo IX, while he accepted the dedication of Peter's work to him, commending Peter for raising the arm of the spirit against such unnatural sexual practices, responded to Peter that it was necessary for a pope to season justice with mercy.[25]

Inevitably the answer to the kind of objections raised by Peter, was to specify in greater detail what the sexual sins were and what penalties were involved. To do so, the newly emerging medieval lawyers turned to the Church Fathers for criteria. Particularly influential in this new generation of legal commentators was Ivo, Bishop of Chartres (1091–1116), who utilized Augustine as his justification for punishing "unnatural" intercourse, defined as using a "member not granted for this."[26] Though Ivo amplified Augustine's definition somewhat, nowhere does he become very precise:

> A use which is natural and lawful in marriage is unlawful in adultery. To act against nature is always unlawful and beyond doubt more flagrant and shameful than to sin by a natural use in fornication or adultery, as the Holy Apostle contends as to both men and women.[27]

In effect, any kind of intercourse not aimed at impregnation was unnatural.[28] The attempts of the early penitential writers to be narrowly precise were replaced by a general category of unnatural intercourse, and it was this ambiguous concept that was adopted by Gratian (d. before 1159), the monk who has been given the title of "Father of the Science of Canon Law."[29] Gratian, who completed his *Concordia discordantium canonum* (*Concordance of Discordant Canons*) about the year 1140, conceived of his work as a universal treatise on the institutions and problems of canon law. He based it upon his researches into Roman law; canons of the Church Councils; papal and royal ordinances; and biblical, liturgical, patristic, and penitential texts. When he came to the question of sexual intercourse, Gratian relied upon both Ivo and Augustine, holding that any act *contra naturam* (against nature) was always unlawful and more shameful and filthy than fornication and adultery.[30] He developed four categories of sexual sins, each progressively more serious: fornication, adultery, incest, and finally, those against nature, which he defined as activities using a member not intended for that purpose.[31] In a later section Gratian also makes a specific reference to the abduction and corruption of boys, a crime deserving of capital punishment if it is *perfectus,* that is, completed.[32] He is suitably ambiguous on precisely what constituted the sin against nature although he might well have had specific activities in mind. This ambiguity proved to be contagious, and Gratian's euphemistic term "sin against nature" became the standard wording for several centuries. The phrase came to be interpreted as forbidding intercourse in any position except with the female on her back; prohibiting any attempt to avoid conception; and interdicting the use of any orifice except the vagina for intercourse, and any instrument but the penis. Though later writers occasionally used the term "sodomy," it is not so much a specific act but rather another euphemism for "unnatural" intercourse. Evidence for this usage of the sins of Sodom comes from the action of the Third Lateran Council held in 1179. One of the canons adopted there was directed against the "incontinence which is against nature," and by reason of which the anger of God came upon the children of disobedience, and consumed five cities by fire. . . ."[33] Similar wording appears in the canons adopted by the Fourth Lateran Council in 1215, and in the supplement to the canon law known as the Decretals.[34] The Decretals remain the final legal word of the Church on the subject until the sixteenth century. Quite clearly the Church was opposed to the sin against nature, but just exactly what this constituted was not always spelled out in detail.[35]

Theological discussion on the subject was also often ambiguous. Peter

Lombard (ca. 1100–1160) referred to the "sin against nature," then proceeded to define it as the use of a member not intended for this purpose. Following earlier categories he classified it as worse than fornication, adultery, or incest.[36] Albertus Magnus, or Albert the Great (1206–1280), was somewhat more precise. Although he held that the procreation of offspring was the natural end of intercourse, he also felt there was a human end of intercourse which he defined as the "end of medicine and of fidelity to bed and of the sacrament."[37] This definition allowed Albert to deviate from Augustine enough to justify intercourse for the sake of pleasure, but he still put limits on the type of sexual activity, some of which involved conduct not only against nature but against reason. Albert did not hesitate to spell out what he meant; on sodomy he was specific, defining it as male lying with male or female with female, and the worst of unnatural sexual activity. He held that sodomy deserved special condemnation for at least four reasons: (1) it proceeded from a burning frenzy that subverted the order of nature, (2) the sin was distinguished by its disgusting foulness, (3) individuals who became addicted to such vices seldom succeeded in freeing themselves, and (4) such vices were contagious and spread rapidly from one to another.[38]

Albert's pupil Thomas Aquinas (1225–1274) took a somewhat more traditional approach. Aquinas classified most sexual sins under the general category of lust, and this included fornication, adultery, seduction, rape, incest, and acts against nature. This last category included masturbation, bestiality, homosexuality, and deviation from the natural manner of coitus, i.e., anything but face-to-face contact with the woman lying on her back. Although by using such a definition Aquinas managed to classify all forms of male and female homosexual practices as contrary to nature, his net also caught a wide range of other sexual activities. Of the sins against nature, Aquinas regarded bestiality as the most grievous, followed by sodomy (defined as male with male or female with female), then intercourse in an unnatural position, while masturbation was the least serious.[39] Aquinas recognized that in many ways the sexual activities he classified as being against nature were not as serious as some of those not against nature, such as adultery, seduction, and rape. He felt that all three of these latter activities injured others and, as such, were contrary to the virtue of charity. Nevertheless, Aquinas argued that since the order of nature had been derived from God, its contravention was always an injury to God because it was contrary to the Divine law.[40] He permitted, however, touching, caressing, or kissing between persons of the same sex, since the intent of such simple acts was not to go counter to God's law. In fact, all contacts that did not arouse venereal excitement were to be permitted.[41] By Aquinas's definition, sins against nature involved ejaculation; without ejaculation there could be no sin against nature even though many of these same activities could be regarded as lustful, which put them into a different category of sin.[42] It was the definitions set forth by Aquinas that dominated later discussion within Catholicism, although some commentators used the term "sodomites" as a euphemism for those who committed crimes or sins against nature.[43] Some also employed the term "onanites," a reference to the biblical Onan who spilled his seed on the ground (Gen. 38:7–10).

In addition to these euphemisms for the sin or crime against nature, another term, "buggery," appeared in the secular law codes of the sixteenth century. The term derived from a group of heretics in southern France who had revived the ancient Manichean beliefs. Since this late medieval heresy was popularly believed to have come from Bulgaria, the term "Bulgar," or in English "Bugger," came to be used to describe them. These medieval Manicheans held the same sexual views as their ancient predecessors, and their complete support for celibacy set them apart from the Christians. This led to their being looked upon not only as socially deviant but sexually perverse; hence "buggery" came to be used as a new term for all types of dark, hidden sex crimes, none of which are known to have been committed by the Manicheans themselves. Long after the Manicheans had been exterminated through the inquisitions and wars, various forms of nonprocreative sexual activity continued to be called buggery. In the sixteenth century, when rulers, such as Henry VIII in England, attempted to extend state control by incorporating matters of sex and morals previously belonging to the ecclesiastical courts into the criminal code, the term "buggery" was used to describe a felony.[44] It became a commonplace description of nonprocreative sex, although the terms "sodomy," "onanism," and "crime against nature" also continued to appear.

Initially in American law there was a preference for using "sodomy" as the catchall term, undoubtedly because the American colonists, particularly those in New England, tried to find biblical justifications for classifying any action as a crime. Both sodomy and adultery were sexual "sins" mentioned in the Bible, although the Scriptures were silent about many other sexual activities including rape, an absence which much distressed the New England commentators of the colonial period as they attempted to implement the sexual code that God would have wanted. Perhaps because of this biblical oversight, later generations of Americans tended to rely less on scriptural sanctions and more on English precedents to guide their legal thinking, and so the term "buggery" entered into the American law code. Most influential in this respect was Sir Edward Coke (1552–1634), the legal commentator whose writings were very influential in forming American attitudes. In 1628 Coke wrote:

> Buggery is a detestable, and abominable sin, amongst Christians not to be named, committed by carnal knowledge against the ordinance of the Creator, and order of nature, by mankind with mankind, or with brute beast, or by womankind with brute beast.[45]

Though Coke's definition (in which sodomy was equated with buggery) required penetration, such specificity soon was clouded with ambiguity.

This is most evident in the work of William Blackstone, whose four-volume *Commentaries on the Laws of England* (1765–1769) was particularly influential on American law in the nineteenth century. Blackstone had conceived of his work as providing a rationale for the common law in history, logic, and "natural law." His discussion of the "crime against nature" was included in the fourth volume of his work which dealt with public wrongs but also included discussions of the crimes of mayhem, forcible abduction, and rape. Here sodomy became the infamous "crime against nature," but with many of the ambiguities that became so much a part of American law:

> What has been here observed, especially with regard to manner of proof, which ought to be more clear in proportion as the crime is the more detestable, may be applied to another offense, of a still deeper malignity; the infamous *crime against nature,* committed either with man or beast. A crime which ought to be strictly and impartially proved, and then as strictly and impartially punished. But it is an offense of so dark a nature, so easily charged, and the negative so difficult to be proved that the accusation should be clearly made out, for, if false, it deserves a punishment inferior only to that of the crime itself.
>
> I will not act so disagreeable a part, to my readers as well as myself, as to dwell any longer upon a subject, the very mention of which is a disgrace to human nature. It will be more eligible to imitate in this respect the delicacy of our English law, which treats it, in its very indictments, as a crime not fit to be named.[46] (Original italics)

Blackstone's discussion never makes clear just what the "crime against nature" was, and although he cited biblical statements and English statutes for his readers to consult, most of the source material was also unclear. This ambiguity continued to plague discussion and law enforcement against same-sex activities in nineteenth-century America. The ambiguity was further compounded because Blackstone also listed "unnatural" crimes under the general category of assault,[47] and in "offenses Against God and Religion."[48] Many of the American states incorporated similarly ambiguous wording. Massachusetts, for example, had a statute which read:

> Every person who shall commit the abominable and detestable crime against nature, either with mankind or with any beast, shall be punished by imprisonment in the State prison, not more than twenty years.

Some states used sodomy or buggery or both as synonyms for the crime against nature, but in such cases sodomy was defined to include almost any form of intercourse not leading to procreation. Pennsylvania, for example, listed both sodomy and buggery without defining or differentiating them, while Virginia listed only buggery.[49]

This lack of precision sometimes led to interesting court decisions. In two nineteenth-century cases (*Fennel* v. *State,* 1869, and *Frazier* v. *State,* 1873), courts in Texas held that since the Texas code did not describe or define what constituted the "crime against nature," it could not be prosecuted. The Texas courts refused to accept English common law definitions because of their ambiguity. Later, anal intercourse was accepted as part of the crime against nature, but in 1893 the Texas court held that oral-genital contacts were not specifically defined as sodomy, and therefore could not be regarded as such. It was only through a series of specific enactments that most areas of sexual conduct were eventually incorporated into the Texas code.[50]

In spite of the Texas example, however, legal commentators, as well as most state statutes, failed to spell out what constituted the crime against nature. It might well be that they feared that if they did spell it out, someone might learn about it and try it; but the result was that judges could often include many forms of sexual behavior under the general category. Edward Livingston, in his *A System of Penal Law for the United States* (1828), goes into detail about such things as the keeping of brothels, procuring or printing obscene materials, adultery, abduction, and rape, but nothing about specific forbidden forms of sexual intercourse.[51] Francis Wharton's *A Treatise on the Criminal Law of the U.S.* went through many editions; although he mentions both sodomy and the crime against nature, it is not until the eighth edition (1880) that he specifically defines it as sexual congress *per anum.* Up to that time Wharton had simply stated that sodomy must be committed in that bodily part where sodomy is "usually committed" to be classified as sodomy.[52] Not everyone followed Wharton's example. Joel Pretiss Bishop's *Commentaries on the Law of Statutory Crimes* (1888) mentions sodomy and bestiality in passing but does not define them in the same kind of detail as he does adultery, fornication, incest, miscegenation, seduction, or rape. The impression left is that all sexual activities not specifically mentioned were included in these catchall categories. Even in his *New Commentaries on Marriage* where Bishop lists sodomy as a "high matrimonial crime," he never defines it.[53] William Oldnall Russell, in his 1877 edition of *A Treatise on Crimes and Misdemeanors,* effectively sums up the prevailing attitudes:

> In treating of the offense of sodomy, *peccatum, illud horrible, inter Christianos non nominandum* [a sin, especially horrible, not to be mentioned among Christians], it is not intended to depart from the reserved and concise mode of statement which has been adopted by other writers.[54]

Toward the last decade of the nineteenth century, there was an attempt to obtain greater specificity in the laws about sex, partly as a result of the generalized crusade against vice in the English-speaking world, and partly as an effort within the legal profession to make laws more scientific—that is, make them more explicit and reduce them to a systematic shape. The leading proponent of this movement in the English-speaking world was the English jurist Sir James Fitzjames Stephen (1829–1894), who has been called the "greatest draftsman codifier of criminal law which Great Britain ever produced."[55]

As we look back, however, Stephen appears not to be a dispassionate investigator but rather a committed believer in Christian values which, when formulated into law, formed the basic pillars of society. Stephen feared that the morality of his own age was being weakened by liberal thought, and to correct the potential decline of society, he felt it essential to develop "emphatic" sermons on just what the law constituted. For a time Stephen attempted to draft a new criminal code for England: though his proposed law code was never adopted, it had great influence and set the foundation for legal codes in many, if not most, parts of the English-speaking world. Most importantly, Stephen not only believed that there were crimes against nature, but felt it essential that such crimes be spelled out in detail. In the United States, his writings either influenced or coincided with an indigenous movement to redefine the criminal law and to make the statute law specific. In California, for example, penal codes were enacted defining the crime against nature to mean "any sexual penetration, however slight," of the anus, and along with this new definitions were enacted against fellatio, cunnilingus, and others sexual activities previously left unmentioned or classified in the general category of "crimes against nature."[56]

In effect, what had once been a catchall category—the crime against nature—and defined not only as sodomy but almost any activity not leading to impregnation, slowly disappeared from the law books and codes, only to be replaced by more specific and detailed language. In the past few decades, however, still another redefinition of "crimes against nature" has taken place, until the majority of states no longer include sodomy among the prohibited sexual acts.

The belief that certain sexual activities were against nature started out as a philosophical concept and then became a theological one, which resulted in various sexual activities being classified as sins. The Church Fathers reinforced the idea of sins against nature by equating them with the sins of Sodom, and interpreting this to mean any sexual activity not leading to procreation. The concepts of the Church Fathers were debated and refined in Canon law which served as a detailed guide for proper Christian conduct. Thus the sins against nature entered into canon law, and from canon law moved over into civil law where they became crimes. English common law also adopted them, and from there they made their passage into American law. In light of the progress in human thought, we should now define what is natural in terms of the scientific findings of today, instead of relying upon ancient observations that were strongly influenced by erroneous assumptions. It might well be that no human sexual activity is really *unnatural.* Certainly some might regard certain sexual activities as undesirable, others as potentially harmful, and still others that many would classify as immoral; but to base our assumptions on ancient Greek philosophy or Jewish mythology is to build a castle on shifting sands.

NOTES

1. Rom. 1:24–27. The translation is from the Authorized Version. The Douay translation, however, differs only slightly, and both use the term "against nature," which also appears in the Latin Vulgate.

2. See, for example, Matthew Black and H. H. Rowley, *Peake's Commentary*

on the Bible (London: Thomas Nelson, 1962), par. 8174b which holds that the passge refers to homosexuality, as does Otto Michel, *Der Brief an die Römer* (Göttingen: Van Hoech & Ruprecht, 1955), p. 59. A much broader interpretation that classifies all sexual activities not leading to procreation as falling under the passage can be found in Herman L. Strack and Paul Billerbeck, *Kommentar zum Neuen Testament auf Talmud und Midrash,* 3d. ed. (Munich: Beck, 1961), III, *Die Brief des Neuen Testament und die Offenbarun Johannis,* pp. 68–69. Gerald Larue, *Sex and the Bible* (Amherst, N.Y.: Prometheus Books, 1983), p. 133, interprets it as referring to homosexuality and lesbianism. John Boswell, *Christianity, Social Tolerance, and Homosexuality* (Chicago: University of Chicago Press, 1980), p. 108, argues that what Paul condemns is homosexual acts committed by apparently heterosexual persons, not homosexuality itself. Moreover, he adds that the reference to homosexuality is simply a mundane analogy to this theological sin and not the crux of the argument: once made it is dropped to go on to the main subject, the orgiastic practices associated with false gods.

3. For Aristotelian ideas about this see Aristotle, *Historia animalium* 608B, translated by D'Arcy W. Thompson in *The Works of Aristotle,* IV (Oxford: Clarendon press 1910), and *Politics* 1.1 (1252B), 7, edited and translated by H. Rackham (London: William Heinemann, 1944). For Stoic ideas see Epictetus, *Encheiridion* 41, in *Discourses,* edited and translated by W. A. Oldfather, 2 vols. (London: William Heinemann, 1956, 1959).

4. Philo, *On the Special Laws* 7.37–42, edited and translated by F. H. Colson (London: William Heinemann, 1958), and also Richard A. Baer, Jr., *Philo's Use of the Categories Male and Female* (Leiden: E. J. Brill, 1970), p. 46.

5. Gen. 9:22–24.

6. See G. A. Baron, "Sodomy," *Encyclopedia of Religion and Ethics,* edited by James Hastings, 13 vols. (New York: Charles Scribner's Sons, 1928), 11:672–74.

7. Derrick Sherwin Bailey, *Homosexuality and the Western Christian Tradition* (London: Longmans, Green and Company, 1955), pp. 1–28. Numerous others have since followed his lead. See, for example, Boswell, *Christianity,* pp. 93–94.

8. Ezek. 16:49–50. Other references appear in Deut. 23:18, 19:23, and 32:32.

9. See also Jubilees 13:17, and 20:5–6. The passages of the pseudepigrapha (called Apocrypha by the Catholics) can be found in vol. 2 of *The Apocrypha and Pseudepigrapha of the Old Testament in English,* edited and translated by R. H. Charles, 2 vols. (Oxford: Clarendon Press, 1913). See also Bailey, *Homosexuality,* pp. 22–23.

10. There is a good dicussion of this in John T. Noonan, *Contraception: A History of Its Treatment by Catholic Theologians* (Cambridge: Belknap Press and Harvard University Press, 1966), pp. 75ff.

11. Clement of Alexandria, *Pedagogue (Instructor)* 2.10, in vol. I of *The Ante-Nicene Fathers,* edited by Alexander Roberts and James Donaldson (American reprint, Grand Rapids: W. B. Eerdmans, 1966), p. 260.

12. Tertullian, *On Modesty* IV, in vol. IV of *The Ante-Nicene Fathers*, p. 77.

13. *Didascalia* or *Apostolic Constitutions*, VI, sec. v. 28, in vol. VIII of *The Ante-Nicene Fathers*, pp. 462–63.

14. Augustine, *Soliloquies* 1.10 (17), translated by Thomas F. Gilligan in vol. 1 of *Fathers of the Church* (New York: Cima Publishing Company, 1948).

15. Augustine, *The Good of Marriage* 16.18, translated by Charles T. Wilcox in vol 15 of *Fathers of the Church*.

16. Ibid., 11.12.

17. Augustine, *Confessions* 3.7, edited and translated by William Watts, 2 vols. (London: William Heinemann, 1950). For further discussion of homosexuality, see chapter 12.

18. *The Theodosian Code* IX, vii, 3, edited and translated by Clyde Pharr (Princeton: Princeton University Press, 1952), pp. 231–32. For enactments of the emperors Theodosius, Valentinian II, and Arcadius II, see sections IX, vii, 6, p. 232. Boswell has argued that the lack of any penalty for noncompliance in the law of 342 indicate that its drafters expected it to meet with popular opposition or neglect. He also holds that it was outlawing gay marriages which he claims previously had been de facto legal. See Boswell, *Christianity*, p. 123, and note 9.

19. *Novella* 77, in *Corpus juris civilis*, 3 vols. (Berlin: Weidman, 1959). This translation is based upon that of Bailey, *Homosexuality*, pp. 73–74. Boswell, who is very interested in defending the Christian Church of taking action against homosexuality, says that the laws were enacted by Justinian without any evidence that the church authorities suggested or supported the legislation. He speculates, following the *Anecdote* of Procopius, a historian contemporary with Justinian, that the emperor acted chiefly to extort money from those threatened with persecution. While the motives of Justinian remain unclear, there is a long history of denunciation of homosexuality by Christian authorities which Boswell ignored.

20. See J. Mansi, *Sacrorum conciliorum* (Florence, 1766), XII, col. 71, and the various Church Councils held under the direction of Charlemagne and his immediate successors, the tects of which are also printed in Mansi, *Capitularium Karoli M et Ludovici Pii libri* VII, Book V, cap. LXXXXIII, in Mansi, XVIIB, col. 839; *Canones Isaac Episcopi Linonensis,* titulus IV, cap. XI, in Mansi, XVI B, col. 1529; *Capitulare octarum anno,* in Mansi XVIIB, col. 412; *Capitulare tertium,* cap. 11, in Mansi, XVIIB, col. 526; *Capitularum Karoli et Ludovici Pii libri VII,* titulus CXLIII, in Mansi, XVIIB, col. 1055; *"additio secunda,"* cap. XXI in Mansi, XVIIB, col. 1143; and *Karoli Magni capitulare primum anni,* titulus XVII, in Mansi, XVIIB, col. 368. For a more detailed analysis of canon law see James Brundage, *Law, Sex, and Christian Society in Medieval Europe* (Chicago: University of Chicago Press, 1987).

21. The quotation is from the *Pseudo-Roman Penitential* by Haltigar, Bishop of Cambrai, and can be found in *Medieval Handbooks of Penance,* edited and translated by John T. McNeill and Helena M. Gamer (New York: Columbia University

Press, 1938), p. 297. For a good overview see Pierre Payer, *Sex and the Penitentials* (Toronto: University of Toronto Press, 1984).

22. McNeill and Gamer, *Medieval Handbooks,* pp. 174–77, see par. nos. 1, 11, 22. The same penitential is found in *The Irish Penitentials,* edited and translated by Ludwig Beiler (Dublin: Dublin Institute for Advanced Studies, 1963), pp. 60–62. Beiler also includes the Latin text.

23. See the various penitentials found in McNeill and Gamer, *Medieval Handbooks;* Beiler, *The Irish Penitentials,* and Payer, *Sex.* Many penitentials have not been translated. A more complete collection can be found in the various compilations by F. W. H. Wasserschleben, particularly in his *Die Bussordnungen der abendlaischen Kirche* (reprint Graz: Akademische Druck-U. Verlagsanstal, 1958).

24. Peter Damian, *Liber Gomorrhianus,* caps. i, xxii in *Opera omnia,* edited by Constantine Cajetan, in J. P. Migne, *Patrologia Latina* (hereafter *PL*) (Paris: Garnier Fratres, 1889) CXLV, cols. 161 and 183. There is an English translation by Pierre Payer, *Book of Gomorrah: An Eleventh-Century Treatise against Clerical Homosexual Practices* (Ontario: Wilfred Laurier University Press, 1982). Though Damian directed his charges against clergy, they clearly applied to the laity as well.

25. For a brief discussion of this see Horace K. Mann, *The Lives of the Popes in the Middle Ages* (London: Kegan Paul, Trench Trubner & Company, 1925), VI:49–53. See also Brundage, *Law,* pp. 212–214.

26. Ivo, *Decretum,* par. IX, cap. 110, 128, in *PL* CLXI, 686, 699. This is the section dealing with activities with activities *contra naturam.* The passage dealing with sins of boys, *De stupratoribus puerorum,* is cap. 109, col. 686. See also Brundage, *Law,* 106–88, 200–204, and *passim.*

27. *Decretum* IX, 106 in *PL* CLXI, 685–86.

28. Noonan, *Contraception,* p. 173.

29. For a brief discussion of the origins of canon law, see Stephen G. Kuttner, *Harmony from Dissonance,* Wimmer Lecture X, St. Vincent College (Latrobe, Pa: The Archabbey Press, 1960).

30. Gratian, *Decretum pars secunda,* Causa XXXII, Question vii, c. 13, in *Corpus juris canonici,* edited by Emil Friedberg, 2 vols. (Leipzig: Bernard Tauchnitz, 1879–1881), I, col. 1144.

31. Ibid., Causa XXXII, Quaestio vii, c. 11, in vol. 2 of *Corpus juris canonici,* col. 1143.

32. Ibid., Causa XXXIII, Quaestio iii, distinctio cap. xv., in vol. 2 of *Corpus juris canonici,* 1161.

33. *Concilium Lateranense,* III, cap. xi, in Mansi, *Sacrorum conciliorum,* XXIII, col. 379. There are many others. The final form was in *Decretales Gregori,* IX, liber V, titulus XXXI, cap. iv, in *Corpus juris canonici,* II, col. 836.

34. See *Concilium Lateranense,* IV (1215), XIV, in Mansi, *Sacrorum conciliorum,* XXII, col. 1003, *Concilium Ramense,* XL, ibid., XXIII, col. 379. There are

many others. The final form was in *Decretales Gregori*, IX, liber V, titulus XXXI, cap. iv, in *Corpus juris canonici*, II, col. 836.

35. For more specific detail on this see Brundage, *Law, passim.*

36. Peter Lombard, *Libri IV sententiarum*, IV, xxxvii, cap. 2, edited by the Fathers of the College of St. Bonaventure, 2d ed., 2 vols. (printed by the College of St. Bonaventure, 1916), 2:970.

37. Albertus Magnus, *Commentaria in IV sententiarum*, Distinctio III, 37, in *Opera omnia*, edited by S. C. A. Bornet, vol. 29 (Paris: Ludovicum Vive, 1895).

38. Albertus Magnus, *Evangelium secundum Lucam*, XVII, 29, in vols. 22 and 23 of *Opera omnia.*

39. Thomas Aquinas, *Summa Theologica*, II–II, Q. cliv, II and 12, translated by the Fathers of the English Dominican Province (New York: Benziger Brothers, 1947).

40. Ibid., II–II, Q. cliv, 12.

41. Ibid., II–II, Q. cliv, 12.

42. Ibid., II–II, Q. cliv, 4.

43. For example, see Bernardine of Siena, *Quadragesimale de Evangelio Aeterno,* Sermo XIX, Articulus II, cap. 4, and Articulus III, cap. 3, in *Opera omnia*, edited by the College of St. Bonaventure (Florence: Collegii S. Bonaventura, 1956), 3:334, 337–38, and Sermo XV, I, 1, in ibid., 3:267–84. See also John Gerson, *Regulae morales*, XCIV, in *Opera omnia*, edited by I. Elliss du Pin (Antwerp, 1706), III, col. 95.

44. For a general discussion of this see Alex K. Gigeroff, *Sexual Deviations in the Criminal Law* (Toronto: University of Toronto Press for the Clarke Institute of Psychiatry, 1968). See also Sir James Fitzjames Stephen, *Digest of Criminal Law (Crimes and Punishments)* (St. Louis: F. H. Thomas and Company, 1878), Articles 168, note x, pp. 115, 377.

45. Edward Coke, *Institutes of the Laws of England*, Part III (reprint London: E. E. Brooke, 1797), chap. X, "Of Buggery, or Sodomy," pp. 58–59. For a brief discussion of the Massachusetts experience see George Lee Haskins, *Law and Authority in Early Massachusetts* (New York: Macmillan, 1960), pp. 146–49.

46. William Blackstone, *Commentaries on the Laws of England*, new edition with notes by Frederick Archibald (London: William Reed, 1811), Book 4, p. 215.

47. Gigeroff, *Sexual Deviation*, p. 17.

48. Blackstone, *Commentaries*, Book 4, pp. 64–65.

49. See for some examples Francis Wharton, *A Treatise on the Criminal Law of the United States*, 4th ed., rev. (Philadelphia: Kay and Brothers, 1857), p. 591.

50. See *Fennel* v. *State*, 32 Texas 378 (1869), Supreme Court of Texas; *Frazier* v. *State*, 39 Texas 390 (1873), Supreme Court of Texas; *Ex Parte* Ed. Bergen, 14 *Texas Criminal Reports* 551 (1893); *Alex Lewis* v. *the State*, 36 *Texas Criminal Reports* 37 (1896); *Algie Adams* v. *the State*, 48 *Texas Criminal Reports* 90 (1905). See also *Vernon's Penal Code of the State of Texas*, annotated (Kansas City, Mo.:

Vernon Law Books) vol. I. Texas has more sodomy cases than almost any other state, perhaps because unlike most states Texas has separate reports on criminal cases in local courts.

51. Edward Livingston, *A System of Penal Law for the United States of America* (Washington, D.C.: Gales and Seaton, 1828), pp. 86–87, 104–105.

52. Wharton, *A Treatise on Criminal Law in the United States.* We consulted the editions of 1857, 1874, and 1880.

53. Joel Prentiss Bishop, *Commentaries on the Law of Statutory Crimes* (Boston: Little, Brown and Company, 1883), pp. 369, 411–14, 437–38, and *New Commentaries on Marriage, Divorce, and Separation,* 2 vols. (Chicago: T. H. Flood and Company, 1891), 1:754–56.

54. Sir William Oldnall Russel and Charles Greaves, *A Treatise on Crimes and Misdemeanors,* 9th American ed. from the 4th London ed. (Philadelphia, 1877).

55. L. Radzinowicz, *Sir James Fitzjames Stephen* (London: Selden Society, 1957), p. 22.

56. *West's Annotated California Codes, Penal Codes Section 211 to 446* (Official California Penal Code Classification, St. Paul, Minn.: West Publishing Col., 1970), section 287, p. 554, and section 288a, p. 624.

4

Masturbation

Masturbation can be defined in various ways, and though it can involve more than one person, the simplest definition is any action of deliberate self-stimulation that brings about sexual arousal. Such stimulation may or may not be pursued to the point of orgasm and it may not even have orgasm as its ultimate objective. The term itself comes from the Latin, although there is some disagreement among etymologists about the root words from which it is derived. In the past, etymologists generally held that the word masturbation had been formed from a combination of the Latin word *manus* (hand) and *stuprare,* meaning to defile. It was this supposed etymology that led some early modern writers on the subject rather pedantically to spell the word *masturpation* because they believed that it was linguistically more correct, since the letters "b" and "p" could be interchanged in Latin. More recent scholarship has been pointed out that the Romans never regarded masturbation as an act of defilement and such an emotionally derogatory connotation cannot be documented in any of the ancient sources. As a result, many have suggested another verb as its source, *turbare,* meaning to agitate or disturb; when combined with the word *manus,* "masturbate" means to disturb or excite by the hand. However, even this definition has been called into question by a new generation of scholars who prefer to see the term as a hybrid derived from the Greek *mezea,* meaning genitals, and *turbare*; hence masturbation would mean "arousing the genitals."

Interestingly, whether this last etymology has any validity or not, it more clearly approaches what we mean by masturbation today. Though the hands or the fingers have undoubtedly been the most common way to masturbate, men, and especially women, have been rather ingenious in ways to stimulate themselves. Japanese women, for example, have long utilized *ben-wa,* a pair of hollow balls, one of which is partially filled with mercury. The two balls are inserted into the vagina, the empty one first; the woman then either lies down or sits in a rocking chair; as she gently rolls her hips, the mercury slides back and forth in the outer ball, constantly nudging the inner ball against the cervix. The vibrations from the balls are transmitted outward to the clitoris and labia and inward to the uterus, enabling a woman to drift from one orgasm to another. Some women have been known to continue their movements for hours. In the West, the same effect has been achieved by vibrators, many of which are shaped in the form of a penis. Both sexes have used a great deal of ingenuity in arousing themselves by rubbing their genitals against various objects, often while fully clothed, or by such activities as horseback riding. We have often wondered, for example, if the traditional emphasis on Western women riding sidesaddle was due not to the difficulty of riding astride a horse with long dresses, but to the fear that the rubbing that ensued from using a regular saddle would prove arousing. The U.S. Army worried that the same thing might happen with their cavalry soldiers; therefore, to lessen the risk of arousal, traditional army saddles were designed with an oval hole in the middle for the penis to fit into and so avoid such rubbing. Ostensibly the justification for this hole was to avoid damage to the testicles, but it was no more protective of them than the traditional saddle used by the working cowboys.

We can say with certainty, however, that the Judeo-Christian religious tradition does not look favorably on masturbation. For example, a passage in Leviticus states:

> And if any man's seed of copulation go out from him, then he shall wash all his flesh in water, and be unclean until the evening. And every garment, and every skin, whereon is the seed of copulation, shall be washed with water, and unclean until the evening.[1]

It is not clear whether this passage refers to a spontaneous emission, premature ejaculation, masturbation, or perhaps even *coitus interruptus,* although it is obvious that the writers of the Jewish Scriptures regarded sexual emission as both sacred and taboo. Normally the purifying ceremonies required short periods of continence.[2]

Nowhere in the Jewish (or Christian) scriptures is there a clear, unchallenged reference to masturbation as distinguished from other nonprocreative sex, although the story in Genesis about the sin of Onan has been often interpreted as a prohibition of masturbation:

> And Judah said unto Onan, Go into thy brother's wife, and marry her, and raise up the seed to thy brother. And Onan knew that the seed should not be his; and it came to pass, when he went in unto his brother's wife, that he spilled it on the ground, lest that he should give seed to his brother. And the thing which he did displeased the Lord; wherefore he slew him also.[3]

A close reading of the passage clearly emphasizes that the activity referred to as the spilling of the seed was *coitus interruptus,* and most modern biblical scholars hold that Onan was punished not for spilling his seed but for his refusal to obey the Levirate requirement that Onan take his dead brother's wife. In spite of such scholarly textual interpretation, there has long been a widespread popular equation of the story with masturbation. In modern Hebrew, for example, the term for masturbation is *onanuth* and one who masturbates is an *onan.* Certainly in the Talmud masturbation is frequently condemned, one Talmudic scholar even classifying it as a capital crime.[4] So great was the fear of males being aroused by accidental touching that Orthodox Jews were urged to avoid touching their penis even while urinating; an exception was allowed for a married man whose wife was readily available for intercourse.[5]

Talmudic commentators were also concerned with female sexuality, particularly that of widows living alone. Such women were prohibited from keeping a pet dog for fear that they would utilize the dog for sexual activity.[6] Widows were also enjoined from acquiring a male slave, probably for the same reason.[7] Interestingly, although female homosexuality was equated with harlotry, and punishable by beating, the rabbis did not put any restriction on private friendships with women, and kept quiet about solitary female masturbation.[8]

Inevitably, with such Jewish attitudes, Christianity expressed considerable fear over masturbation, a fear given sanction by the Church Fathers such as St. Augustine, who regarded any nonprocreative sex as sin. Early Christian penitentials are full of warnings about self-arousal. Often the penance was as harsh for the masturbator as it was for the fornicator.[9] Such attitudes in the penitentials and theological writings carried over into canon law. In the eyes of some commentators, masturbation constituted grounds for divorce just as homosexuality did.[10]

Medical and scientific writers before the eighteenth century generally either ignored the subject of masturbation or mentioned it only in passing. Galen, one of the great medical authorities of antiquity, for example, recommended that women masturbate in order to avoid hysteria. Such advice was believed necessary because Galen taught that females had a secretion similar to the male semen, produced in the uterus, and the retention of the substance through sexual abstinence led to spoilage and the corruption of blood, which, in turn, resulted in a cooling of the body and an irritation of the nerves, causing hysteria.[11] His solution to the difficulty was to apply warm substances to the uterus and to use digital manipulation. Galen illustrated with a case study:

> Following the warmth of the remedies and arising from the touch of the genital organs required by the treatment there followed twitchings accompanied at the same time by pain and pleasure after which she emitted turbid and abundant sperm. Thus it seemed to me that retention of a sperm impregnated with evil essence had—in causing damage throughout the body—a much greater power than that of the retention of the menses.[12]

Galen recognized that a similar syndrome existed in males; in fact he taught that the retention of sperm had a much more noxious influence upon the male body than the retention of the menses upon the female.[13] The fact that Galen failed to mention masturbation as a remedy might well be that he felt his male readers knew enough to solve the problem on their own without turning to him for advise.

By the eighteenth century many of the sexual activities previously regarded as a matter of faith and morals, had come to be regarded as important subjects for medical and scientific investigation. This is because eighteenth-century medical theories assumed that good health was the result of a kind of equilibrium which could be thrown out of kilter by certain activities, thus causing a drain on the body. Equilibrium could be restored either by avoiding such activities or by taking other kinds of strengthening measures. While theorists disagreed in their assumptions about how the body worked, they all emphasized the need to keep the body in balance. Sexual activity of any kind was thought to endanger the body's equilibrium. Two factors contributed to such an assumption: One is the observable phenomenon that orgasm in the male results not only in the ejaculation of semen but also in a brief feeling of lassitude. This led many, if not most, physicians to believe that the rash expenditure of semen could result in growing feebleness, even insanity. Adding to this assumption was a second observation, namely, that many sexually promiscuous individuals also contracted syphilis, which in its tertiary stage results in insanity or various other physical debilities.

Since it was not shown until late in the nineteenth century that syphilis, usually after a long period of quiescence, had a third phase, these debilities were associated with sexual intercourse itself, and taken as proof of the dangers of sexual activity.

Particularly influential in focusing medical attention on masturbation as a causal factor in disease was the Lausanne, Switzerland, physician S. A. D. Tissot (1728–1797), one of the more important medical writers of the eighteenth century.[14] In observing that sexual intercourse, like any other forms of exercise, increased the peripheral circulation, Tissot concluded that all sexual activity was potentially dangerous because it caused blood to rush to the head. Such a rush of blood, he believed, starved the nerves, making them more susceptible to damage, thereby increasing the likelihood of insanity. Tissot, in effect, incorporated the Augustinian view of sex into medicine, making what had been a sin into a causal factor for disease. Since his emphasis on the dangers of sexual activity conformed so closely to Christian belief patterns, Tissot's "scientific" conclusions came to be widely accepted. Tissot, however, went further than the Church Fathers in emphasizing the evils of masturbation. For him, the very worst kind of sexual activity was the solitary orgasm, since it could be indulged in so conveniently and at such a tender age that excess was inevitable and the resulting nerve damage irreparable. Moreover, the dangers of masturbation were made worse because masturbators realized they were committing a sin, a recognition that made their nervous system more vulnerable to damages. All this misinformation appeared in Tissot's influential treatise *L'Onanisme, dissertation sur les maladies produites par la masturbation* (*Onanism, Dissertation on the Maladies Brought On by Masturbation*), which was quickly translated into English and other languages.[15]

While Tissot's ideas seem to have been inspired as much by religious pamphleteering as by real scientific proof,[16] his influence on the medical profession was profound. During the rest of the eighteenth century and throughout the nineteenth century, treatise after treatise pointed to the dangers of masturbation, and the whole era might well be called the age of masturbatory insanity.

In the United State, Benjamin Rush, the physician-signer of the Declaration of Independence, and a formative figure in American medicine, threw his influence behind the belief that masturbation was one of the inciting causes of insanity. If the pamphlet literature is any indication, large numbers of Americans believed him. Rush taught that the overuse of sexual power, typical of the masturbator, caused seminal weakness, impotence, dysury [painful urination], tabes dorsalis [destruction of the posterior column of the spinal cord], syphilis, pulmonary consumption, dyspepsia, dimness of sight, vertigo, epilepsy, hypochondriasis [morbid anxiety over one's health], loss of memory, manalgia [ulcers], fatuity, and death.

Rush, however, was not entirely anti-sex. He believed that most sexual activity was less harmful than masturbation. Moreover, he held, abnormal restraint from sexual activity was also dangerous since it could lead to "tremors, a flushing of the face, sighing, nocturnal pollutions, hysteria, hypochondriasis, and in women *furor uterinus* [i.e., hysteria]."[17]

With only a few exceptions, nineteenth-century American physicians believed in and taught the dangers of masturbation. Some extended the meaning of masturbation to include all sexual activity not resulting in procreation, all of which, they proclaimed, debilitated the patient's physical and mental capacities, causing him or her to succumb more easily to grave physical and mental illness. As further evidence for such assertions, physicians offered their observations that a large proportion of patients in the growing number of mental institutions masturbated. From this they then concluded that it was such practices that originally had caused these people to become ill. Inevitably when physicians could find no other cause for insanity, they looked to masturbation. Numerous tracts were written warning young men and women of its perils. Some were more cautious than others but the conclusions were the same. Thomas L. Nicholas, for example, a nineteenth-century hydropathic practitioner, believed that some people might be more hereditarily predisposed toward insanity than others. Still, the risk to everyone was increased by exhaustion from masturbation, disappointments in love, grief, and disorder of the passions.[18]

The nineteenth century also began to be marked by an official prudery notable for its reluctance to discuss sexual matters directly. Some physicians, who believed in the dangers of masturbatory insanity, hesitated to mention masturbation openly, fearful that the mere mention of the subject might encourage people to try it. William Acton, a prominent British physician who usually adhered to the proper standards of decorum in matters about sex, urged his colleagues not to be reticient in discussing masturbation in order to overcome the misinformation given out by by quacks. Acton justified his own writing as necessary in order to correct this deficiency in the medical profession, but his ideas were the same as those of the people he called quacks, namely, that masturbation was a causal factor in insanity.[19]

Masturbation not only caused mental illness, but was regarded by many as a root cause for all kinds of sickness. Alfred Hitchcock, an American physician who reported on the evil effects of masturbation among his own patients, included the case of a twenty-three-year-old man who died after six years of habitual masturbation.[20] The famed Abraham Jacobi (1830–1919), considered the founder of pediatrics in the United States, was simply reflecting current medical ideology when he blamed infantile paralysis and rheumatism in children on masturbation.[21] Those physicians who were skeptical of such claims were chastised by what had come to be the medical establishment. Allen W. Hagenbach, who had studied some eight hundred "insane" males at Cook County Hospital in Chicago, explained that while there might have been some exaggeration of the effects of masturbation, the dangers were such that it was difficult to overrate them. Inevitably Hagenbach's passionate belief in the evil effects of masturbation led him to ignore any contrary data. For example, he claimed that the penis of the typical male masturbator was "enormously enlarged," when elsewhere in his own study he reported that after measuring the genitalia of twenty-six "insane" masturbators, he could find only five with enlarged penises; eighteen were classed as normal, and three had "atrophied" appendages, whatever that might mean.[22]

Increasingly, discussions of masturbation went far beyond self-stimulation, including almost all nonprocreative sex. Several of the cases described by Hagenbach involve homosexual relationships. Later Joseph W. Howe flatly stated that pederasts were diseased individuals whose problems stemmed from youthful masturbation. It was masturbation which had led men to separate further and further from women, and to put themselves in a peculiarly "unnatural relation to them."[23] He was seconded by James Foster Scott who lumped together *coitus interruptus, coitus in os* (oral sex), *coitus inter femora* (interfemoral copulation), pederasty, bestiality, mutual stimulation, and "self-pollutions" as masturbation. Scott went so far as to claim that a child conceived by any method of perverted coition would have a malformed sexual instinct.[34] It was the growing fear resulting from the antimasturbatory propagandists that led two states, Indiana and Wyoming, to put statutes on their books making it a crime to encourage a person to masturbate.

American beliefs were only reflections of continental trends. Richard Freiherr von Krafft-Ebing (1840–1902), probably the major sex researcher of the last part of the nineteenth century, subscribed to masturbation as a causal factor of what he called *psychopathia sexualis* as well as other ills. According to Krafft-Ebing,

Nothing is so prone to contaminate—under certain circumstances, even to exhaust—the source of all noble and ideal sentiments, which arise of themselves from a normally developing sexual instinct, as the practice of masturbation in early years. It despoils the unfolding bud of perfume and beauty and leaves behind only the coarse, animal desire for sexual satisfaction. If an individual spoiled in this manner, reaches an age of maturity, there is wanting in him that aesthetic, ideal, pure, and free impulse which draws one toward the opposite sex. Thus the glow of sensual sensibility wanes, and the inclination toward the opposite sex becomes weakened. This defect influences the morals, character, fancy, feeling, and instinct of the youthful masturbator, male or female, in an unfavorable way. . . .
But too early and perverse sexual satisfaction injures not merely the mind, but also the body, inasmuch as it induces neuroses of the sexual apparatus (irritable weakness of the centers governing erection and ejaculation, defective pleasurable feeling in coitus).[25]

One particularly horrifying story Krafft-Ebing told was of a woman who began to masturbate as a child and continued to do so in her marriage, even during her twelve pregnancies. As a result of the woman's activities, he said, five of her children died early, four of them were hydrocephalic, and two of the boys began to masturbate at early ages. Krafft-Ebing left unrecorded the fate of the twelfth child, but the implication was clear: masturbation was dangerous. Often, he added, even heroic medical intervention failed to discourage degenerate child masturbators. As an illustration, Krafft-Ebing cited the "disgusting story" of a girl who began to masturbate at seven, and by the age of ten was given to the most "revolting" vices, although what these were was not mentioned. Treatment included applying a white hot iron to the girl's clitoris, which, he sadly reported, had no effect in overcoming the practice.

It was not only physicians and medical professionals who wrote about the dangers of masturbation; it was a topic about which everyone could recount horror stories. One influential writer was Mrs. Elizabeth Osgood Goodrich Willard, who, we believe, was the first to use the term "sexology" to describe writing about sex. Willard, following Tissot, held that all sexual activity was debilitating since it resulted in a waste of a person's strength. She compared regular sexual activity in a man to piling up bricks and then throwing them down, or to a man beating the wind with his fist. "A sexual orgasm," Willard wrote, "is much more debilitating to the system than a whole day's work."

It is this constant abuse of the sexual organs, producing constant failures and the most loathsome disease; it is this ridiculous farce of a strong man putting forth all the nervous energy of his system, till he is perfectly prostrated by the effort, without one worthy motive, purpose or end; it is this which has so disgraced the act of impregnation. When human beings are generated under such conditions, it is no wonder they go through life as criminals, without a single good purpose or deed, and where all sense of shame is not lost, hanging their heads as if ashamed of their existence.

She adds:

We must stop this waste through the sexual organs, if we would have health and strength of body. Just as sure as that the excessive abuse of the sexual organs destroys their power and use, producing inflammation, disease and corruption, just so sure is it that a less amount of abuse in the same relative proportion injures the parental function of the organs, and impairs the health and strength of the whole system. Abnormal action is abuse.[26]

For Willard, it seems, almost every sexual activity was debilitating.

Under the influence of such ideology, worried parents anxiously inspected their children for any signs of masturbation. John Harvey Kellogg, whose Battle Creek Sanitarium in Michigan introduced new breakfast foods to the world, listed the suspicious signs exhibited by the child masturbator. These included a general debility; consumption-like symptoms; premature and defective development; sudden changes in disposition; lassitude; sleeplessness; failure of mental capacity; fickleness; untrustworthiness; love of solitude; bashfulness; unnatural boldness; mock piety; being easily frightened; confusion of ideas; aversion to girls in boys but a decided liking for boys in girls; round shoulders; weak backs and stiffness of the joints; paralysis of the lower extremities; unnatural gait; bad position in bed; lack of breast development in females; capricious appetite; fondness for unnatural and hurtful or irritating articles (such as salt, pepper, spice, vinegar, mustard, clay, slate pencils, plaster, and chalk); disgust at simple foods; use of tobacco; unnatural paleness; acne or pimples; biting of fingernails; shifty eyes; moist cold hands; palpitation of the heart; hysteria in females; chlorosis or the green sickness; epileptic fits; bed-wetting; and the use of obscene words and phrases. The dangers were terrible to behold, since genital excitement produced intense congestion and led to urethral irritation, enlarged prostate in males, bladder and kidney infection, priapism, piles and prolapse of the rectum, atrophy of the testes, varicocele (varicose enlargement of the veins of the spermatic cord), nocturnal emissions, and general exhaustion. The ultimate nervous shock of continuing masturbation was so profound that insanity would result.[27]

Once a child masturbator was recognized and diagnosed, parents were advised to take action. To help them there were a number of devices. Gloves were made for children to wear to bed so that they could not touch themselves, and parents were advised to encourage their children to sleep with their hands outside the covers. For more difficult cases, special belts were made, often called chastity girdles. These devices were designed to prevent individuals from touching, looking at, or examining their genitals. John Moodie described in 1848 some of his own inventions in this line: For girls he had designed a girdle of padded cushions to fit around the labia with a special mesh grating made of either ivory or bone to allow urine to pass through. The whole apparatus was hooked together by means of belts to a pair of tight-fitting drawers and secured by a padlock with a secret flap containing the keyhole. Moodie claimed that his device prevented girls not only from masturbating but also from being seduced. For males he had designed a belt made of strong woven material in which a metal container shaped generally to the outlines of the male genitals was attached. The tube was perforated at the end for the purpose of urination, and along the side for ventilation, but it also was locked in place in back.[28]

A number of these devices received patents from the U.S. Patent Office while others were patented in other countries. One of the male devices patented in 1897 consisted of a metal shield shaped to the abdomen and held in place around the waist by a belt with a lock in back. The lower portion of the plate was fashioned into a tube through which, according to the wording of the application, "the male organ is based." The tube was adjustable in size and protruding on the inside of the tube were a number of pricking points that pierced the penis if it became erect. The patent application stated that when

> from any cause, expansion in this organ begins, it will come in contact with the pricking points and the necessary pain or warning sensation will result. If the person wearing the device be asleep he will be awakened or recalled to his senses in time to prevent further expansion.

However,

If through forgetfulness or any other cause his thoughts should be running in lascivious channels (in waking hours), these will be diverted by the pain from the pricking points on the inside. Voluntary self-gratification will be checked as the wearer cannot find relief without removing the appliance.[29]

When even these devices seemed to be ineffective, the dutiful and loving parents, wanting to preserve their child's health and sanity at all costs, could turn to even more drastic means. In England, for example, Dr. Isaac Baker Brown performed clitoridectomies, i.e., the removal of the clitoris to cut down on female masturbation. By 1866 he had performed forty-eight such operations, although the subsequent publication of his book on the topic caused his London Surgical House, where he performed such operations, to be shut down. For males, the most extreme procedure was castration. According to one investigator, R. A. Spitz, who surveyed standard American medical textbooks dating from the turn of the century, the standard treatment, particularly in mental hospitals, was cauterization of the genitals.[30]

For a time the medical preoccupation with masturbation led to a short lived specialty group which emphasized orificial surgery, a euphemism for circumcision in boys and excision of the hood of the clitoris in girls, although it also included removal of hemorrhoids in the rectum of both sexes. The society was founded by Dr. E. H. Pratt, who held that this kind of surgery cured a number of illnesses, including epilepsy and masturbation. Pratt advanced the theory that health began below the belt (i.e., in the genitals) because the irritation of the lower terminals of the sympathetic nervous system effected the emotional, moral, and religious side of humankind far more than did those of the upper terminals.[31]

Some of Pratt's followers turned to drastic measures. In a particularly troublesome case of nervousness, an Ohio physician first attempted to cure an especially fractious masturbator by cauterizing her clitoris. When this failed to stop the child from touching her genitals, a surgeon was called in to bury the clitoris with silver wire sutures. When the child tore the wires out and continued to masturbate, the clitoris itself was removed. Later the patient reported that she no longer touched her genitals because there was nothing left for her to touch.[32] Such were the medical wonders of the orificial surgeons.

One of the long-lasting effects of the concern of American physicians with the dangers of masturbation, was widespread circumcision of male infants, to such an extent that circumcision came to be a distinguishing characteristic of the American male just as it traditionally had been for

Jews. Nominally it was done for reasons of preventive health, to cut down urinary infections in infant males and to avoid the problems of cleaning the penis, which causes the penis to become erect and thereby, it was believed, imprints a love of masturbation in the infant. The practice of circumcision has become so much the norm in this country that when a special task force of the American Academy of Pediatrics indicated in 1975 that there was no absolute medical indication for routine circumcision,[33] it occasioned a great deal of surprise and a series of debates that is still ongoing. Despite the support given to the pediatricians' action by the American College of Obstetricians and Gynecologists as well as the College of Urologists, changes in procedures were slow. Some argued that male circumcision prevented cancer of the cervix (an idea later proved to be erroneous); that it prevented penile cancer (a rare malignancy); and that it prevented phimosis, a narrowing of the external orifice of the penis. The prevention of phimosis is much better documented, although this is comparatively rare and if phimosis does occur, it can be dealt with surgically. However, the majority of infant males are still being circumcised simply because parents do not want their children to be different from others, and once a custom is established, even if based on mythical assumptions, it often continues. The operation, however, is no longer routine and it has to be requested by the parents.

Probably the first major sex researcher to examine the evidence on masturbation objectively was Havelock Ellis (1859–1939), who, between 1896 and 1928, published a series of books on sex which were collected into a seven-volume work titled *Studies on the Psychology of Sex.* By the time Ellis wrote, the effects of third-stage syphilis were well known; therefore, some of the misinformation about the dangers of masturbation had already been disproved. Ellis's major contribution was to document that masturbation had been found among people of nearly every race regardless of the condition under which they lived.[34] Though Ellis himself still remained somewhat fearful of the consequences of masturbation, others began to speak out more forcibly. Among them was Ralcy Husted Bell, a physician who, in 1929, stated that masturbation, by

> every known law of nature, according to clinical data, according to the plainest commonsense . . . is not more harmful than the co-operative act between mates. Why should it be? Certainly, if it were, the race would have destroyed itself ages and ages ago. The act, as a physiological function, is not in any sense an outlaw, physiologically considered.[35]

Perhaps the most important evidence on the topic was that gathered by Kinsey et al., who found that 92 percent of their male sample and 62 percent of their female sample had masturbated at some time in their life, most of them to the point of orgasm (1 percent of the males and 4 percent of the females had not achieved orgasm). Males, as a rule, began masturbating at puberty and the incidence decreased after that as they turned to other forms of sexual activity. Females, on the other hand, were slower to begin masturbation but continued to masturbate longer. According to Kinsey, masturbation to orgasm in females was more common among women in middle age than among girls in their teens.[36]

A 1973–74 survey conducted by the Playboy Foundation found that among 2,026 individuals, every other married male and one out of three married females had masturbated during the preceding year. The highest rates were in the twenty-five-to-thirty-four age group for both males and females, although the prevalence among eighteen- to twenty-four-year-olds was almost as high. After age thirty-four there was a steady decline until by age fifty-five (and over) only 20 percent of males and 20 percent of females still engaged in masturbation. The *Playboy* study also found that attitudes toward masturbation had become more liberal since the time of Kinsey, although many still remained ambivalent. Generally the more education a person had the more he or she was likely to masturbate, in part because the many traditional taboos about masturbation tend to impress the less educated, and in part because premarital coitus at the time was more common among the less educated than among the better educated. Masturbation in this sense served as an alternative. Although many of these class differences, particularly concerning premarital coitus, are beginning to disappear, they still remain a significant factor. A rather high percentage of people still feel that masturbation is wrong; however, there is greater inclination among young people than among their elders to accept masturbation as normal, so the trend toward acceptability seems to be on the rise.[37] The most recent sexual survey, however, shows that a disparity continues to exist and that men are more likely than women to engage in autoerotic practices.[38]

Interestingly, in light of this tendency, one of the most outspoken advocates of masturbation has been sexologist Betty Dodson, who emphasizes that

> Masturbation is a primary form of sexual expression. It's not just for kids or for those in-between lovers or for old people who end up alone.

> Masturbation is the ongoing love affair that each of us has with ourselves through our lifetime.[39]

In her book Dodson recounts her own sexual history, including her initial struggle to accept masturbation as sex rather than sin. Once a person overcomes the inhibitions, she argues, masturbation can be a vital form of self-expression. Dodson has traveled around the country with her Bodysex Workshops, at which she has taught thousands of women and men to feel comfortable with solo sex.

Masturbation was a key methodology for William Masters and Virginia Johnson, as well as for William Hartman and Marilyn Fithian in their studies of the human sexual response. One of Masters and Johnson's discoveries was that of the most pleasurable way for women to masturbate. Contrary to mythology it was not by direct rubbing of the clitoris but rather by manipulating the side of the clitoris or stimulating the entire mons area rather than concentrating on the clitoral body. Masters and Johnson emphasized, however, that no two women had been observed to masturbate in exactly the same way.[40]

Sex therapists such as Joseph LoPiccolo, Helen Singer Kaplan, and Lonny Barbach have emphasized that a program of directed masturbation is effective in treating primary orgasmic dysfunction, although they often find it necessary to relieve a client's fear or anxieties about such practices.[41] Shere Hite even went so far as to claim that masturbation may be the key to sexual enjoyment for women. In her study of a self-selected sample of women, only 30 percent of participants were able to "orgasm" as a result of heterosexual intercourse. A significant portion who reported they could reach orgasm only with masturbation had not shared this information with their sex partners—evidence both of the continued hold of ancient taboos and the lack of communication about matters sexual.[42]

In retrospect, it seems clear that masturbatory insanity was a disease created by physicians and perpetuated by pseudoscientific assumptions which fitted into the antisexual traditions of Western culture. Consequently, generations of children were brought up believing that masturbation might well send them to a mental institution and that their acne, bad breath, body odors, and numerous other symptoms were all evidence of their secret sin. Although no medically trained or scientifically oriented person today would subscribe to the ideas advanced by Tissot and his followers, some hidden fears about masturbation continue to linger. Evidence for this is the reluctance to change patterns of male circumcision. Perhaps we can hold such strong attitudes because condemning masturbation, which is usually difficult to detect or observe, has provided such a simple solution to societal problems. While only a small number today would publicly claim that by eliminating the masturbator, there would be no mental illness, no poverty, no juvenile delinquency, it still takes a long time for new scientific assumptions to catch up with old mythologies that once had such a strong emotional appeal. Such beliefs still lurk in the unconscious of many. In fact, the 1994 sex survey conducted out of the University of Chicago reported that masturbation was the most sensitive of all topics on which information was sought. So reluctant were those interviewed to talk about their own experience that they gave their answers in writing, and the interviewer herself did not know their responses. No other sexual qustion was treated so cautiously.[43]

All we can hope for is that the new scientific assumptions will ultimately replace the old. This will happen only if we continue to challenge and to modify and accept what we find. This, however, has proven difficult in terms of human sexuality; unfortunately science in the past has often only added to the anxieties about sex.

NOTES

1. Lev. 15:16–18.
2. Exod. 19:14–15.
3. Gen. 38:8–10. The quote is from the Revised Standard Version.
4. Niddah, 13a, translated into English by Israel W. Slotki, in the *Babylonian Talmud,* edited by J. Epstein (London: Soncino Press, 1948).
5. Ibid.
6. Abodah Zarah, 22b, translated by A. Mishcon and A. Cohen, in the *Babylonian Talmud.* See also Lev. 20:16.
7. Bab Mezia, 71a, translated into English by Salis Daiches and H. Freeman, in the *Babylonian Talmud.*
8. See Louis H. Epstein, *Sex Laws and Customs in Judaism* (New York: Bloch Publishing Company, 1948), p. 138.
9. See, for example, the translations of the various penitentials by John T. McNeill and Helena M. Gamer in *Medieval Handbooks of Penance* (New York: Columbia Univeristy Press, 1938), *passim,* and the discussion by Pierre Payer, *Sex and the Penitentials: The Development of a Sexual Code 550–1150* (Toronto: University of Toronto Press, 1984), pp. 46–47, and *passim.*
10. For a variety of interpretations in canon law see James Brundage, *Law,*

Sex, and Christian Society in Medieval Europe (Chicago: University of Chicago Press, 1987). See the references in the index under the term "masturbation."

11. Galen, *De locis affectis,* VI (Venice: Juntas, 1586), II, 39. The passage is discussed by Henri Cresbron, *Histoire critique de l'hysterie* (Paris: Asslin & Houzen, 1909), p. 41, and in some detail by Ilza Veith, *Hysteria: The History of a Disease* (Chicago: University of Chicago Press, 1965), pp. 31–39.

12. Cresbon, *Histoire critique,* p. 44.

13. Ibid., p. 42.

14. For a biography see Antoinette Emch-Dériaz, *Tissot: Physician of the Enlightenment,* American University Studies, Ser. 9, no. 126 (New York: Peter Lang, 1992).

15. It went through many editions and translations. Particularly influential on the English-speaking world was *Onanism: A Treastise Upon the Disorders produced by Masturbation,* translated by A. Hume (London: J. Pridden, 1766). This particular edition was reprinted by Garland in a series on *Marriage, Sex, and The Family in England 1660–1800,* edited by Randolph Trumbach (New York: Garland, 1985). It had been preceded in the English-speaking world by an anonymous book titled *Onania; or, the Heinous Sin of Self-Pollution* which went through several editions. See the eighth edition (London: Elizabeth Rumball, for Thomas Crouch, 1723), a work which aroused considerable controversy.

16. See Alex Comfort, *The Anxiety Makers* (New York: Dell Publishing Company, 1969), pp. 74ff.; E. H. Hare, "Masturbatory Insanity: The History of an Idea," *Journal of Mental Science* 108 (1962): 1–25; R. H. MacDonald, "The Frightful Consequences of Onanism," *Journal of the History of Ideas* 28 (1967): 423–31; Rene A. Spitz, "Authority and Masturbation," *The Psychoanalytic Quarterly* 21 (1952): 490–527; Vern L. Bullough and Martha Voght, "Homosexuality and Its Confusion with the 'Secret Sin' in Pre-Freudian America," *Journal of the History of Medicine* 28 (1973): 143–55.

17. Both quotes are from Benjamin Rush, *Medical Inquiries and Observations upon the Diseases of the Mind* (Philadelphia: 1812), p. 347.

18. Norman Dain, *Concepts of Insanity in the United States, 1789–1865* (New Brunswick, N.J.: Rutgers University Press, 1964), p. 160.

19. Steven Marcus, "Mr. Acton of Queen Anne Street, or, the Wisdom of Our Ancestors," *Partisan Review* 31 (1964): 201–30.

20. Alfred Hitchcock, "Insanity and Death from Masturbation," *Boston Medical and Surgical Journal* 26 (1842): 283–86.

21. Abraham Jacobi, "On Masturbation and Hysteria in Young Children," *American Journal of Obstetrics* 8 (1876): 595–96; 9 (1876): 218–38.

22. Allen W. Hagenbach, "Masturbation as a Cause of Insanity," *Journal of Nervous and Mental Diseases* 6 (1879): 603–12.

23. Joseph W. Howe, *Excessive Venery, Masturbation and Continence* (New York: Bermingham and Co., 1889), pp. 113–15.

24. James Foster Scott, *The Sexual Instinct* (New York; E. B. Treat & Co., 1899), pp. 419-27.

25. Richard von Krafft-Ebing, *Psychopathia Sexualis,* translated into English by Charles Gilbert Chaddock from the seventh German edition (Philadelphia: F. A. Davis, 1894), pp. 188-89. Another English translation, based on the twelfth German edition, was done by Franklin S. Klaf (New York: Bell Publishing Company, 1965). Pagination in this edition is very similar to that in the Chaddock translation.

26. Elizabeth Osgood Goodrich Willard, *Sexology as the Philosophy of Life* (Chicago: J. R. Walsh, 1867), pp. 306-308.

27. J. H. Kellogg, *Plain Facts for Old and Young* (Burlingame, Iowa: I. F. Senger, 1882), pp. 332-44. The book has often been reprinted, including one edited by Vern L. Bullough (Buffalo, N.Y.: Heritage Press, 1974).

28. John Moodie, *A Medical Treatise: With Principles and Observations to Preserve Chastity and Morality,* quoted in Eric John Dingwall, *The Girdle of Chastity* (New York: The Macaulay Company, n.d.), pp. 122-28.

29. See Vern L. Bullough, "Technology for the Prevention of 'Les Maladies Produites par la Masturbation,' " *Technology and Culture* 28 (1987): 828-32. See also "Chastity Belts for Men," *Sexology,* March 1972, pp. 68-70, which is the source of the quote. We found several dozen such inventions in an examination of the published records of the U.S. Patent Office for the last two decades of the nineteenth century and first decade of the twentieth.

30. See Spitz, "Authority and Masturbation," pp. 490-527.

31. E. H. Pratt, *Orificial Surgery and Its Application to the Treatment of Chronic Diseases* (Chicago: Halsey Brothers, 1890).

32. See Spitz, "Authority and Masturbation."

33. "Report of the Ad Hoc Task Force on Circumcision from the Committee on Fetus and Newborn of the AAP," *Pediatrics* 56, no. 4 (October 1975).

34. Havelock Ellis, "Auto-Eroticism," part 1, *Studies in the Psychology of Sex,* 2 vols. (reprint New York: Random House, 1936), 1:166.

35. Ralcy Husted Bell, *Self-Amusement and Its Spectres* (reprint New York: The Big Dollar Books Company, 1932), p. 35.

36. Alfred C. Kinsey, Wardell B. Pomeroy, and Clyde Martin, *Sexual Behavior in the Human Male* (Philadelphia: W. B. Saunders, 1948), pp. 499ff., and Kinsey, Pomeroy, Martin, and Paul H. Gebhard, *Sexual Behavior in the Human Female* (Philadelphia: W. B. Saunders, 1953), pp. 142ff.

37. See Morton M. Hunt, *Sexual Behavior in the 1970s* (Chicago: Playboy Press, 1974). Individual articles appeared in the October, November and December 1973 issues and the January and February 1974 issues of *Playboy.*

38. Edward O. Lauman, John H. Gagnon, Robert T. Michael, and Stuart Michaels, *The Social Organization of Sexuality: Sexual Practices in the United States* (Chicago; University of Chicago Press, 1994), p. 135.

39. Betty Dodson, *Sex for One: The Joy of Selfloving* (New York: Harmony

Books, 1987), p. 3. Earlier version were called *Selflove* (1974) and *Orgasm and Liberating Masturbation* (1983).

40. William H. Masters and Virginia E. Johnson, *Human Sexual Response* (Boston: Little, Brown and Company, 1966), pp. 635–65.

41. Joseph LoPiccolo and W. Charles Lobitz, "The Role of Masturbation in the Treatment of Orgasm Dysfunction," *Archives of Sexual Behavior* 2 (1973): 163–71. See also Helen Singer Kaplan, *The New Sex Therapy* (New York: Brunner/Mazel, Inc. 1974), pp. 330–31, 388–94, and *passim*, and Lonnie Barbach, "Group Treatment of Preorgasmic Women," *Journal of Sex and Martial Therapy* 1 (1974): 139–45.

42. Shere Hite, *The Hite Report: A Nationwide Study of Female Sexuality* (New York: Macmillan, 1976).

43. Lauman et al., *The Social Organization of Sexuality,* p. 64.

5

Sex and Gender

In the past, whenever a woman acted particularly aggressive, she was likely to be described as being masculine or as attempting to play a man's role. Despite many changes in sexual stereotyping since the 1960s, the stereotypes still remain. That is why, even today, if a man tends to act tender or nurturing, he is likely to be labeled as effeminate.

On the whole, our society has tolerated the "masculine" woman better than the "feminine" man, perhaps because the male has traditionally been looked upon as the more important sex.[1] Thus, we accept it as more or less natural for women to try to achieve male status by becoming more masculine themselves, provided they do not overdo it. Conversely, a male who shows a "feminine" side loses status and is thereby deserving of derision. If either sex trespasses too far into the role of the other, however, he or she is in for a difficult time.

This strict dichotomy of sexual roles is easily illustrated by an examination of standard dictionary definitions of masculinity and femininity. Almost every dictionary up to 1990 (there have been some slight changes since) tended to equate masculinity with virility, robustness, strength, and vigor, while femininity was defined in terms of tenderness, nurturing, pliability, softness, and receptivity. Inherent in such stereotypes is the belief that sexual behavior and sexual attitudes are genetically determined, and that once a person is found to be male or female there is only one possible kind of action. It is from such rigid stereotypes that much of our Western attitudes about sexual roles derive.

Biologically, males have a penis and testicles and the equipment to manufacture and deposit semen, while females have a uterus and ovaries and can manufacture ova, receive the semen, and bear children. Associated with the difference in sex organs are secondary sexual characteristics such as beards, breasts, muscular structure, and fat distribution. Do such obvious biological differences necessarily preclude women from becoming truck drivers or men from doing needlepoint? Clearly the answer is no, and vast numbers of tasks that society has defined in terms of being masculine or feminine have little or nothing to do with biology. Some evidence of this is that cultures and peoples do not agree upon which tasks are male and which female. Moreover, a woman who is aggressive is no less a female than a woman who is passive, while a man who is tender and loving is no less a male than a man who is rough and hostile. To go further, it becomes essential to distinguish biological sex, that is, the reproductive apparatus associated with being male and female, from gender, the conduct and self-identity associated with masculinity and femininity.

The term "gender" is used carelessly today by many as both a synonym and an antonym of sex. It first appeared in the language of sexuality in 1955 when sexologist John Money adopted it from philosophy and linguistics to serve as an umbrella concept describing the manliness or womanliness of persons born with sexually indeterminate genitals.[2] Money, however, continued to expand on its meaning; he currently holds that *sex* is a person's status as male, female, or intersex, while *gender* is one's identity as masculine or feminine, according to somatic and behavioral criteria. In spite of recent attempts to equate sex with gender, it is this more technical usage that we employ here.

The concept proved useful in challenging traditional ideas about male or female behavior. When psychologists first began examining these differences in the first part of the twentieth century, they based their definition of what was masculine or feminine on simplistic empirical differences based on the assumption that males and females are opposite. At its most mindless, this dichotomy equated "masculinity" with men's preference for taking showers, working as building contractors, and reading magazines such as *Popular Mechanics,* while femininity was equated with preferences for taking baths, work as seamstresses, and reading magazines such as *Good Housekeeping.*

Encouraged by Money's attempt to separate sex from gender, psychologists attempted to develop more sophisticated measures. Two such tests appeared in 1974: Sandra Bem's *Bem Sex Role Inventory* and Janet Spence and Robert Helmreich's *Personal Attributes Questionnaire,* both of which divided masculinity and femininity into two separate dimensions. Both measures demonstrated that each sex shared personal characteristics usually attributed either to one or the other, and the composition varied according to the individual.[3]

Though these tests still remained simple measurements and were not based upon any comprehensive theory of gender differences, they emphasized what was perhaps always known, namely, that certain activities were labeled as masculine or feminine simply because of societal stereotypes of what a male or female should be. Closely related to the qualities associated with gender is the nature of the gender identity that a person has. Such identity starts with the knowledge and awareness of sexual differences, long before the infant is conscious that such differences exist. This is because society, particularly in the twentieth century, has felt it important to label infants as boys or girls and to dress and treat them differently. Before this, both boys and girls were kept in dresses until past the toddler stage and toilet training. With the development of cotton diapers, modern indoor plumbing, washing machines, and color-fast fabrics not only separate clothes but separate colors were developed so we could easily recognize the boys from the girls. Different countries adopted different color schemes. In fact, there were heated arguments over colors in the American popular press, with one side maintaining that pink was a more masculine color than light blue. Despite these arguments, pink came to be adopted for girls and blue for boys in the United States, primarily because of the publicity given Thomas Gainsborough's painting *Blue Boy* and Sir Thomas Lawrence's *Pinkie* when the American Henry Edwards Huntington paid a small fortune, the highest price then paid for works of art, to bring these paintings to his San Marino museum early in the twentieth century.

One reason color schemes are so important is that researchers have found that Western parents usually handle boy babies differently than girls, treating the girls as if they were much more delicate. They also tend to worry more if their boy acts feminine than if their girl is a tomboy. Usually boys are given toy trucks and sports equipment, while girls are given dolls and doll furniture, although this is less true now than a generation ago.

Gender identity itself is complicated by the fact that a person can visualize himself or herself in a number of different gender roles, some of which society classifies as abnormal or deviant. Thus a man can see himself as any one of a number of different kinds of men—an aggressive man, a gentle man, an effeminate man, or even fantasize himself as a woman. On the other hand, a woman may envision herself as gentle and submissive, determined, "manly," or even as a man. Gender identity affects the gender role, that is, the overt behavior that a person displays in society. Usually in most people sex, gender, gender identity, and gender role are synonymous or compatible with societal expectation, but in others they are at variance, and this variance is believed to be a causal explanation for homosexuality, transvestism, and transsexualism.[4]

In recent years there has been considerable scholarly investigation into gender and sex roles in an effort to determine whether they are a result of nature or nurture, i.e., whether they are biological or social-psychological. Hermaphrodites provided one of the natural research samples: it was the study of these individuals that led John Money to adopt the term "gender." Money, Joan Hampson, and John Hampson originally studied 105 hermaphrodites using five biological determinants of sex: (1) chromosomal sex, (2) gonadal sex, (3) hormonal sex, (4) internal accessory reproductive structures, and (5) external glands. Thirty individuals had a sex assignment differing from at least one of the above five biological determinants but only five of the group had a gender role identity or an erotic orientation different from their assigned sex.[5] Money, Hampson, and Hampson concluded that psychosexuality was neutral at birth and determined almost entirely by socialization; they also held that the critical period for development of gender identity took place before twenty-seven months of age.

Demonstrating greater complexity was the case of two identical twin boys who, at the age of seven months, were circumcised by electrocautery. During the procedure an accident occurred whereby the penis of one twin was burned off. After considerable emotional upheaval, the parents, on the advice of a physician, decided to raise the mutilated boy as a girl. At seventeen months the boy had his name, clothing, and hairstyle changed, and underwent the initial steps toward genital reconstruction as a female, although surgery to make an artificial vagina was postponed until after puberty.[6]

Initial reports indicated that the boy was becoming more feminine, and the case was publicized as demonstrating just how much of our gender behavior is social-psychological. Matters, however, were not so simple: despite the efforts of the family and therapists to have the child adjust to this situation, the sex switch was recognized as not successful by the time the child reached his (or her) teens. As soon as he was able, the individual sought reconstructive surgery to fashion a penis. As of this writing, he lives as a male and seeks females as erotic companions.[7]

Giving further support to the importance of biological factors was the study by Julianne Imperator-McGinley and her colleagues in the Dominican Republic. Here, due to a genetic quirk, some males in the village of Salinas were born without apparent penises; but then, in early adolescence, a penis and scrotum emerged from the genital slit and they developed normal male secondary characteristics. Thirty-three such persons were known by the researchers, nineteen of whom had been raised as girls before the village recognized such a possibility and labeled them as "penis at twelve" children. Only eighteen of those raised as girls could be located, and sixteen of them had changed their sex to male and adopted male gender patterns and erotic interests. One changed his gender identity and thought of himself as a man with male erotic interests, but remained in a female work role. Only one retained both the gender identity and role of a woman.[8] While these cases seemed to emphasize the importance of biological factors, they were challenged by additional studies emphasizing that it was not a matter exclusively of nature or nurture. This is because after the first few such children were born, the village recognized the possibility that such a change might recur; hence they imparted this information to the families of other boys born without penises about symptoms that might lead to these children's growing a penis at twelve. Thus their ambivalent status as neither male nor female probably enhanced the boys' later ability to adjust to their male role.[9]

Further complicating the issue is the study of those whom psychologists label as gender dysphoric individuals, whom we in our own studies simply call cross-dressers. A significant number of these individuals adopt the gender identity of the other sex through transvestism, all or part of the time. Some don only certain items of clothing associated with the opposite sex while others go so far as to seek a surgical change of sex. Many of those who cross-dress are heterosexuals while some are homosexuals. Complicating things still further is that many of those who undergo surgery and actually change their sex organs end up being attracted to members of their newly assigned sex, while others prefer partners from the sex they have left; that is, the change leads to classifying individuals who regarded themselves as heterosexual before surgery, as homosexual or lesbian afterwards.

TRANSVESTISM

Transvestism is a term coined by the German sexologist Magnus Hirschfeld in 1910 and publicized by him in a book titled *Die Transvestiten* (*Transvestites*). This was a series of case studies on individuals who regularly (some permanently) cross-dressed, sixteen men and one women, most of whom were heterosexual; but there were some whom Hirschfeld classed as monosexual ("auto-erotic") and a few were homosexual. By classifying these people as transvestites, Hirschfeld gave a name to a phenomenon widely known throughout history,[11] thus inaugurating a change in public opinion which moved the cross-dresser from the category of eccentric to one deserving medical and psychiatric study. Adding to Hirschfeld's groundbreaking work was Havelock Ellis, another major twentieth-century sex researcher, who in 1913 described the same phenomenon as sexo-aesthetic inversion and described four cases.[12] As a result of conversations and discussion following his paper, Ellis concluded that to use the word "inversion" to describe this phenomenon was misleading, since it suggested homosexuality which he felt was not the case; instead Ellis adopted the word *eonism,* derived from Chevalier d'Éon, an eighteenth-century cross-dresser.[13] Ellis did not consider eonism to be a particularly troublesome problem, since most of the people he studied were able to lead lives they found satisfactory and they did not harm others. He made no proposal to change the individuals involved, and neither did Hirschfeld. Neither regarded transvestism as necessarily a sign of homosexuality. These researchers' toleration of cross-dressing, however, had little influence on later psychiatrists and others who adopted Hirschfeld's nomenclature but not his tolerance. Part of the difficulty is that there has long been societal hostility toward males dressing and acting as women unless they did so in a comic setting.

The ancient source of Western hostility to cross-dressing is not so much Greek as Jewish, a prejudice that was carried over into Western culture through Christianity. A passage in Deuteronomy (22–25) states:

> The woman shall not wear that which pertaineth unto a man, neither shall
> a man put on a woman's garment; for all that do so are an abomination
> unto the Lord thy God.

In spite of this prohibition, Christianity generally has tolerated cross-dressing at festivals such as Halloween, or under certain conditions, as in the theater where the actor's real sex is known to the audience. It also looked more favorably upon women trying to be like men and even dressing like men. Christianity has, however, been suspicious of the motives of the serious male transvestite who tries to pass as a woman. The toleration today of the female cross-dresser and the ability of women to adopt what traditionally has been regarded as men's clothing, helps account for the small number of modern female cross-dressers. In fact so-called unisex clothing is basically men's clothing which women wear, and is so ubiquitous that only the most extreme cases could be called transvestites. The historical record, however, is full of women who lived and worked as men, and who were discovered only after they had died or decided to resume their traditional dress and role.

Undoubtedly the hostility to male cross-dressers comes from the Western assumption that women are inferior to men. Though Christianity has always insisted that women were as much a special creation of God as men were, the Christian Church tended to look upon women as weaker vessels. This view was effectively summed up by the thirteenth-century theologian Thomas Aquinas, who, after admitting the special creation of women, stated:

> Good order would have been wanting in the human family if some were not governed by others wiser than themselves. So by such a kind of subjection woman is naturally subject to man, because in man the discretion of reason predominates.[14]

Tied in with this was a kind of mystic view of the inferiority of females, which emphasized that the male was superior to the female because he represented the more rational parts of the soul, while the female represented the less rational. This attitude was exemplified by the Alexandrian philosopher Philo, who taught that progress for the female meant giving up her female gender—the material, passive, corporeal, and sense-perceptive world—and taking up the active, rational world of mind and thought, the world of the male. He felt women could do this by denying their sexuality and remaining virgins—in effect giving up that part of them which was most female.[15]

With such attitudes underlying basic Christian concepts it would follow, then, that a female who wore men's clothes, who adopted the role of the male, would be trying to imitate the superior sex, thus becoming more rational; while the male who wore women's clothes, who tried to take on the gender attributes of the female, would be losing status, becoming less rational, and less likely of achieving salvation. Indeed, this seems to have been precisely the attitude of Jerome in the fourth century, who held that as

> long as woman is for birth and children, she is different from a man as body is from soul. But when she wishes to serve Christ more than the world, then she will cease to be a woman and will be called man.[16]

A similar sentiment was expressed by Jerome's contemporary, Ambrose:

> She who does not believe is a woman and should be designated by the name of her sex, whereas she who believes progresses to perfect manhood, to the measure of the adulthood of Christ. She then dispenses with the name of her sex, the seductiveness of youth, the garrulousness of old age.[17]

With the sanction of the Church Fathers behind them, inevitably a number of early devoted Christian women donned the garb of males, lived as men, and achieved sainthood. It was only after they had died that their true sex was revealed, and their ability to pass and live as devoted men tended to enhance their saintliness. Probably the archetype of the female transvestite saint was Pelagia. Her story is confused and contradictory, probably because the legends of her life incorporated several different individuals. According to the more or less standardized versions accepted today, Pelagia was a beautiful dancing girl and prostitute in Antioch. Repenting of her life, she converted to Christianity; but not wishing to be identified with her past, Pelagia left Antioch dressed as a man, a role she continued to play for the rest of her life. After much travel she found refuge on Mount Olive in Jerusalem, where, as the monk Pelagius, she acquired a great reputation for holiness. It was not until Pelagia's death that her true sex was revealed, whereupon her mourners are said to have cried out: "Glory be to thee, Lord Jesus, for thou hast many hidden treasures on earth, as well female as male."[18] Similar stories are told about a number of other women, some of whom were even said to have fathered children. Only when they died was their true sex revealed and their fellow monks came to realize how truly devoted these women had been.[19]

On the other hand, male transvestism was likely to be regarded either as a comedic interlude or associated with witchcraft or with attempts to penetrate the company of women in order to commit fornication.[20] Since there were so many limitations placed on where women might go and what they might do, men could officially cross gender boundaries in situations where a "woman" was needed. One such situation was the theater. Even in Church dramas, the forerunner of the later secular theater, female roles were taken by males, usually young clerics, since women were forbidden access to the altar area. Using males in female roles under such conditions was the lesser of two evils.[21] It was only in the last part of the seventeenth century in England that women were finally allowed to play themselves on stage. What was true of the stage was also true of opera, where European society turned to *castrati,* castrated males, to sing the woman's roles, a custom that continued into the nineteenth century.[22]

Generally, however, male transvestism, except under these conditions, was a forbidden activity, although the rich and powerful were not always bound by conventional restrictions. One of the best documented examples of historical cross-dressing is that of François-Timoleon de Choisy, better known as the Abbé de Choisy (1644–1724). He offers an interesting example because his role as a woman was one that he had grown up in. He was dressed in girl's clothes at a very tender age, although historians are not sure of the reason. Some feel his mother wanted a daughter, others that it was a political decision by his parents to ingratiate themselves with the queen whose second son, Philippe d'Orléans, the younger brother of Louis XIV, was dressed in girl's clothes, apparently in an effort to discourage him from mounting a challenge to his brother's power. Both de Choisy and Philippe continued to dress in women's clothes as adults although Philippe never acted particularly feminine in them. De Choisy, however, tried for a time to live and pass as a woman. Between the ages of fifteen and eighteen he lived the life of a young girl, accompanying his mother to the theater, receptions, and dances. This episode ended in 1662 with the death of Madame de Choisy, but the rigid corsets de Choisy had been forced to wear during his youth had given his body such feminine contours that he continued to be mistaken for a girl in boy's clothing. He soon decided to return to his skirts and live the life of a woman. De Choisy's great wealth allowed him to move to a rural area where he pretended to be a countess, and soon dominated the local social life. He took particular joy in training the daughters of the village residents in the art of being ladies, training which involved considerable fondling. When one of his young charges became pregnant, de Choisy decided to return to Paris where he publicly resumed the role of a male, but dressed privately as a woman. He also had another period of living as a woman but eventually reverted to his masculine persona and became a diplomat and an author. In the later part of his life de Choisy wrote an account (now partly lost) of his adventures in women's clothes, and it is this memoir which gives us most of our information about him.[23]

Several factors associated today with transvestism are evident in the abbé's account, namely, the early approval he received for his feminine role-playing and his delight in cross-dressing, yet with all his awareness that he was a male in woman's clothes and the periodic purges during which he tried to rid himself of his habit. De Choisy's case is quite different from that of Charles-Geneviève-Louis-Augusta-André-Timotheé d'Éon de Beaumont (1728–1810), after whom Havelock Ellis patterned his description of eonism. In the light of present-day psychological assumptions, in fact, it is not clear that d'Éon was a transvestite since he might well have been a hermaphrodite. D'Éon lived during the reign of Louis XV, and for a time served in the king's own secret service. One of his assignments was to Russia where he apparently cross-dressed and in this role became a favorite of Catherine the Great.

Later, in 1763, d'Éon was attached to the French embassy in London to help negotiate a peace treaty, after which he stayed as King George III's personal representative and then, during a hiatus between ambassadors, as minister plenipotentiary. When the French eventually named a new ambassador, d'Éon soon found himself involved in a disastrous quarrel with him. The ambassador publicly questioned d'Éon's masculinity and d'Éon responded by threatening to publish secret correspondence dealing with French wartime plans for England during the Seven Years' War that was just ending. The threat, undoubtedly made in anger, threw the whole weight of the French bureaucracy against d'Éon. Moreover, his longtime patron, Louis XV, was dead, and the new king, Louis XVI, had been antagonized by his threat to expose French secrets. The issue was complicated by two other factors: (1) d'Éon had fallen heavily in debt while in England and desperately needed to pay off his creditors, and (2) the charges of the French ambassador had led to large wagers being placed about his sex. Seeking a way out, d'Éon announced he was a woman, and when the gamblers took the issue to court, two physicians, apparently bribed, testified he was indeed a woman. Apparently d'Éon's confession endeared him to the king; thereupon he returned to France where he was offered a pension by the king, provided he give up his manly ways and live as a woman. After things quieted down, the king allowed "her" to return to England to settle some business, and d'Éon was stranded there by the outbreak of the French Revolution. This meant that d'Éon lost his French pension; although he could now have reverted to the masculine role, he feared that if he did so, his life would be in danger. Instead, to survive, d'Éon turned to staging fencing exhibitions dressed in proper women's attire. Seriously wounded in an exhibition in 1796, he lived off the charity of friends, dying in poverty in 1810. As d'Éon was being prepared for burial, he was found to be a man after all, a revelation somewhat shocking to the woman who had taken care of him for the last fourteen years of his life. A cast taken of his body at death showed a plump bosom, rounded limbs with small hands and feet. His most masculine feature, other than his genitals, were his muscular forearms.[24] Though it does not really matter whether or not d'Éon was a hermaphrodite or a transvestite, his station in life and his abrupt change of clothing in later years made him the subject of numerous stories, many of them pure fabrications, which, however, continue to circulate to this day.

Interestingly de Choisy and d'Éon are the only male cross-dressers who attracted much attention before the twentieth century, but many female transvestites are known. In almost every war women have served in the army disguised as men since there were virtually no physical exams before the twentieth century. Many soldiers were discovered to be women only when they were wounded or killed, while others only revealed their true sex many years later. Many others simply cross-dressed as males because it gave them greater freedom and economic opportunity. One such individual was James Barry (1795–1865) who served as a surgeon in the British army, reaching the rank of Inspector General of Hospitals. Little is known about Barry's early childhood, but it is believed she was either the niece or illegitimate daughter of James Barry, an influential English artist. Apparently she was raised as a boy and as such attended medical school at the University of Edinburgh, which did not then accept female students. After receiving "his" medical degree, James entered the army medical service. His military career was marked by numerous quarrels, with both superiors and subordinates, but in spite of this he moved up the professional ladder until his retirement in 1859. Barry was not particularly masculine-looking, being described as a peppery little figure with dyed red hair, a high-pitched voice, and tiny white hands, who looked absurd in the full-dress uniform with cockaded hat and huge sword; but in spite of this, and in spite of the fact that his masculinity had been often questioned, Barry was accepted as a man. It was not until his death that he was found to be a female.[25]

Colonel Barker, née Valerie Arkell-Smith, perhaps explained the motivation of many women for cross-dressing when she stated:

> [T]rousers make a wonderful difference in the outlook on life. I know that dressed as a man I did not, as I do now I am wearing skirts again, feel hopeless and helpless. Today when the whole world knows my secret I feel more a man than a woman. I want to up and do those things that men do to earn a living rather than to spend my days as a friendless woman.[26]

Arkell-Smith was born on the island of Jersey in 1895, the daughter of a gentleman farmer and a woman of independent means. The family moved to England in 1897, but Valerie spent much of her childhood attending a convent school in Brussels. After her coming-out party, Valerie took up war work during World War I, first as a nurse, then as an ambulance driver, and finally as a member of the Women's Auxiliary Air Force. In 1918, she married Lieutenant Harold Arkell-Smith, an Australian officer, but the marriage lasted only six weeks. She then became involved with another Australian, Ernest Pearce-Crouch, with whom she lived until 1923 and by whom she had two children. She then left him to assume her new identity as Victor Barker and, as such, married Elfrida Howard in 1923.

Posing as a retired military official, "Colonel" Barker made little attempt to keep out of the limelight and became a member of the National Fascisti, a military breakaway group from the British Fascist party. She took over responsibility for the organization's boxing program, training members for "combat," and organizing demonstrations against the Communists and left-wingers. She was exposed as a woman in 1929 through her connection to a bankruptcy case, and remanded to prison, in part for committing perjury by claiming to be a man when she married Elfrida Howard. During the trial Howard claimed she did not know her husband was a woman, only that "he" had a war injury which prevented "normal" sexual relations.[27] This statement was probably not true since the two had met while Valerie was still living as a woman; but by denying sexual relations both partners could escape charges of being lesbians, much more damaging for a woman than simply cross-dressing. There are hundreds of other women transvestites, most of whom seemed more interested in playing the role of men rather than simply wearing their clothing. Some others were quite clearly lesbians who felt they could survive in society only by passing as men.[28]

TRANSSEXUALISM

Transsexualism is a diagnostic category that is the result not of any theoretical breakthrough but of the development of surgical treatment. Ordinarily, a diagnosis is made independent of the planned treatment, but in the case of transsexuals, the treatment becomes the diagnosis. Public awareness of transsexualism was primarily due to Christine Jorgensen, an ex-GI who underwent surgery in Denmark in 1953 to become a woman. The publicity given Jorgensen caused a major rethinking about gender issues. Though Hirschfeld included the case of a person who might today be described as a transsexual, the term itself was not in common use until after the Jorgensen case. In fact, the surgeon who removed Jorgensen's penis and testicles called him a transvestite.[29] Harry Benjamin, who popularized the term "transsexual," believed he had originally coined the word in a 1953 lecture at the New York Academy of Medicine. He later found that the term "psychopathia transexualis" (spelled with one "s") had earlier been used by D. O. Cauldwell to describe the case of a girl who wanted to be a boy.[30]

Christine Jorgensen, moreover, was not the first person to change sex.

An earlier case, which achieved notoriety in the 1920s, was that of the Danish painter Einar Wagener, who became known as Lili Elbe. She died of a cardiac condition shortly after surgery, and no official record of the case has been published.[31] In any event, it is doubtful that the same results would have been achieved as was done in the case of Jorgensen simply because research into hormones was in its infancy and even after they were isolated, it was only in the late 1940s that enough hormones could be manufactured to give Jorgensen the female curves and appearance she so desired. Surgical removal of both testicles and penis was an ancient operation, although most eunuchs (the technical term for a castrated male), only had their testes removed. It was not until much later that surgical procedures had progressed enough that there was an attempt to give Jorgensen a vagina.[32]

The news about Jorgensen's sex change led many others to try to change their sex as well, but surgeons were cautious in going further; for a long time the barriers to such operations called for drastic action by those men who wanted to become women. Charles (Charlotte) McLeod, the second American to undergo a sex change (also in Denmark), was only allowed to have the operation performed after he had started to cut off his own penis.[33] Ultimately, however, several universities such as Stanford and Johns Hopkins became interested in the question of transsexualism, and a number of independent surgeons began performing the operation. Most surgeons, however, refused to do it without a psychiatric workup and required their clients to live in the role of the sex to which they wanted to be assigned for a year before completing the surgery. Although the early cases were male to female (M/F), they were soon followed by a number of female to male (F/M). There is still, however, a disproportionate number of males who change sex as compared to females.

In simple terms, a transsexual is a person who feels that he or she belongs to a sex different from his or her biological one. They want to remove the external evidence of this "wrongful" sex, such as genitalia or mammary glands, which continually reminds them that they are in the wrong body. It is not enough to cross-dress, or even live the role of the opposite sex; they want but to become a member of the desired sex. Most want to become as biologically female or male as possible, although not all those who have undergone surgery in recent years fit into such categorical absolutes.

POSSIBLE EXPLANATIONS FOR GENDER CONFUSION

What transvestites and transsexuals emphasize is that there are a number of variables at work in forming a person's gender identity. The twin whose penis was burned off and who was unsuccessfully raised as a girl would indicate perhaps the strong pull of biology, but the case of transvestites and transsexuals indicates that other psychosocial variables might be involved as well. While society has always recognized that there are individuals known as hermaphrodites, with at least some of the characteristics of both sexes, the full extent of nature's confusion is only now just becoming apparent. On a simple visual basis, it is estimated that in the past one infant out of every thousand could be classed as a hermaphrodite, that is, as having genitalia that were somewhat ambiguous. Since visual classification was the only means of sex assignment we have had, many people throughout history were not correctly classified. Surgical exploration became possible in the twentieth century, but this was painful and resorted to only in extreme cases. Matters were made easier in 1949 when Murray L. Barr and E. G. Bertram proposed the chromatin test. They had found that cells from a female mammal possessed a small mass of chromatin in the nuclei, which cells in the male lacked. Thus by scraping the *buccal mucosa* off the inside of the cheeks, cells could be obtained which, when stained, showed a distinctive spot of color in the female.[34] One of the first publicized uses of the new test was during the Olympic Games where women athletes were required to prove their femaleness. The women objected to this discrimination, and rightly so, since male athletes were not required to take the test. Nonetheless, there have been several individuals in past Olympic Games who competed as women and later had their sex reclassified as male. The assumption of the Olympic committee was that the male muscular structure of these pseudo-hermaphrodites had given them an advantage over other biological females. Most such "women" athletes, however, had thought they were females and had been reared as women, and their sudden "transformation" must have been particularly traumatic.

Genetic sex also proved complicated. One of the major breakthroughs came with the discovery by J. H. Tijio and A. Levan that there were forty-six chromosomes in the human cell instead of the forty-eight previously hypothesized.[35] This discovery made it possible to count the existence of chromosomes with certainty for the first time, and one of the earliest findings was that there were genetic variations. Since the initial discovery of chromosomes, it had been assumed that sex was determined by the existence of the sex-determining chromosomes, labeled X and Y. Two X chromosomes (XX) in the egg fertilized by the sperm led to the eventual birth of a female, while an X chromosome plus a Y (XY) led to a male infant. The matter proved to be somewhat more complicated because it was found that among the viable genetic possibilities are not only XX and XY but X, XXX, XXY, XYY. There is also a condition known as *mosaicism*, in which some of the cells, though not all, of a given individual have either a supernumerary or a missing chromosome. A single Y chromosome is not viable although the combination of Y or part of a Y in any combination of Xs will cause the embryo to differentiate as a male.

When there is a single X chromosome, a condition known as *Turner's syndrome*, the individual has a female body, but the ovaries are either nonfunctional or have degenerated entirely. This ovarian deficiency prevents the child from developing normally at puberty. It also has a growth-inhibiting effect: people with Turner's syndrome seldom grow to five feet. They may also have other congenital defects as well as intellectual disabilities. Fortunately, if the condition is diagnosed early enough, the deficiency can be alleviated by the administration of estrogen, the female sex hormone, although even after treatment the individual will remain somewhat shorter than average and will be sterile.

Those with the XXX condition develop a normal female body, although fertility may be diminished and there is a greater possibility of mental retardation. The XYY body type is male, abnormally tall, and is also usually sterile or suffers from genital anomalies. It is now believed that certain behavior disorders might be more likely to occur with this genetic inheritance, although the case for this is not fully demonstrated. XXY individuals have what is known as *Klinefelter's syndrome*. The penises are usually small, the testes in the adult are shrunken, and the output of androgen is low, which results in female breast formation, although there are variations from individual to individual.[36]

Even with a normal chromosomal pattern, other things can occur to influence sex development in the fetus. We now believe that the male gonads, that is, the testes, begin to develop at about the sixth week after fertilization if the child is to be a male, while the ovarian differentiation does not occur until the twelfth week if the child is to be female. In experiments on animals it has been shown that if the embryonic gonads are removed prior to the critical period when the sexual anatomy is formed, then the embryo will proceed to differentiate as a female, regardless of cellular sex. This seems to imply that to be masculine it is necessary to add something. Once the testes of the fetus begin to develop, they secrete a *Müllerian-inhibiting* substance, so called because it suppresses further development of the primitive Müllerian ducts which in the female form the uterus, fallopian tubes, and upper segment of the vagina. If for some reason this substance fails to be secreted in a genetically male embryo, a boy is born with a uterus and fallopian tubes in addition to normal internal and external male organs. The male organs are normal except for *cryptorchidism,* i.e., undescended testicles.[37]

In addition to secreting the Müllerian-inhibiting substance, the testes release testosterone, the male sex hormone, which promotes the proliferation of the *Wolffian ducts* to form the internal male reproductive structure. Later, by circulating in the bloodstream, the testosterone reaches the embryonic sexual organs and affects their development. The genital tubercle becomes a penis instead of a clitoris, the skin folds wrap around the penis on both sides of the genital slit and fuse in the midline, forming the urethral tube and foreskin, in place of the bilateral *minor labia* and the clitoral hood. The outer swellings of either side of the genital slit fuse in the midline to form the scrotum to receive the testes. In the female this swelling becomes the *labia majora.*

If testosterone is added to the bloodstream of a genetic female fetus during a critical period in development, the girl will be born with either a grossly enlarged clitoris or, in rare instances, a normal-looking penis but with an empty scrotum. In human beings such masculinization can occur in the fetus as a result of an abnormal function of the cortex of the adrenal glands. It may also occur if the pregnant mother has a tumor which induces her to produce male hormones, or any other condition causing a large number of male hormones to be present. For a brief period in recent history the condition was much more common than it statistically ought to have been because the synthetic pregnancy-saving hormone, *progestin,* led to masculinization of the fetus.[38]

Embryologically the external organs are the last stage of sexual development to be completed. This means that it is not uncommon for the external genitalia to be left unfinished, neither fully masculinized nor feminized. Since the unfinished state of either sex looks remarkably like that of the other in infants,[39] this has caused great difficulties with infant sexual identification in the past. In countries where having a male child was emphasized, all such doubtful cases were assigned to the male category, which caused considerable trauma in many of the individuals when they reached puberty and began to menstruate. Several such cases came to our attention during a year-long stay in Egypt: all the doubtful cases had been raised as males.

Fortunately, most of the human race has no genetic or other complications in their biological sexual development, and their gender identity and sex identity agree. There are, however, a number of individuals whose gender identity does not agree with their biological or genetic sex. Transvestism and transsexualism are two such examples, although there might well be others that have not yet been explored. There are various levels of transvestism or transsexualism, and there are even organizations and foundations devoted to assisting them. As far as transvestism is concerned, at one extreme are the men who have learned the woman's role so well that they can and do pass successfully in society as women. A number of such individuals are known to us, and several of them have lived as women for much of their adult life. What is true for men is also true for women, and we have known a few women who have dressed and been taken to be men for many years. At the other end of the transvestite scale is the intermittent male cross-dresser who emphasizes that he is always masculine, even when indulging in cross-dressing. He does not wish to look like a woman, feel like a woman, or pass as a woman but is simply a person who gets sexually excited by wearing women's clothes. Some would call such a person a fetishist; this kind of transvestism is more frequent among males than females. The psychologist Richard Docter has developed a scale on which he places various types of cross-dressers, with transsexuals at one extreme and occasional cross-dressers at the other.[40]

It is only in the past thirty years or so that transvestites have been able to be studied in any kind of statistical way. This has been due in large part to the growth of organized clubs of cross-dressers, most of them for heterosexual males, which started through the activities of Virginia Prince in 1960. Prince set the pattern for the clubs as well as the emphasis on heterosexuality, although many of the newer organizations are much more receptive to bisexuals, homosexuals, and transsexuals.

In spite of their desire to pass as members of the opposite sex, transvestites usually do not wish to sacrifice the external genitalia or any aspect of their biological sex. The overwhelming majority of transvestites are male, and most of those in transvestite organizations classify themselves as heterosexual. Many of them are married with children; their wives express varying degrees of hostility or enthusiasm for their husband's "habit."[41] Some male transvestites go to rather extreme lengths in their efforts to impersonate females—taking female hormones, undergoing beard removal, retraining themselves to speak at a higher pitch, and so forth[42]—perhaps the only distinction between these extremes and the transsexual is the preservation of the male genitalia.

Still the classification of many remains ambiguous, and many longtime cross-dressers initially were determined to undergo surgery when the Christine Jorgensen case first hit the papers. Most eventually decided not to because they also valued their male selves. Transsexuals are simply not satisfied with cross-dressing; they emphasize that it is not clothes that make the woman or man, but the sex organs. Interestingly, however, perhaps because the surgery for the F/M is both more complicated and less successful (at least as far as penile construction is concerned) most F/Ms do not go all the way. Many females have their breasts removed and undergo a hysterectomy but use a prosthesis of one sort or another as a penis.

Obviously there is a great deal yet to be explored in the field of gender and sexual identity, and at present we do not have any real explanation as to why a person might become a transvestite, a transsexual, a homosexual, or for that matter a heterosexual. Certainly most of us are programmed to be heterosexual since this is what has assured human survival, but, as indicated, many biological complications can occur. Moreover, childhood conditioning, particularly early on, seems to be of importance, but as everywhere else there are many variables. In short we can say with some certainty that there are biological, social-psychological, and cultural variables involved, but we are not certain what all of them are or how they interact. In the past, individuals have suffered through their problems. Some of them, however, managed to overcome handicaps and become influential, as did James Barry or the Abbé de Choisy, but their lot may not have been a happy one, if only because of the constant fear of exposure. Perhaps such individuals will be happier in the future as we continue to emphasize that biology is not necessarily destiny. Females will continue to conceive and bear children and males to impregnate, but beyond that there is a lot of variation.

NOTES

1. We developed these ideas at considerable length in Vern L. Bullough and Bonnie Bullough, *The Subordinate Sex: A History of Attitudes toward Women* (Urbana, Ill.: University of Illinois Press, 1973), and in an update by Vern L. Bullough, Brenda Shelton, and Sarah Slavin, *The Subordinated Sex: A History of Attitudes toward Women* (Athens, Ga.: University of Georgia Press, 1988).

2. See John Money and Anke A. Ehrhardt, *Man and Woman, Boy and Girl* (Baltimore: Johns Hopkins University Press, 1972).

3. See Sandra S. I. Bem, "The Measurement of Psychological Androgyny," *Journal of Consulting and Clinical Psychology* 42 (1974): 155–62; J. T. Spence and R. J. Helmreich, *Masculinity and Femininity: Their Psychological Dimensions, Correlates and Antecedents* (Austin: University of Texas Press, 1978). For discussion see Donald L. Mosher, "Gender: Psychological Measurements of Masculinity and Femininity," in *Human Sexuality: An Encyclopedia,* edited by Vern L. Bullough and Bonnie Bullough (New York: Garland, 1994), pp. 237–42.

4. For a discussion of this see Vern L. Bullough and Bonnie Bullough, *Cross-Dressing, Sex, and Gender* (Philadelphia: University of Pennsylvania Press, 1993), pp. 312–38. Consult the bibliography to those pages for further references.

5. John Money, Joan Hampson, and John Hampson, "Imprinting and the Establishment of Gender Role," *Archives for Neurology and Psychiatry* 77 (1957): 333–36.

6. Money and Ehrhardt, *Man and Woman,* pp. 118–20.

7. Milton Diamond, "Sexual Identity, Monozygotic Twins Reared in Discordant Sex Roles and a BBC Follow-Up," *Archives of Sexual Behavior* 11, no. 2: 181–85, and Milton Diamond, "Genetic Considerations in the Development of Sexual Orientation," in *The Development of Sex Differences and Similarities in Behavior,* edited by M. Haug, R. E. Whale, C. Aron, and K. L. Olsen (Dordrecht: Kluwer Academic Publishers, 1993).

8. J. Imperato-McGinley and R. E. Peterson, "Male Pseudohermaphroditism: the Complexities of Male Phenotypic Development," *American Journal of Medicine* 61 (1976): 251–72; J. Imperator-McGinley, R. E. Peterson, T. Gautier, and E. Sturia, "Androgen and Evolution of Male-Gender Identity among Male Pseudohermaphrodites with 5A-Reductase Deficiency," *New England Journal of Medicine* 300 (1979): 1233–37.

9. L. Gooren, E. Fliers, and K. Courtney, "Biological Determinants of Sexual Orientation," *Annual Review of Sex Research,* edited by J. Bancroft, 1 (1990): 175–96.

10. Magnus Hirschfeld, *Die Transvestiten* (Leipzig: Max Spohr, 1910). This was translated into English by Michael Lombardi-Nash, *The Transvestites* (Amherst, N.Y.: Prometheus Books, 1991). Hirschfeld published a second edition of his study (Berlin: Spohr Verlag, 1925).

11. See Bullough Bonnie Bullough, *Cross-Dressing, Sex, and Gender.*

12. Havelock Ellis, "Sexo-Aesthetic Inversion," *Alienist and Neurologist* 34, part 1 (May 1913): 3–14; part 2 (August 1913): 1–31.

13. Havelock Ellis, "Eonism," in *Studies in the Psychology of Sex,* vol. 2, part 2 (reprint 7 vols. in 2, New York: Random House, 1936), pp. 1–120.

14. Thomas Aquinas, *Summa Theologica* (New York: Benziger Brothers, 1947), part I, 92, "The Production of Women," I, ii.

15. Philo, *On the Creation,* edited and translated by F. H. Colson and G. H.

Whittaker (London: William Heinemann, 1963), pp. 69–70, 151, 162; *Questions and Answers on Genesis,* edited and translated by Ralph Marcus (London: William Heinemann, 1961), I, 40. See also Richard A. Baer, Jr., *Philo's Use of the Categories Male and Female* (Leiden: E. J. Brill, 1970), pp. 46, 51.

16. Jerome, *Commentarius in Epistolam ad Ephesios* III, bk. 16, col. 567, in J. P. Migne, *Patrologia Latina* (hereafter *PL*) (Paris: Garnier Fratres, 1887) XXVI, 1938.

17. Ambrose, *Expositiones in Evangelium secundum Lucum libri X,* bk. 16, in *PL* XV, col. 1938.

18. See A. Butler, *Butler's Lives of the Saints,* edited, revised, and supplemented by Herbert Thurston and Donald Atwater, 4 vols. (New York: P. J. Kennedy & Sons, 1956), 4: 59–61, and Helen Waddell, *The Desert Fathers* (reprint Ann Arbor: University of Michigan Press, 1957), pp. 171–88. More complete accounts can be found in *Acta sanctorum* (Antwerp, 1643, in progress).

19. For a discussion of these see Bullough and Bullough, *Cross-Dressing,* pp. 52–57, and Vern L. Bullough, "Transvestism in the Middle Ages: A Sociological Analysis," *American Journal of Sociology* 79 (1974): 1381–94; John Anson, "The Female Transvestite in Early Monasticism: The Origin and Development of a Motif," *Viator* 5 (1974): 1–32; Valerie R. Hotchkiss, "Clothes Make the Man: Female Transvestism in the Middle Ages," unpublished Ph.D. dissertation, Yale University, 1990.

20. See Bullough and Bullough, *Cross-Dressing,* pp. 61–64.

21. For female impersonation on stage see Roger Baker, *Drag: A History of Female Impersonation on the Stage* (London: Triton Books, 1968), and C. J. Bulliet, *Venus Castina* (1928, reprint New York: Bonanza Books, 1956).

22. Angus Heriot, *The Castrati in Opera* (London: Secker and Warburg, 1956).

23. This was republished under the title *Mémoires de l'abbé Choisy habillé en femme,* edited by George Mongredin (Paris: Mercure de France, 1966). The original edition was published in 1735. It was translated into English as *The Transvestite Memoirs of the Abbé de Choisy,* trans. R. H. F. Scott (London: Peter Owen, 1973).

24. There is a vast literature on the chevalier. The two best books are Cynthia Cox, *The Enigma of the Age: The Strange Story of the Chevalier d'Éon* (London: Longmans, Green and Company, 1966), and Edna Nixon, *Royal Spy, The Strange Case of the Chevalier d'Éon* (New York: Renal and Company, 1965). Both are based on primary source materials. Earlier works include F. Gaillardet, *Mémoires du Chevalier d'Éon* (Paris: Ladvocat, 1836), which is highly unreliable and was corrected by Gaillardet thirty years later under the same title (Paris: E. Dentu, 1866); J. B. Telfer, *The Strange Career of the Chevalier d Éon de Beaumont* (London: Longmans, Green and Company, 1885) is also reliable, but E. A. Vizetelly, *The True Story of the Chevalier d'Éon* (London: Tylston and Edwards, 1895) has many inaccuracies and Telfer wrote a book to correct it: *Chevalier d'Éon de Beaumont: A Treatise* (1896). There are numerous works in French as well. For further information see Bullough and Bullough, *Cross-Dressing,* pp. 126–32.

25. Isobel Ray, *The Strange Story of Dr. James Barry: Army Surgeon, Inspector General of Hospitals, Discovered on Death to be a Woman* (London: Longmans, Greens, and Co., 1958); see also Percival R. Kirby, "Dr. James Barry, Controversial South African Figure: A Recent Evaluation of His Life and Sex," *South African Medical Journal*, April 25, 1970, pp. 506–16.

26. *The Sunday Dispatch,* March 31, 1929, and quoted by Julie Wheelwright, *Amazons and Military Maids: Women Who Dressed as Men in the Pursuit of Life, Liberty and Happiness* (London: Pandora, 1990), p. 50.

27. The British press had a field day with the case and the London newspaper published several stories: *The Times,* March 28, April 26, 1929; *Daily Express,* March 6, March 28, 1929; *Daily Sketch,* March 6, March 28, April 14, 1929. There are many others.

28. Bullough and Bullough, *Cross-Dressing,* pp. 94–173.

29. Christian Hamburger, George K. Sturup, and E. Dahl-Iversen, "Transvestism: Hormonal, Psychiatric, and Surgical Treatment," *Journal of the American Medical Association* 152 (May 30, 1953): 391–96.

30. David O. Cauldwell, "Psychopathia Transexualis," *Sexology* 16 (December 1949), 274–80.

31. Nels Hoyer, *Man into Woman: An Authentic Record of a Change of Sex* (New York: E. P. Dutton, 1933).

32. See Christine Jorgensen, *A Personal Autobiography* (New York: Paul S. Eriksson, 1967).

33. Personal testimony to the authors by Charlotte McLeod who was then living in California. We have since lost contact with her.

34. M. L. Barr and E. G. Bertram, "A Morphological Distinction between Neurones of the Male and Female, and the Behavior of the Nucleolar Satellite during Accelerated Nucleo-Protein Synthesis," *Nature* 163 (1949): 676–77; Murray L. Barr, "Cytologic Tests of Chromosomal Sex," *Progress in Gynecology* 3 (1957): 131–41; and K. L. Moore, ed., *The Sex Chromatin* (Philadelphia: W. B. Saunders, 1966).

35. J. H. Tijio and A. Levan, "The Chromosome Number of Man," *Hereditas* 42 (1956): 1–6.

36. Money and Ehrhardt, *Man, Woman, Boy, Girl,* pp. 28–33. See also H. F. Klinefelter, I. C. Reifenstein, and F. Albright, *Journal of Clinical Endocrinology* 2 (1942): 615.

37. Money and Ehrhardt, *Man, Woman, Boy, Girl,* pp. 6–7.

38. Ibid., pp. 7–8.

39. John Money, *Sex Errors of the Body* (Baltimore: Johns Hopkins University Press, 1968), p. 41.

40. Richard F. Docter, *Transvestites and Transsexuals: Toward a Theory of Gender Behavior* (New York: Plenum Press, 1988), pp. 121–65.

41. Vern L. Bullough and Thomas W. Weinberg, "Women Married to Transvestites: Problems and Adjustments," *Journal of Psychology and Human Sexuality*

1 (1988): 83–104; Thomas S. Weinberg and Vern L. Bullough, "Alienation, Self-Image, and the Importance of Support Groups for the Wives of Transvestites," *Journal of Sex Research* 24 (1988): 262–68.

42. Virginia Prince, *How to Be a Woman Though Male* (Los Angeles: Chevalier Publications, 1971).

6

Menstruation

"Menstruation" is derived from the Latin word for month (*mensis*). In the past, menstruation was a dark secret which somehow contaminated women and made them impure.[1] Since the most common and well-known cycle of twenty-eight days is the same as that of the moon, women traditionally have been regarded as being under the influence of the lunar cycle. It is only in the twentieth century that we have finally arrived at a scientific understanding of the process, while developments such as the sanitary napkin and tampons have simplified women's lives.

In most primitive societies women were isolated and confined to specially designed menstrual huts during their menses. Intercourse with a menstruating woman was thought to cause great harm to men, and food prepared by them would cause illness for anyone who ate it.[2] Pliny the Elder (23-79 C.E.), in his *Natural History,* reported that menstrual blood would turn new wine sour, dry seeds, make fruit fall, and rust bronze and iron. Dogs who ate menstrual blood would be driven mad and their bites infected with an incurable poison.[3]

The Bible held that a menstruating women was unclean for seven days and that everything that touched her was also considered unclean.[4] "And if any man lie with her at all, and her flowers be upon him he shall be unclean seven days and all the bed whereupon he lieth shall be unclean."[5] Even today in orthodox Judaism, a woman has to go through a special cleansing process at the end of her menstrual period. For a long time Christians believed that menstruation was a curse inflicted upon women because of the sins of Eve, a belief that retains currency through the use of such euphemisms as "the curse" as short for "the curse of Eve." Some of the earlier Church fathers urged women to fast during their menses, a suggestion that would have only added to the possibility of becoming anemic, a condition which in the past helped keep women subordinate.

Undoubtedly in the past, menstruation was a more untidy process than it is today. Even those women determined to be active during the menses found it somewhat awkward to do so, particularly if the flow was heavy or if they suffered from menstrual cramps. Much of the excess clothing women were burdened with was worn because they menstruated. Since they did not want to signal the onset of their periods they wore heavy petticoats all the time to hide the bulges and odors of menstruation.

Perhaps the most dramatic "modern" example of reticence about this physiologic process appears in the story of Lizzy Borden from Fall River, Massachusetts, who allegedly "took an axe" and gave her aged father "forty whacks," then bludgeoned her stepmother to death. Her trial in 1892 became part of our national folklore, and her life and actions have been the subject of poems, ballads, novels, scholarly studies, and even a ballet. Most Americans, however, do not know that Lizzie was acquitted of the charge of murder, in part because she was menstruating at the time the crime was committed. Her alibi, taken in secret testimony before the judge, was that she was in the basement at the very instant of the murders washing out her menstrual rags, a common enough procedure before the development of disposable sanitary napkins. The judge and both the prosecuting and defense attorneys felt that to mention this biological function would be improper. By implication they seemed to accept the fact that no women would confess to such a female secret unless, in fact, this was what had actually happened. None of the evidence offered by the prosecution was sufficient to overcome this assumption.[6] America was not alone in its attitudes toward open discussion of menstruation. As late as 1965, the Lord Chamberlain of England refused to allow reference to menstruation in the play *Creditors*.[7]

Menstruation became much easier to handle with the invention of Kotex®, an accidental byproduct of the First World War. During the war, Kimberly-Clark produced surgical cellulose pads made from wood fibers instead of cotton because the resulting product offered both greater absorbency than cotton and was more resistent to infestation by lice. Nurses seized upon the product to make menstrual pads for themselves, a fact which led the company, deprived of the wartime market for their bandages, to decide in 1920 to manufacture Kotex®. Early in that year the company marketed the first disposable sanitary napkin. It consisted of several layers of wadding cut into a rectangular shape and wrapped with gauze. It was touted to have five times the absorbency of cotton, an advantage to which women responded quickly.

The problem was how to market the product. Stores were reluctant to display Kotex®, arguing that it would antagonize or embarrass customers. Even when store managers were persuaded, they sometimes found their worst fears realized. An F. W. Woolworth store in San Francisco was directed by a men's organization to dismantle its window display fronting on Market Street. Commercial magazines also proved reluctant; the first advertisement for the product, in the *Ladies Home Journal,* did not appear until 1924. In spite of a costly sixty cents for six napkins, sales quickly escalated. Montgomery Ward accepted a listing for sanitary napkins in its mail order catalogue in 1926, and by the end of the decade advertisements appeared in a variety of magazines. By then a number of rival products had also appeared, and the forbidden subject of menstruation did not seem to be such an embarrassing secret.[8] The development of effective sanitary pads allowed women to discard their multiple petticoats, raise their hemlines, and gain more physical freedom than they had enjoyed before. Other feminine products, including tampons, further increased that freedom.

Technically menstruation is a phase in the reproductive cycle; indeed, it symbolizes the thwarting of that cycle, since the onset of the menses usually signifies that pregnancy has not occurred. During the menstrual cycle the lining of the uterus, called the *endometrium,* thickens in preparation for the implantation of a fertilized egg or ovum. If fertilization and implantation do not occur, the specially prepared endometrium is shed along with the blood in its engorged vessels. As soon as this takes place the process begins again. Usually the cycle takes about twenty-eight days, although cycles from twenty-five to thirty-four days are accepted as normal, with wider ranges of normal accepted if there are no symptoms suggesting a problem.[9]

Many of the technical terms dealing with menstruation have been coined in the past hundred years, indicating how recent the scientific consideration of the process is. The term "menarche," for example, used to describe a girl's first period, was coined by the physician Heinrich Kisch in the late nineteenth century from the Latin *mensis* (month) and the Greek *arche,* meaning "beginning."[10] In many societies menarche was regarded as the dividing line between childhood and adult status, and girls often married shortly after their first period. Many primitive societies have puberty rites associated with menarche, with the young women being segregated from the rest of the tribe, living in a special hut, and eating and bathing in a special manner. Some cultures believe that the young woman has supernatural powers at the onset of menstruation. Menarche usually occurs between the ages of nine and seventeen, although younger and older ages have been reported depending on diet and other factors. The crucial factor related to the onset of menstruation seems to relate to body weight and fat content. When the adolescent female achieves a fat content of approximately 28 percent (enough to support pregnancy), menarche usually occurs. At the present time in North America the average age at menarche is 12.5 years. This is approximately one year younger than the average or normative age of past centuries.

Roman law assumed that females were mature at the age of twelve and classical writers described menarche as taking place between the ages of twelve and fourteen. Medieval writers usually placed it between thirteen and fourteen.[11] In Islamic countries it was a criminal act to have sexual relations with a girl before she had menstruated. Before a marriage could be consummated, village or neighborhood women were to examine the girl to see that she was physically prepared, and Arabic law set the time for this examination between twelve and thirteen years of age.[12]

Some English and other northern European medical writers of the nineteenth and early twentieth centuries indicated a later age at menarche, with an average of between fourteen and fifteen years.[13] Edward B. Foote, a popular medical writer of the nineteenth century, placed the average age at menarche for American girls between twelve and fourteen,[14] while a statistical study done in 1905 led to an estimate of fourteen years.[15] The fact that the current average is only 12.5 years suggests a significant improvement in the diet of the industrialized world, but there is no reason to believe that the average will significantly diminish, because extra fat in addition to necessary minimum of 28 percent of body fat, does not change the calendar of events, which are also controlled by hormonal and other growth factors.

The onset of menstruation is marked by irregularity, but by the end of the first year a regular pattern has been established. Most women feel some discomfort during the menses, with bloating and abdominal cramps, but only a minority of women find these symptoms debilitating. The pain is caused by contractions of the uterus, which is under hormonal control; cramps do not ordinarily occur if there is no ovulation. The most common *anovulatory cycle* is that experienced by women on birth control pills, so oral contraceptives are often used in the treatment of *dysmenorrhea*. Other factors may be implicated, such as a very small cervical opening, a condition that disappears after one delivery. Occasional cases of severe dysmenorrhea are caused by *endometriosis,* a condition characterized by small implants of endometrial tissue outside the uterus in the *peritoneum.* Since this tissue responds to the same hormonal stimulation as the uterine lining, it bleeds with the menstrual cycle but the blood cannot escape, causing severe pain. Surgical or laser treatment is called for in this condition. Ordinary and even severe dysmenorrhea has been made more tolerable by the development of nonsteroidal anti-arthritis medications, including, most particularly, ibuprofen.[16]

An often overlooked consequence of menstruation is anemia. The loss of approximately an ounce of blood each month does not sound like much but it can be significant for people who do not have adequate iron and protein in their diets. This was the case among many women in the past; it is also a common problem today for women in underdeveloped countries, anorexics, and women who diet almost continually to lose weight. These women are likely to be tired and listless, and to recover slowly from deliveries or illnesses. In the past, when transfusions were not available and many women existed on subsistence diets, any trauma involving substantial blood loss could be fatal to a severely anemic woman.[17]

There are also mood swings and symptoms associated with the menstrual cycle. The days just before ovulation have been associated with a sense of well-being, high energy levels, and heightened sexuality.[18] However, the days just before menstruation are sometimes marked by depression, irritability, and lowered self-esteem. These symptoms may be accompanied by a feeling of being bloated or fluid retention. This constellation of symptoms has been called the *premenstrual syndrome* (PMS). However, the condition is not yet well understood and medical treatment is not always effective. Various approaches, including progestins, diuretics, dietary regimens, and vitamin B, have been used with only partial success.[19]

Toward the end of a woman's reproductive life the menstrual cycle tends to become irregular, and somewhere between the ages of forty-five and fifty-five it ceases for most women. The *menopause,* or cessation of menses, was a term coined in 1875 to describe the process. Although pregnancy after age forty-seven is rare, it occasionally does happen and pregnancy even in the early sixties has been recorded. The incidence of certain fetal abnormalities, including Down's syndrome, is more common among pregnancies occurring after age thirty-five. Very little attention has been paid to menopause in the past, primarily because the symptoms were vague and because of a general disinterest in "female problems." The most well-known symptom is the "hot flash" or "hot flush," an experience of waves of heat spreading over the face and upper half of the body. Other symptoms include depression, joint pains, and headaches, which are often most severe in the premenopausal years when the hormones may be out of balance. Estrogen replacement therapy (ERT) was considered controversial in the 1970s because of studies linking it with uterine cancer.[30] Some feminists were also wary of ERT because they viewed menopause as a normal process and generally mistrusted medical intervention. However, it has now been realized that the cancer danger can be eliminated if progestin (synthetic progesterone) is given concomitantly with the estrogen. The progestin prevents proliferation of the endometrium and thus virtually eliminates the cancer risk. In addition ERT has been shown to lessen the incidence of coronary heart disease, which is the leading cause of death in older women, and to slow the progress of *osteoporosis,* the thinning of the bones which is also a major cause of disability and death in older women.[21] There are now many women well past menopause who are taking a combination of estrogen and progestin.

As indicated earlier in this chapter, the scientific study of menstruation is very recent, limited mostly to the twentieth century. Although nineteenth-century physicians and other medical writers wrote extensively about menstruation, this cannot be considered the beginning of any real scientific effort. Rather it may well have been a frantic effort to stop the beginning steps being taken by women to seek college educations and responsible jobs. Menstruation, with all of its mystery and taboos, lent itself well to this campaign to halt all progress for women.

One of the most backward and unscientific beliefs about menstruation was promulgated in the *American Journal of Obstetrics* in 1875 by a physician named A. F. A. King, who argued that menstruation was pathological. He was undoubtedly influenced by the Victorian disgust at all sexual and reproductive processes as well as by his strong belief that in Paradise humans had reproduced asexually. It was only when man had fallen due to Eve's tempting him with the apple, that perfection had been replaced with the evil of sex. King believed that intercourse during the menses was forbidden because it would result in gonorrhea. Yet he also held that conception was most likely to occur when intercourse took place during the menses. Since menstruation therefore stood in the way of fruitful coitus, it obviously was contrary to nature and not ordained by God, since God would not have made women fruitful at the same time they were contagious.[22]

King's concept was radically different from the view put forth by earlier popular sex manuals such as the pseudonymous *Aristotle's Masterpiece,* which looked at menstruation as a casting out of blood that would have nourished the embryo had pregnancy occurred.[23] Instead King was extending, albeit in a very unscientific way, the findings of a German physician, E. F. W. Pflüger, who in 1861 had demonstrated that a woman whose ovaries had been removed did not menstruate. In trying to explain his findings Pflüger hypothesized that the growth of the follicle in the ovary at a certain stage produced a mechanical stimulation of the nerves that triggered menstrual bleeding and ovulation. From this he came to believe that menstruation and ovulation occurred simultaneously.[24] It was not until the twentieth century that the hormonal involvement in the timing of ovulation was fully understood. In the meantime many physicians accepted Pflüger's theory that nervous stimulation triggered menstruation. It was this erroneous belief in the association of menstruation with the nervous system that led a number of physicians to express opposition to any emancipation of women.

Probably the most influential spokesman for the continued subordination of women was Edward H. Clarke, professor of *materia medica* at Harvard University and Fellow of the American Academy of Arts and Sciences. In 1873 he wrote his classic *Sex Education: or, A Fair Chance for Girls,* in which he stated:

> Woman, in the interest of the race, is endowed with a set of organs peculiar to herself, whose complexity, delicacy, sympathies, and force are among the marvels of creation. If properly nurtured and cared for, they are a source of strength and power to her. If neglected and mismanaged, they retaliate upon their possessor with weakness and disease, as well of the mind as the body.[25]

Clarke then went on to argue that the one thing the female could not do if she was to retain good health was to be educated using the pattern or model of man. This was because the male developed steadily and gradually from birth to manhood, while the female, at puberty, underwent a sudden and unique period of growth during which time her whole reproductive system developed.[26] If such development did not take place at puberty, it would never occur; moreover, since the system could never do "two things at the same time," females between twelve and twenty must concentrate on developing their reproductive system at the expense of all other pursuits.

Dr. Clarke expounded further on his belief that the body could not do two things at the same time, arguing that the muscles and the brain cannot function optimally at the same moment. Thus he argued that it was impossible to meditate on a poem and drive a saw, do brain work and digest a dinner, or to stimulate the brain and at the same time achieve physical growth. For this reason the female between twelve and twenty had to concentrate all of her energy on developing her reproductive system. If she tried to do brain work it would overload the system, resulting in signals from the developing organs of reproduction being neglected in favor of those coming from the overactive brain. This would lead to dire consequences. Even after puberty women should not exercise their minds without restriction because of their monthly cycles. During the menstrual cycle it was vital that women allow the physiological processes of their bodies to be carried out without restriction. Any mental activity during the time of the menses, which Clarke called the "catamenial week," interfered with ovulation and menstruation.[27]

To prove his point that higher education left its female adherents in poor health for life, Clarke reported a number of case studies from his own practice. One case was that of a young woman who had entered a female seminary at fifteen in good health, but within a year intensive study had caused her to be pale and tired "every fourth week." A summer's rest temporarily restored her, but by the end of the second year she was not only pale but suffered from an "uncontrollable twitching of a rhythmical sort" in the muscles of her face. She was cured by taking a year off from school to travel in Europe; however, she unfortunately returned to school where she studied without regard to her menstrual periods and, though she graduated at nineteen as valedictorian, she was an invalid. It took two years in Europe for her to recover. Her illness, the doctor reported, was caused by making her body do two things at once.

Clarke recounted the case of another young woman, a student at Vassar who began to have fainting spells during her menses, which were painful and sparse. She graduated at nineteen, an invalid suffering from chronic headaches. Dr. Clarke held that this was because she suffered from arrested development of her reproductive organs due to her concentration on education. Further evidence of the woman's arrested development was the fact that she was flat-chested. Another young college woman with a history of diminishing menstrual flow, constant headaches, depression, acne, and rough skin proved to be so far gone that Dr. Clarke had her committed to a mental institution.[28]

The situation, Clarke felt, had reached a critical juncture: unless America stopped allowing its young women to be educated the ranks of possible mothers would be so depleted that within fifty years "the wives who are to be mothers in our republic must be drawn from trans-Atlantic homes," where there was no need for girls to be educated.[29] Dr. Clarke also expressed concern for young girls who had to go to work, especially in domestic service or in factories. Having seen considerable evidence of ill health among these women due to the stresses of their work, Clarke concluded that labor in a factory or at a loom was also damaging to a woman. However, it did far less harm than education, because factory work kept only the body busy but not the brain. It was primarily brain work that destroyed feminine capabilities.[30]

Clarke argued that women who chose to pursue their educational ambitions would lose their "maternal instincts," and become coarse and forceful. By educating women, he stated, we were creating a class of sexless humans analogous to eunuchs. To solve this alarming problem Clarke recommended strict separation of the sexes during the educational process; he urged all girls' schools to provide periodic rest periods for students and give them brief vacations during their menstrual periods. Young women should never study as hard as young men since they were by nature weaker and less able to cope:

> A girl cannot spend more than four, or, in occasional instances, five hours of force daily upon her studies, and leave sufficient margin for the general physical growth that she must make. . . . If she puts as much force into her brain education as a boy, the brain or the special apparatus [the reproductive system] will suffer.[31]

Although there was at the time unfavorable criticism of Clarke's thesis, his book became very popular: it went through seventeen editions in thirteen years and his concepts were widely circulated. Clarke's opponents scored some telling points, all of which he ignored. They pointed out that Clarke had done no scientific study on the matter, and that he generalized from a few clinical case studies from his own practice. One pair of enlightened critics pointed out that "Dr. Clarke has thrown out to a popular audience a hypothesis of his own which has no place in physiological or medical science. . . . His whole reasoning is singularly unsound.[32] From our current vantage point it seems that Clarke's book may have been motivated by a desire to prevent Harvard from admitting female students. If this was the case, he was successful. Harvard resisted proposals to admit women; instead Radcliffe College for women opened in 1879 to provide education using the Harvard pattern but keeping women segregated. Harvard did not admit female students until well into the twentieth century.

Clarke had many disciples who spread his misguided ideas about women.

T. S. Clouston, an Edinburgh physician, wrote a lengthy series for the American *Popular Science Monthly* in order to prove the dangers of education for females, based on Clarke's erroneous assumptions. Clouston added a few more bits of misinformation. He pointed out, for example, that it was medically accepted that the "female organism" was much more delicate than that of the male and "not fitted for the regular grind that man can keep up." Overstimulation of the female brain caused stunted growth, nervousness, headaches, neuralgia, difficult childbirth, hysteria, inflammation of the brain, and insanity. The female character was likewise altered by education; the educated woman might become more cultured but she was also more unsympathetic and selfish. Clouston admitted that his conclusions were not founded on any real scientific collection of "collated statistical facts," but rather on the observations of physicians, which he felt were nonetheless true. He at least had the humility to urge others to gather research about the matter even though he thought new research would not change his basic interpretation.[33]

Noted philosopher and educator John Dewey attempted to rebut Clouston's arguments about the harmful effects of education for women by using statistics gathered by the Massachusetts Labor Bureau on the health of American college women, but his evidence was more or less ignored.[34] The Massachusetts study had found that of 705 college women questioned, 78 percent were in good or excellent health. The study concluded that there were no significant differences between the health of women who attended college and those who did not.[35]

We can see, then, that despite sound evidence to the contrary, the belief persisted that menstruation made women unable to deal with intellectual matters. In 1884, Henry Maudsley wrote that the concurrence of puberty and higher education in girls meant that mental development could be achieved only at the expense of physical development. Maudsley would not cut out education for girls altogether, but rather emphasize the type of schooling that would prepare them for their proper sphere, as "the conceivers, mothers and nurses of children."[36] Even those physicians who disagreed with the theory that nervous stimulation triggered the menstrual mechanism were caught up in the belief in female inferiority. John Goodman, a Louisville physician, held that the female body was governed by "a law of monthly periodicity," setting loose a "menstrual wave" that affected the entire female being and from whose dictates women could not escape.[37] Obviously this "wave" made them unsuitable for anything other than motherhood.

J. H. Kellogg, whose *Plain Facts for Old and Young* was responsible for inculcating vast numbers of Americans with the idea that masturbation led to insanity, also added to the public fund of misinformation about menstruation. Although somewhat more cautious than Clarke, Kellogg argued that menstruation rendered a woman especially susceptible to morbid influences and liable to serious derangements. Young women in particular had to be carefully watched to make sure they did not study excessively during their menstrual periods.[38]

It seems, superficially at least, that as the demands for female emancipation grew the rhetoric of male physicians about the frailties of females increased. In 1905 F. W. Van Dyke, the president of the Oregon Medical Society, claimed that hard study took away women's beauty, brought on hysteria, neurasthenia, dyspepsia, astigmatism, and dysmenorrhea, and killed the sexual desires. Educated women could not bear children with ease, because their studies had arrested the development of the pelvis while at the same time increasing the size of the fetus's brain and head. The result was that childbirth caused extensive suffering in educated women. Van Dyke concluded with a plea to women to abandon education since the names of such good mothers and faithful wives as Penelope, Cornelia, and St. Elizabeth would be remembered long after the last "graduate of a woman's college" had faded from the recollection of men.[39] Along the same lines, Dr. Ralph W. Parsons wrote in the *New York Medical Journal* in 1907 that college women suffered from digestive disorders as well as nervous and mental diseases:

> The delicate organism and sensitive and highly developed nervous system of our girls was never intended by the Creator to undergo the stress and strain of the modern system of higher education and the baneful results are becoming more apparent as the years go by.[40]

For "proof" he offered the fact that 42 percent of the women admitted to the New York "insane" asylums in 1902 were well educated, while only 16 percent of the men admitted had gone beyond grade school. Obviously women "who have undergone the strain of the modern system of education are much more likely to become victims of insanity than men of the same class." Parsons also worried that education would modify the so-called feminine traits of mind and make women more masculine. He reported that educated women had loud voices, laughed with gusto, and even used slang and profanity. Parson's solution to the problem was to prohibit girls from learning Latin, Greek, civics, political economy, or higher mathematics, for these subjects could be of no use to them in their proper sphere. They should have shorter school hours than boys, spending most of their time in home economics classes.[41]

As so often happens in the field of sex research, many of the so-called experts who were arousing such fears ignored the research data. During the 1890s Mary Roberts Smith had carried out a longterm study comparing the health of college women, not to the so-called average woman of the census, as past projects had done, but to a control group of noncollege women composed of the relatives and friends of the college group. The results indicated that though college women married two years later than noncollege women, there was a growing tendency in both groups to marry at a somewhat later age. Noncollege women had more children but college women had more children per years of married life. Not surprisingly there were no differences in the problems related to pregnancy or mortality of children among the two groups. Also, there were no significant differences in the health of the two groups or the health of their children.[42]

Yet again, such studies were ignored and the unproven theories of Clarke and others were adopted because they fit the prejudices of the day. G. Stanley Hall, regarded as one of the outstanding American psychologists of the early twentieth century, dismissed as inaccurate the statistical studies of investigators like Mary Roberts Smith simply because he believed that the woman's place was in the home. The most accurate information, he felt, came from the physicians who treated overeducated women and were thus able to see the true circumstances of imposing education upon a menstrual-rhythm-wracked body. Inevitably Hall's classic publication *Adolescence* repeated all of the outmoded fears about the danger of education for menstruating women. Hall noted the fact that the average age of menarche was slightly lower in United States than Europe and attributed this to the stimulation of education, arguing that this trend was harming American girls.[43] He proposed that instead of a weekly sabbath women should have a monthly sabbath when they rested for four days at a time. It was during this period that women were more inclined to piety and dependence, accounting for the "fact" (at least in Hall's mind) that women were more religious than men.[44]

Such opinions however, finally came to be challenged by women themselves. Martha Carey Thomas, president of Bryn Mawr College, attacked Hall's report on periodicity as "sickening sentimentality" and "pseudoscientific." She held that Hall's work was one of the most degrading to womanhood ever written. To emphasize the dangers of such claptrap Thomas wrote that when she was a student she was "terror struck lest I and every other woman with me" become "doomed to live as pathological invalids in a universe merciless to women as a sex." Thomas added that she knew, as did most other educated women, that it was not women who were pathological creatures but rather the men who believed such things about them. Such a man as Hall was "himself pathological, blinded by the neurotic mists of sex, unable to see that women form one-half of the kindly race of normal healthy human creatures in the world."[45]

Other women used physiological research to dispel anxieties about menstruation. Leta Stetter Hollingworth, an educational researcher, found that none of the efficiency curves of female students correlated with menstrual cycles and that males had varying efficiency scores similar to females. She felt that the whole mumbo jumbo about menstruation had come about because scientific and medical writers partially subscribed to the romantic notion that the woman was a "mysterious being, half hysteric, half angel," and had seized upon the menstrual cycle as the source of the alleged mystery of womanhood. Once formulated it had become a dogma cited by each succeeding authority, none of whom made an attempt to check it. Hollingworth also argued that few physicians knew anything about the average woman; they simply generalized from a few cases of female hysteria or mental illness in order to posit an entire thesis that suited their own prejudices.[46]

Celia Mosher, whose research into menstruation among college women spanned several generations between 1890 and 1920, found that the girls in the earlier part of her study experienced greater menstrual difficulties than those in the later part of the study. At first she hypothesized that this was because nineteenth-century girls had been taught they were going to be sick during their periods, while those of the twentieth century thought themselves a little more sophisticated, and that both prophesies were self-fulfilling. Mosher likewise found a correlation between dress and menstrual problems. During the 1890s and the early years of the twentieth century most girls were put into tight corsets at the age of six or seven, and after that they wore tight waists and heavy unsupported skirts. Mosher believed that such clothing interfered with respiration, made the abdominal muscles flabby, restricted physical activity, and deformed the body in much the same way that foot-binding maimed the women of China. She believed there was a chronic misplacement of the pelvic organs which encouraged menstrual problems. Mosher prepared tables correlating menstrual pain among college women with the width and weight of their skirts and the measurements of their waists. Her figures showed that as the skirt grew shorter and skimpier, and the waist larger, the functional health of the women improved.[47]

Such studies did much to improve the level of knowledge about menstruation. Reassurance also came from the increasing numbers of college-educated and career women who seemed none the worse for their years of hard study or work. Unfortunately, not every physician adjusted his or her thinking to correspond with the scientific findings. As late as 1970, Edgar Berman, a friend and physician of Minnesota Senator Hubert H. Humphrey, stated that women could not fill leadership roles, because of the influence of periodicity on their thinking. This statement cost him a position in the Democratic party and made Humphrey an object of attack by Patsy Mink, a member of Congress from Hawaii.[48] Contemporary researchers find little support for nineteenth-century beliefs in the harmful effects of academic study, or inferior performance, or public instability. Although menstrual-related pain or psychological issues represent legitimate needs for health care for some women, there is little evidence that women's public performance is diminished.[49]

Part of the problem is that on many issues physicians do not revise their thinking much after they have finished their formal education, so that what they are taught in medical school and residency training remains influential. Sociologists Diane Scully and Pauline Bart did an analysis of twenty-seven gynecology textbooks published between 1943 and 1973. The stance of the physician authors toward the female patients portrayed in these books was, with few exceptions, paternalistic and even condescending. Women were described as anatomically destined for motherhood, able to be fulfilled only by reproducing, mothering, and attending to their husbands.[50] At a later date Scully did an observational study of the residency training for gynecologists. She reported that the major focus of the training was on surgical approaches to treatment. Dysmenorrhea was usually dismissed as psychogenic in origin, although the female residents were more likely to take their patients with this complaint more seriously than the male residents.[51] Fortunately, the rise of feminism has made medicine and science more conscious of women's issues. The number of women coming into medicine has significantly increased in recent years, so that along with the increasing numbers of nurse practitioners in women's health care, it is now possible for a woman with dysmenorrhea or PMS, or one who does not want to focus her life on motherhood, to find a sympathetic health care provider.

NOTES

1. *Black Magic: The Anthropology of Menstruation,* edited by Thomas Buckley and Alma Gottlieb (Berkeley and Los Angeles: University of California Press, 1988).

2. Janice Delaney, Mary Jane Lupton, and Emily Toth, *The Curse: A Cultural History of Menstruation,* rev. ed. (Urbana and Chicago: University of Illinois Press, 1988), pp. 7–17.

3. Pliny, *Natural History,* translated by H. Rackham (Cambridge, Mass.: Harvard University Press, 1942), 7. 549.

4. Lev. 15:24

5. Lev. 20:18

6. Edward D. Radin, *Lizzie Borden; The Untold Story* (New York: Simon and Shuster, 1961), p. 288.

7. Michael Meyer, *Times Literary Supplement,* June 11, 1976, p. 694.

8. Vern L. Bullough, "Merchandising the Sanitary Napkin," *Signs* 10 (1985): 317–32.

9. Stephanie A. Sanders and June M. Reinisch, "Psychological Correlates of Normal and Abnormal Menstrual Cycle Length," *Menstrual Health in Women's Lives* (Urbana and Chicago: University of Chicago Press, 1992), p. 134.

10. Heinrich Kisch, *The Sexual Life of Woman,* translated by M. Eden Paul (reprint New York: Allied Book Company, 1928), pp. 33ff. The original German edition appeared at least as early as 1904.

11. Vern Bullough and Cameron Campbell, "Female Longevity and Diet in the Middle Ages," *Speculum* 55 (1980): 324.

12. Koran II (The Cow), 234; Ali ibn abu-Bakr, *The Hedaya or Guide: A Commentary on Mussulman Laws,* C. Hamilton, editor and translator (reprint Lahore, West Pakistan: 1957), book 7, chap. 2, p. 186; R. Levy, *The Social Structure of Islam* (Cambridge, England: Cambridge University Press, 1957), p. 17.

13. Vern L. Bullough, "Age at Menarche: A Misunderstanding," *Science* 213 (July 17, 1981): 365–66.

14. E. B. Foote, *Plain Home Talk . . . Embracing Medical Common Sense* (Wells, N.Y., 1871), p. 454.

15. C. A. Mills, *Human Biology* 9 (1937): 43.

16. R. Lichtman and S. Paperce, *Gynecology: Well Women Care* (Norwalk, Conn.: Appleton and Lange, 1990).

17. Bullough and Campbell, "Female Longevity," pp. 317–25; Vern L. Bullough, "Nutrition, Women and Sex," *Perspectives in Biology and Medicine* 30 (Spring 1987): 450–80.

18. Elizabeth Rice Allgeier and Albert Richard Allgeier, *Sexual Interactions,* 3rd ed. (Lexington, Mass.: D. C. Heath, 1991), p. 487.

19. Paula Weideger, *Menstruation and Menopause: The Physiology and Psychology, the Myth and the Reality,* rev. ed. (New York: Delta, 1977), pp. 47–58.

20. Patricia A. Kaufert and Sonja M. McKinlay, "Estrogen-Replacement Therapy: The Production of Medical Knowledge and the Emergence of Policy," *Women, Health, and Healing: Toward a New Perspective,* edited by Ellen Lewin and Virginia Olesen (New York: Tavistock Publications, 1985), pp. 113–38.

21. Lisa Monagle, "Menopause," in *Human Sexuality: An Encyclopedia,* edited by Vern L. Bullough and Bonnie Bullough (New York: Garland Publishing Company, 1994), pp. 393–95; K. Martin and M. Freeman, "Postmenopausal Hormone-Replacement Therapy," *New England Journal of Medicine* 328 (April 1993): 115–17; A. Nabulski, A. Folsom, A. White, G. Heiss, K. Wu, and M. Szklo. "Association of Hormone Replacement Therapy with Various Cardiovascular Risk Factors in Postmenopausal Women," *New England Journal of Medicine* 328 (April 1993): 1069–75.

22. A. F. A. King, "A New Basis for Uterine Pathology," *American Journal of Obstetrics* 8 (1875–1876): 242–43.

23. Aristotle (pseud.), *The Works of Aristotle in four Parts, Containing I. His Complete Masterpiece . . . II. His Experienced Midwife . . . III. His Book of Problems . . . IV. His Last Legacy . . .* (London: published for the bookseller, 1808), p. 126.

24. E. F. W. *Pflüger, Über die Eierstoche der Säugethiere und des Menschen* (Leipzig: Engelmann, 1863).

25. Edward H. Clarke, *Sex in Education: or, Fair Chance for Girls* (Boston: James R. Osgood and Company, 1873), p. 33. This book was reprinted by Arno Press in 1972 as a part of the series *Medicine and Society in America,* edited by Charles E. Rosenberg.

26. Ibid., pp. 37–38.

27. Ibid., pp. 40–41.

28. Ibid., pp. 65–72.

29. Ibid., p. 63.

30. Ibid., p. 133.

31. Ibid., pp. 156–57.

32. George F. and Anna Manning Comfort, *Woman's Education and Woman's Health* (Syracuse: Thomas W. Durston & Company, 1874), p. 154.

33. T. S. Clouston, "Female Education from a Medical Point of View," *Popular Science Monthly* 24 (December 1883–January 1884): 332–33.

34. John Dewey, "Health and Sex in Higher Education," *Popular Science Monthly* 28 (March 1886): 606–11.

35. Anne G. Howes et al., *Health Statistics of Women College Graduates: Report of a Special Committee of the Association of Collegiate Alumnae* (Boston: Wright and Potter, 1885), p. 9.

36. Henry Maudsley, *Sex in Mind and in Education* (Syracuse: C. W. Bardeen, 1884), p. 14.

37. John Goodman, "The Menstrual Cycle," *Transactions, American Gynecological Society* 2 (1877): 650–62.

38. J. H. Kellogg, *Plain Facts for Old and Young* (Burlington, Iowa: I .F. Segner, 1882), pp. 83–86.

39. F. W. Van Dyke, "Higher Education a Cause of Physical Decay in Women," *Medical Records* 48 (1905): 296–98.

40. Ralph Wait Parsons, "The American Girl versus Higher Education Considered from a Medical Point of View," *Medical Records* 47 (1905): 296–98.

41. Ibid., p. 119.

42. Mary Roberts Smith, "Statistics of College and Non-College Women," *Publications,* American Statistical Association, 7, nos. 49–56 (1900–1901): 1–26.

43. G. Stanley Hall, *Adolescence, Its Psychology and Its relationship to Physiology, Anthropology, Sociology, Sex, Crime, Religion and Education,* 2 vols. (New York: D. Appleton and Company, 1904), 1: 478.

44. Ibid., 1: 511, 2: 639.

45. M. Carey Thomas, "Present Tendencies in Women's College and University Education," February 1908, in William O'Neill, ed., *The Woman Movement: Feminism in the United States and England* (Chicago: Quadrangle Books, 1969), p. 168.

46. Leta Stetter Hollingworth, *Functional Periodicity: An Experimental Study of the Mental and Motor Ability of Women during Menstruation,* Teachers College Columbia University Contributions to Education, No. 69 (New York: Columbia University, 1914), pp. 44, 66, 93, 95.

47. Clelia Duel Mosher, "Normal Menstruation and Some of the Factors Modifying It," *Johns Hopkins Hospital Bulletin* 12 (1901): 178–79; Clelia Duel Mosher, *Women's Physical Freedom* (New York: The Women's Press, 1923), pp. 1–29.

48. *New York Times,* July 26, 1970; *Los Angeles Times* February 21, 1972.

49. Karen E. Hood, "Contextual Determinants of Menstrual Cycle Effects in Observations of Social Interactions," in *Menstrual Health in Women's Lives,* edited by Alice J. Dan and Linda L. Lewis (Urbana and Chicago: University of Chicago Press, 1992), pp. 84–95.

50. Diane Scully and Pauline Bart, "A Funny Thing Happened on the Way to the Orifice: Women in Gynecology Texts," *American Journal of Sociology* 78 (1973): 1045–51.

51. Diane Scully, *Men Who Control Women's Health* (Boston: Houghton Mifflin Company, 1980), pp. 94–95.

7

Contraception

Theoretically when a couple engages in intercourse without using any method of birth control, there is a 3 percent chance that pregnancy will occur. This means that a pregnancy occurs approximately once in every thirty-three incidents of coitus. It is also estimated that the average woman could become pregnant every other year during her reproductive life, which is roughly between ages fifteen and forty-five. This adds up to an average of fifteen children, unless there are multiple births which increase the total number. The largest number of births recorded for any one woman is sixty-nine by the first wife of Feodor Vassilyev (her name does not appear in the records), a peasant woman from the village of Shula, 150 miles east of Moscow. She had twenty-seven pregnancies, including sixteen pairs of twins, seven sets of triplets and four sets of quadruplets, between 1725 and 1765. Almost all of these offspring survived beyond their first year. The most prolific mother of the twentieth century to date is Leontina Espinosa Albina (b. 1925), who had fifty-nine children, including five sets of triplets, Forty of her children were alive in 1994.[1]

If a man conceived children every time he engaged in sexual intercourse, he could impregnate thousands of women and presumably father as many babies. The male who is reported to have the most children was the polygamous Moulay Ismail (1622–1727), the last Sharfan Emperor of Morocco. He was said to have had 525 sons and 242 daughters by 1705, and in 1721 he recorded the birth of his seven-hundredth son. The Western male with the most progeny was probably Augustus the Strong, King of Poland and Elector of Saxony (1670–1733). His nickname came from his ability in the bed chamber rather than his military skills. He fathered 365 children, only one of whom was legitimate.[2]

In studying potential rates of increase, demographers use the married Hutterite women as their standard for maximum potential. The Hutterites are members of a communal religious group that first settled in North Dakota between 1874 and 1877. They now live in over a hundred different religious colonies in the United States and Canada. They do not use any method of family planning. While their living standard is not luxurious, their food supply is more than adequate and they are regarded as very healthy. The average number of children born to Hutterite women in the early part of the twentieth century was 10.6, although the rate has now declined somewhat.[3] The Hutterite rate is considered the maximum for a totally uninhibited rate of fertility.

No known society has reached the theoretical potential of 10.6 per woman. The fertility rate for the Ashanti of Africa was estimated at six, for the Sioux Indians at approximately eight, and for certain Eskimo groups at five. Only a minority of peoples of the past ever reached a rate as high as ten.[4] Modern fertility rates in such Third World countries as Pakistan, Indonesia, and Kenya average between six and eight; these rates, like most of those from the past, are lower than the early twentieth-century Hutterite rate partly because the women are not as healthy or well-nourished, but also because of customs and practices that control fertility. It seems clear that many factors worked to control population growth in the past. Some of these were consciously developed practices, but many others were unconscious factors.

An important limit on population was the high infant mortality rate. Although statistics from the past are difficult to obtain, it is estimated that somewhere between 30 and 40 percent of the infants born prior to the nineteenth century did not live beyond their first year. In England, where data are available for the decade 1731–1740, 437 infants out of every 1,000 born alive died before reaching their first year. During the decade 1791–1800, the death rate was 240 per 1,000 births.[5]

Celibacy is one of the oldest methods for limiting births, both at the individual and the societal level. When large armies were raised and sent off for protracted campaigns, most of the common soldiers were forced by circumstances to be celibate. While it is true that camp followers sold their services as prostitutes during many wars, very often the common foot soldier could not afford the prostitute. The Catholic church maintained celibacy for priests, monks, and nuns. Celibacy could also be fostered by raising the marital age not only in the obvious case of women but also for men. This is because the frequency of intercourse for men tends to decline with age, and frequency itself has an effect on the pregnancy rate. Although we have little data on the frequency of intercourse in the past, Kinsey and his associates found that the period of greatest sexual activity in married American males occurred between the ages of sixteen and twenty. These younger males engaged in coitus more than three times a week, compared to 1.7 times a week for those aged forty-one to forty-five.[6]

A temporary postponement of marriage can clearly lower fertility rates, as happened during the mid-nineteenth-century potato famine in Ireland, when the average age at marriage went up by almost a decade for both men and women. Short periods of continence were also used by many societies. These include, for example, prohibitions against sexual intercourse during Lent, various feast days, or during certain periods of a woman's life such as lactation or menstruation. It is highly unlikely that such prohibitions were originally established as birth-control measures, although they undoubtedly cut down the fertility rate. The modern rhythm method is a deliberate effort to utilize temporary periods of continence to control pregnancies.[7]

Polygamy also tends to limit the number of children simply because the incidence of coitus for each woman is lower.[8] The impact of homosexuality on birth rates of the past is a largely unexplored variable. However, even when the norms forced marriage, gay men and lesbians undoubtedly sought heterosexual intercourse much less often than heterosexuals; therefore, this was a de facto measure of birth control.

Prolonged lactation was an important factor in delaying pregnancy in times past and still is in some Third World countries. Lactation and the stimulus of the infant suckling ordinarily suppress ovulation and cause amenorrhea. It is highly effective as a birth control mechanism only when the total food supply of the infant is breast milk, or when abstinence during lactation is the norm, which was often the case in primitive societies. As soon as partial weaning takes place—and this could be as early as four to six months after birth—the menstrual cycle returns in most women who are adequately nourished, and pregnancy is again possible.[9]

Venereal disease has served as an involuntary limit to population growth by causing sterility in one or both partners. Although its historical role in causing infertility is not completely known, we do know that presently venereal disease is a major cause of infertility; therefore, we may assume that it has played a similar role throughout history. Gonorrhea was probably the most likely cause of sterility. With the advent of antibiotics in the 1940s, gonorrhea was almost eradicated and public health measures aimed at controlling it were abandoned. However, with the development of antibiotic-resistant strains of gonorrhea it has now returned with an incidence of approximately 700,000 cases a year in the United States.

Throughout history people have also tried to utilize artificial means of preventing conception, although only a few have been particularly effective. Contemporary peoples who still live in tribal or nomadic societies, for example, are known to use douches and drugs, to practice withdrawal, and to insert tampons and pessaries to avoid pregnancies. Subincision is also practiced in some groups and has a long history, although it is not clear whether it was originally done for ritualistic reasons or contraceptive purposes. Subincision is an operation that creates a hole in the male urethra at the base of the penis near the scrotum, so that during ejaculation semen dribbles out over the scrotum instead of entering the vagina. A more normal ejaculation can be obtained by covering the hole with a finger, which allows the semen to follow its original path. The same procedure facilitates urination through the penis.[10]

The earliest known prescriptions for contraceptives come from Egypt of the second millennium B.C.E. Written on papyrus scrolls, they called for substances such as crocodile dung, honey, and gumlike substances to be inserted into the vagina to block the path of the sperm. Crocodile dung was probably not a good choice, since its alkalinity would neutralize the acidity of the vagina, creating optimum conditions for sperm. Other recipes utilizing elephant dung would be more effective because of its acidity. Honey, gumlike substances and oils have long been known for their contraceptive value because they serve as mechanical barriers to the sperm. The ancient Greeks inserted olive oil which also serves as a mechanical barrier. One of the gums often used in ancient times was gathered from the tips of the acacia shrub; it contained lactic acid, an ingredient used in some current contraceptive gels.[11] A sponge soaked in vinegar is mentioned in the Talmud.

Intrauterine devices were also used. Books attributed to Hippocrates, the great Greek physician, mention their existence in classical Greece. On a more practical level, Arab camel drivers were accustomed to inserting a round stone into the uterus of the female camel before departing on a long journey in order to prevent her impregnation during the trip.

Coitus interruptus, the term describing the withdrawal of the penis from the vagina before ejaculation occurs, is known to have been used in ancient times because it was condemned by Jewish, Christian, and Islamic writers alike. They argued that the male seed was too precious to waste. *Coitus interruptus* was also used on a broad scale in France at the end of the eighteenth century, causing a population decline of significant proportions. Induced abortions, discussed in chapter 8, have also been widely practiced as a method of controlling births.

An important development supporting the birth control movement was the realization that untrammeled population growth could be harmful to the environment and to human beings themselves. The first serious consideration of this point of view was with the publication in 1798 of *An Essay on the Principle of Population* by The Reverend Thomas Robert Malthus. Malthus argued that while population growth occurred in geometric steps, doubling every generation, food supply tended to grow only in numerical steps; therefore, without major catastrophes such as war or plagues, famine would be inevitable. He was against any mechanical restraints to conception, but instead urged men to restrain their sex instincts and to marry as late as possible.[12]

Although his predictions were often borne out on local levels, such as the famine in Ireland in the nineteenth century, the worldwide implications of Malthus's theory only became apparent in the twentieth century, as advances in sanitation and health allowed many people to live longer and the real dimensions of the population problem started to emerge. Between 1650 and 1850 the number of people living on earth approximately doubled, from about 500 million to a little over one billion, but the population doubled again in the one hundred years between 1850 and 1950, when it reached two billion. Since 1950 the world's population has been increasing at an even faster rate, so that it will soon reach the four billion mark.[13] Most of the earth's people are now hungry, and life-threatening famines have become common in many parts of the world.

Since Malthus was opposed to contraception, those who adopted his premise regarding uncontrolled population growth but supported contraception were called Neo-Malthusians. Most of the early publications about contraception were published as throwaway tracts designed to reach the widest possible audience. The proposals of the English tailor Francis Place (1771–1854) are generally acknowledged to be the starting point for the modern contraceptive movement in the English-speaking countries. Place's *Illustrations and Proofs of the Principles of Population,* published in 1822, urged the use of "precautionary means," but he did not go into detail.[14] To remedy this Place made up handbills in 1823 addressed to "The Married of Both Sexes," advocating the use of a moist piece of sponge which was to be placed in the vagina before intercourse.[15]

The next phase of the birth-control movement emerged in the United States with the publication in 1830 of a booklet titled *Moral Philosophy* by Robert Dale Owens. Most of the booklet was devoted to the social and eugenic arguments for birth control and advocated that one of three methods be used: *coitus interruptus,* the vaginal sponge, or the condom.[16]

More controversial was the booklet *Fruits of Philosophy* by the Massachusetts physician Charles Knowlton in 1832. He advocated douching immediately following intercourse with a solution of alum with astringent vegetable substances such as white oak, hemlock bark, green tea, or raspberry leaves. In some cases Knowlton suggested a solution of zinc sulfate, which would be even less effective than douching with the alum solution.[17] In spite of the fact that we now know that douching was not as effective as the methods suggested by Owen, Knowlton's was the most influential of the tracts of its kind.

Knowlton, however, is remembered not so much for his contraceptive advice as for the difficulties he had disseminating it. In 1832, he was charged with obscenity and fined at Tauton, Massachusetts, and in 1833 he was jailed for three months in Cambridge for distributing his book. A third attempt to convict him in Greenfield, Massachusetts, led to disagreement between two different juries and so the case was dropped. The publicity, however, served to increase sales of Knowlton's book; as a result, by 1839 it had sold over 10,000 copies.

One of the most popular nineteenth-century contraception tracts was the *Elements of Social Science* by George Drysdale, published in England in 1854 while Drysdale was still a medical student. Most of the work focused on establishing the case for birth control although contraceptive methods were covered briefly (five pages in the original work). Drysdale preferred the sponge in combination with a douche of tepid water. He also recognized a sterile period, placing it from two days before the menstrual period until eight days after. However, Drysdale felt that *coitus interruptus* caused nervous disorders and he considered the sheath unaesthetic and deleterious to enjoyment.[18]

The growth of the eugenics movement contributed to a renewed interest in birth control in the last part of the nineteenth century. Eugenics defined itself as an applied biological science concerned with increasing the proportion of persons with better-than-average eugenic endowment from one generation to the next. The word was coined by Francis Galton (1822–1911), a cousin of Charles Darwin. Galton was a great believer in heredity. Unfortunately he also had many of the prejudices of an upper-class Englishman with regard to social class and race.[19] Some of Galton's hypotheses were carried to extremes by Karl Pearson (1857–1936), the first holder of the chair of eugenics, which Galton endowed at the University of London. Pearson, who was one of the founders of modern statistics, believed that the high birth rate of the poor was a threat to civilization, and that it was the duty of members of the "higher" races to supplant the "lower" races.[20] Although Pearson's views were eventually opposed by the English Eugenics Society, the American Eugenic Society, founded in 1905 and much more racist than the English group, adopted Pearson's ideas wholeheartedly. Ultimately Pearson's arguments were used by Adolf Hitler to justify his racial policies, which tainted the whole eugenic movement for most people, and created a burden for advocates of contraception and abortion.

However, even without this burden the birth control movement found it difficult to reach the public with its message. One reason for this was that in the English-speaking world the mere dissemination of birth control information came to be considered obscene. In England this was tied up with Victorian prudery. In America the censorship of sex-related information was intensified by fears over the growth of large cities and the gathering together of vast numbers of young people who no longer appeared to have the same values as their elders. In a sense the American movement for censorship represented a generation gap; however, it was also related to a socioeconomic gap, with the establishment worried about the morals of immigrants and other working men and women in the cities. It was to provide moral guidance to these young people that reformers gathered in groups in the large cities to establish organizations aimed at combatting obscenity. The New York City group, established in 1872, was called the Society for the Suppression of Vice; the Boston organization was the Watch and Ward Society, and other local groups used variants of these names. One of the first accomplishments of these organizations was to tighten the postal obscenity law and to support the appointment of Anthony Comstock, the secretary of the New York Society, as a special postal agent. For the next forty years Comstock acted as a moral censor for material originating in New York City and disseminated through the mail.[21]

One of the first American works on birth control to run afoul of Comstock was a pamphlet by Edward Bliss Foote which discussed contraceptive methods. Foote was prosecuted in 1876 and fined $3000.[22] With his prosecution, discussion and practice of birth control information went underground, and was confined primarily to persons of high socioeconomic status.

A change in the situation in the twentieth century was brought about by Margaret Sanger, an American nurse. Her first effort, a pamphlet, ran afoul of Comstock and she was forced to flee to Europe to avoid prosecution. While in Europe Sanger explored various methods of birth control and finally brought the diaphragm to the United States in 1916. The death of Comstock eventually resulted in the dismissal of the charges against her.

Still determined to help poor and immigrant women, Sanger established a clinic on the lower east side of New York City, Her well-publicized activities offended the authorities: she, her sister Ethyl, and Fania Mindell were jailed for opening the clinic. Sanger went on a hunger strike and was pardoned by the governor of New York, with the expectation that the clinic would close. Nevertheless, she persisted with singleminded fervor to make family planning services available to women who needed them, and the court of appeals ruled that she could disseminate information for "the cure and prevention of disease."[23] This odd ruling allowed the clinics in New York and some other states to continue operating by conceptualizing pregnancy as an illness. Sanger's work went on; she helped found several organizations that continue this day, including Planned Parenthood. In Britain, the first birth control clinic was opened in 1921 by Dr. Marie Stopes and her husband, H. V. Roe.[24]

The first modern contraceptive device was not, however, the diaphragm but the condom, which had first been described in the sixteenth century by Fallopius. He probably did not actually invent the condom; rather he was describing a device that had long been in use. Fallopius did, however, popularize a linen sheath shaped to fit the erect penis which could be soaked with chemicals and serve as an effective barrier to sperm as well as to infectious organisms.[25] The sheaths of this period were also made of animal intestines and fish bladders. They were used primarily as prophylactic devices to cut down the possibility of contracting venereal disease rather than as methods of birth control, although their contraceptive properties were known. Because they had to be individually crafted they were a luxury item used only by well-to-do men. In England the sheath was named the condom for reasons that are unknown. There are stories told about a mythical Dr. Condom who was supposedly a physician in the king's court, but no actual records of him have been discovered.

The discovery of the process of making liquid latex in 1844 made the production of rubber condoms possible, although they did not actually appear on the market until 1870. The quality of the new product was so poor that condoms made of animal membranes were probably still superior in quality. The first latex condoms were designed to fit only the tip of the penis, but the design was soon extended to cover the entire penile shaft. Seamless condoms were developed in the early twentieth century.[26] Early condoms were often sold in brothels and barber shops. Since state laws against contraception prevented their being sold for that purpose, their prophylactic use was emphasized. In 1920, Merle Young, a drugstore products salesman, started Young Rubber Company. He marketed condoms to drugstores and successfully challenged the laws against the dissemination of condoms as contraceptives.

Unfortunately, however, the quality control of condoms was poor. A survey done by the National Committee on Maternal Health in 1938 found that 40 percent of the rubber condoms sold in the United States had small holes or other defects.[27] This led to the Food and Drug Administration (FDA) being assigned the task of controlling the quality of condoms sold in interstate trade.[28]

For those who use condoms consistently the failure rates are low, between 1 and 3 percent; but for inexperienced and occasional users the rate is higher, almost 10 percent. However, condoms used with a spermicide also prevent the spread of most venereal diseases, including AIDS, syphilis, gonorrhea, chlamydia, herpes, and human papilloma virus, so they are now highly recommended.[29] Prevention of each of these diseases is important, but some of them are more of a threat than others: AIDS is fatal, human papilloma virus has been linked to cervical cancer, and chlamydia is a leading cause of infertility. Because of the serious nature of these diseases, condoms have emerged as one of the most important contraceptive devices. Certainly condoms are the contraceptive of choice for anyone who has had or plans to have more than one sex partner in a lifetime.[30]

Condoms for women are now on the market. The Reality® vaginal pouch looks somewhat like a large male condom with a rubber ring at the bottom which fits into the vagina like a diaphragm. The polyurethane sheath latex covers the labia and lines the inside of the vagina. The more recent bikini condom, which is still in clinical trials, includes a latex perianal shield with an attached vaginal pouch.[31]

The vulcanization of rubber also led to the development of diaphragms and cervical caps. *Pessaries,* designed in the nineteenth century to support a prolapsed uterus, are ringlike structures inserted into the vagina and pushed up to fit around the cervix. Some of the pessaries blocked the opening of the cervix so they could also be used as a birth control device, although this added effect was not publicly stated to avoid the stigma of contraception.[32] Several of these devices were patented in the nineteenth century; the device that turned into the popular diaphragm used in the twentieth century was developed by C. Hasse, a German physician who used the pseudonym Wilhelm P. J. Mensigna to protect himself from the stigma of dealing with a sexual product. The Mensigna diaphragm included a latex covering for the cervix, which was held in place by a coiled spring that fit behind the pubic bone and over the cervix at the back of the vagina.[33] Arleta Jacobs, a student of Hasse (Mensigna), opened a contraceptive clinic in the Netherlands, where she was visited by Margaret Sanger.

Diaphragms and *cervical caps* block the passage of sperm before they reach the cervix, so that they cannot make it up through the uterus and into the fallopian tubes where fertilization takes place. The diaphragm consists of a circular spring with a dome made of rubber. Contraceptive jelly (about one teaspoon) is smeared inside the dome, and the diaphragm is inserted inside the vagina in a position which covers the cervix and the front portion of the vagina. Diaphragms are sized to fit the individual woman so a new diaphragm must be fitted by a competent practitioner such as a physician, nurse practitioner, or physician's assistant. The diaphragm should be inserted before coitus, but it can safely stay in place for several hours before the sex act if that is convenient. Indeed, it should be left in place for at least six hours after intercourse, but for less than twenty-four hours to avoid the possibility of toxic shock syndrome.[34]

The failure rate of diaphragms is calculated at somewhat less than 10 percent, or in medical jargon, ten per one hundred woman-years of use. This means that for every one hundred women using the diaphragm with a spermicide for one year, fewer than ten will become pregnant. Failures are most likely to occur among new users. More experienced users tend to have failure rates as low as two or three per one hundred woman-years.[15] When the diaphragm is properly fitted and inserted neither partner is particularly aware of its presence. Negative side effects are rare, although a few women develop cystitis (an inflammation or infection of the bladder) because the diaphragm creates pressure on the bladder. A few people are also allergic to rubber; however, plastic diaphragms are available.

The *cervical cap* is a small thimble-shaped cup that fits over the cervix. A smaller device than the diaphragm, it was widely used at the beginning of the twentieth century in Europe but much less so in United States, probably because Margaret Sanger chose to introduce the diaphragm instead. This may have been because the cervical cap is more difficult to fit and to learn to insert, although once inserted it is comfortable, safe, and can be left in place for several days. The cervical cap gained new popularity in the 1970s, when several feminist groups advocated its being made available to American consumers to give them an additional choice of contraceptives. By this time, however, rigid government standards for devices had been put in place; the cervical cap had to go though a long testing procedure by the FDA and was finally approved in 1988.[36]

All the barrier contraceptives (condoms, diaphragms, cervical caps, and sponges) are used with *spermicides* for full effectiveness. As indicated earlier, ancient people had experimented with various types of spermicidal preparations long before the invention of the microscope made it possible to visualize sperm. The most effective of the early preparations included a paste, gum, oil, or wax that was combined with an acid. Research sponsored by the Rockefeller Foundation in the 1920s helped to develop improved spermicides. In 1937 phenylmercuric acid was produced under the trade name Volpar®. While an effective spermicide, it has been removed from the American market because of concerns about the safety of the mercury that it contained. A breakthrough came in the 1950s with the introduction of the surficants. These agents act primarily by disrupting the integrity of the sperm membrane. Since they are not strongly acetic they rarely irritate the vagina or penis. Spermicide containing nonoxynol-9 dominate the market now. It is a surficant spermicide which is effective as both a contraceptive and germicide.[37]

Spermicides can be purchased as jellies, creams, foaming tablets, or suppositories. The jelly is best for use with diaphragms, cervical caps, or condoms because oils destroy the latex.[38] The other preparations can be used alone. The failure rate for spermicide alone is about fifteen per one hundred woman-years. Although they prevent most venereal diseases, spermicides are not as effective alone as when used in combination with a barrier method.

Since they are mentioned in the Talmud, sea sponges soaked in vinegar, lemon juice, or other acidic fluids were a traditional folk method of birth control. However, the modern commercial contraceptive sponge dates only from the mid-1970s, when it was developed by an Arizona research group with a grant from the federal government. The original plan was that the sponge be washed and reused; however, this tended to wash out the spermicide so the failure rate was high. As a result, for several years a sponge with the trademark Today® was on the market. It was a mushroom-shaped polyethylene sponge impregnated with the spermicide nonoxynol-9. The user was instructed to moisten it and insert it before the sex act occurred. Although marketed for one-time use, it could be left in place up to twenty-four hours and used for more than one sex act. The disadvantage of the sponge was its relatively high failure rate (twenty-four per one hundred woman-years among older women who have had several pregnancies, and fourteen per one hundred woman-years with younger women). This disadvantage outweighed its accessibility and the manufacturer ceased production early in 1995.[39]

Oral contraceptives are synthetic hormones that prevent pregnancy. They were first approved by the FDA in 1960. While FDA approval was not then necessary for mechanical or barrier devices, it was for medications, so the pill was the first method of birth control to go through the full FDA approval process. The research that finally culminated in the pill had begun three decades earlier as an effort to control menstrual pain. This led to the realization that progesterone could prevent ovulation. Ovulation is the process by which the egg ripens and ruptures out of the ovary. If ovulation does not occur there can be no pregnancy; therefore, researchers realized that these hormones could also be effective as contraceptives. Continued research found that a combination of estrogen and progesterone was more effective in preventing ovulation and dysmenorrhea than either hormone alone.[40]

Synthetic progesterone (called progestin) was developed by Carl Djerassi at the Syntex laboratories in Mexico; this breakthrough led to the development of other synthetic hormones, including estrogen. The synthetic products were needed because both the progesterone and estrogen derived from animals were expensive and easily destroyed by enzymes in the human body.

Gregory Pincus, the medical director and vice president of the Planned Parenthood Federation, provided leadership in using these discoveries to develop the first oral contraceptives. He received support in this effort from Margaret Sanger, who secured funds for the research from Katherine Dexter McCormick (1875-1967), a longtime supporter of the planned parenthood movement.[41] The experimental trials testing the pill were done in Puerto Rico under the direction of Pincus. A group of 265 women were given pills containing a combination of synthetic progesterone and estrogen. Before the trial the pregnancy rate in Puerto Rico was sixty-three per one hundred woman-years (a very high rate). The results were remarkable. No woman who took the pills faithfully for twenty days of each cycle became pregnant during the two years of the study. However, the doses of both hormones were high and some women dropped out of the study complaining of nausea, vomiting, dizziness, and pelvic pain. This was also true of those women who took Enovid®, the first pill marketed for general use in 1960. However, it was soon realized that the doses of hormone could be reduced markedly, so that by 1980 significant side effects had been eliminated for most women.[42] Oral contraceptives function by interfering with the hormonal control of the female reproductive system. They create a false signaling system so that the brain and the pituitary gland do not send the usual messages to the ovaries. Consequently ovulation does not occur. In addition, the oral contraceptives also interfere with the work of the fallopian tubes that push the egg through the tubes to reach the uterus; they alter the lining of the uterus to make it unfriendly terrain for an egg, and they make the cervical mucous too thick for sperm to penetrate easily.

There are three types of oral contraceptives: *combination pills,* which include both estrogen and progestin; *triphasic pills,* which include these same two elements but in different proportions throughout the menstrual cycle; and *low-dose progestin pills,* sometimes called *mini-pills.* The combination pills are the most common. They are taken from the first day of the cycle until the twenty-first day, and discontinued for seven days during which time the menstrual period occurs. They come in a package that marks off the days of the cycle. Some packages include an additional seven pills of some inert substance so that the user can take a pill every day. Manufacturers of the triphasic pills, which came on the market in the 1980s, claim that they have even fewer side effects than the regular pills. Some women report this to be true while others see no difference. The mini-pills containing only progestin are preferred for mothers who are nursing babies, because too much estrogen is not good for the child.[43]

Possible side effects of the oral contraceptives include weight gain, swelling, nausea, headaches, rash, and sterility for several months after they are discontinued. The progestin-only pills can sometimes cause heavy bleeding. Side effects can often be controlled by changing to a different pill, since response tends to be individualized. However, with the current low dosages most women have no negative side effects after the first couple of months.

Although the incidence is low, serious cardiovascular problems, including strokes and heart attacks, have been related to oral contraceptives. For this reason women with a history of stroke, heart attack, diabetes, or other blood vessel problems should not take the pill. These complications are more likely to occur in older women, particularly those who smoke, because smoking damages blood vessels. For this reason the pill is ordinarily not given to women over thirty who are smokers. The smoking itself is actually the most dangerous practice, and some clinicians are prescribing oral contraceptives up to forty-five years.[44] The theoretical effectiveness of the oral contraceptives is 100 percent. In actual fact there are between four and ten failures per one hundred woman-years because people either forget to take their pills or don't take them on schedule.

The social impact of the pill is difficult to overestimate. For the first time in history it gave women the power to control their lives by deciding when and if they would be pregnant. Moreover, the contraceptive was being taken at a time unrelated to coitus, which somehow made many women feel more comfortable. The development of the pill is thus clearly an important factor in the revolutionary advances made by women in the last part of the twentieth century.

There are now two long-lasting progestin contraceptives on the market: Norplant®, a progestin implant which releases small amount of hormone over a period of three to five years; and three monthly injections of Depo-Provera®. While both these preparations have been used throughout the world for at least two decades, the FDA did not allow their use in the United States, because early trials with large doses of progestin caused breast cancer in dogs. It is now known that large doses of any progestational agent will cause breast cancer in dogs.[45] Improved testing indicated the safety of both methods of delivery of progestins, and both products have now been approved by the FDA.

Norplant is packaged as five-year progestin implants in six hollow capsules made of silicone rubber (silastic); the three-year implants use two solid silastic rods. They are injected under the skin on the inside of the upper arm where they gradually release a small amount of progestin which prevents conception by stopping implantation in the uterus. If the user decides she wants to become pregnant before the implants have spent their hormones, they can be removed early; otherwise they are removed at the end of the designated time period and new implants can be inserted.

The injectable Depo-Provera® is given within five days after the start of the menses, when the woman is known not to be pregnant. This timing also prevents ovulation during the first month so no second contraceptive is needed. The failure rate for both Norplant® and Depo-Provera® is about 0.3 percent. Both often cause irregular menses at first but the bleeding diminishes over time, and some women stop menstruating altogether after a year or so.[46] Los Angeles nurse practitioners report that women whose husbands disapprove of contraception are frequent users of the three-month Depo-Provera® injections because its use cannot be detected at home.

Intrauterine devices (IUDs) made out of a variety of materials have been tried sporadically throughout the ages, because almost any foreign body in the uterus will prevent conception. However, foreign bodies can also cause an infection; therefore, before the infectious disease process was understood and antibiotics developed, IUDs were too dangerous to be popular. The first IUD to be widely used was a ring of gut and silver wire developed in the 1920s by Ernst Graafenberg, a German gynecologist and sex researcher.[47] In 1934, Tenrei Ota of Japan introduced gold-plated silver intrauterine rings.[48] Jack Lippes, a Buffalo, New York, gynecologist, used the basic design developed by these researchers, but in 1962 introduced a loop made of plastic with an attached thread that fell into the vagina for easy checking or removal.[49] More recent IUD designs use copper, which has some contraceptive properties itself, or else a reservoir of progestin. These IUDs have proven safe and effective contraceptives; in addition, they are an effective treatment for heavy bleeding in some women, thus obviating the need for a hysterectomy.[50] IUDs are now one of the most effective contraceptives available, with a failure rate of less than one per one hundred woman-years. They act by inhibiting the passage of the sperm and preventing implantation in the uterus. They must be inserted and removed by a health-care provider, but once in place they can remain for several years. They should be avoided by women who are sexually active with multiple partners because they are likely to contract sexually transmitted diseases, and the IUD increases the likelihood of the infection traveling up into the pelvis. IUDs work best for women who have already had at least one child, so they are ideal for the time span between the end of child-bearing and menopause.

Unfortunately, an IUD called the Dalcon shield, marketed in the 1970s, was poorly designed, not tested, and it caused serious infections. By 1976 seventeen deaths could be linked to its use; however, the pharmaceutical company that had developed it took no steps to notify the public or health-care providers of the danger until 1980. This led to a large number of lawsuits; the company declared bankruptcy and the other IUD companies took their products off the market because of the fear of litigation.[51]

This disaster occurred partly because IUDs are devices instead of drugs, and as such they were not then controlled by the FDA. This situation changed in the aftermath of the Dalcon shield incident, but even with FDA approval IUDs are not used as often as they could be in the United States because of the fear caused by the Dalcon shield incident.[52]

As knowledge of reproductive physiology improved, it became possible to prevent conception using periodic abstinence. Formerly called the rhythm method, this approach is now called *natural family planning*. It is the only form of birth control that is not frowned upon by the Catholic Church. In order to be successful with natural family planning the couple must be able to identify or calculate when ovulation occurs, and abstain from intercourse for several days before and after the expected date of ovulation. While this ordinarily occurs fourteen days before the next menstrual period, it is not always possible to know exactly when the next menstrual period is scheduled to begin. This is particularly true if the woman has irregular menses. To improve the calculations some women take their temperature each day. It usually starts to rise mid-cycle at the time of ovulation. Two Australian physicians, John and Evelyn Billings, developed a method of periodic abstinence based on combining all the various indicators of ovulation with an emphasis on the changes in the cervical mucous. The mucous at the time of ovulation is thin and slippery, while it is thick at other times.[53]

Natural family planning is without risk to the body, but the failure rate is high among people with irregular menstrual cycles as well as those who are not conscientious about measuring and assessing the various clues that signal ovulation. The failure rate is approximately twenty per one hundred woman-years, although careful use of the method employing multiple indicators of ovulation can lower this figure to eight per one hundred woman-years.[54]

Contraceptive sterilization has become the most widely used method of family planning in the world. Since healthy women are fertile until about age fifty or fifty-one and men may remain fertile throughout their lives, many people who have finished bearing their desired number of children are now seeking voluntary sterilization. Since 1970 approximately one million sterilizations have been performed annually in the United States. Vasectomies were for a time the most popular approach, but now tubectomies outnumber vasectomies by about a two-to-one ratio.[55]

The lower rate of vasectomies relative to tubal ligation is undoubtedly related to the myth of impotence and the confusion with castration in the minds of many men. They can still ejaculate but the semen, which comes from the prostate, lacks sperm. Vasectomies are actually less dangerous and easier to perform than tubal ligations. The procedure involves cutting the vas deferens which is the tube that carries the sperm from the testes. Since it takes about six weeks to clear all the sperm from the system, intercourse should be delayed until then, or a condom should be used. The ejaculate should be examined under a microscope to make sure it is clear of sperm before the couple resumes intercourse.

Women are sterilized by cutting and tying the fallopian tubes. Since 1960 a simplified procedure has been possible using a laparoscope (a tube like a telescope). The surgeon works through the tube to locate, cut and tie off each fallopian tube.

Sterilization is also possible by removing the uterus and/or ovaries. One of these procedures might be chosen if the operation was done at the time of a Caesarean section, or if there are problems involving the reproductive tract.[56]

The newest contraceptive, RU-486, now in the process of clinical trials, looks promising as both a contraceptive and a morning-after pill for women with unprotected coitus, as well as an abortifacient. The details of this product will be discussed in the following chapter on abortion.

Also on the horizon are vaccines against pregnancy, several of which are in various stages of testing. They act by mobilizing body defense systems against some aspect of the reproductive process. The most advanced of the various vaccines induces antibodies against human chorionic gonadotropin. In addition to creating an immunity against pregnancy this particular vaccine also immunizes against tetanus. which may be an important feature in the developing countries. Early clinical trials in India look promising.[57]

This brief history of the birth control movement indicates what an uphill struggle it has been. Ancient beliefs that the male element was either the only or the most important factor in reproduction prevented effective contraception until modern physiological developments clarified the picture. However, even with an understanding of reproduction there were other obstacles to overcome. Nineteenth-century Americans proclaimed birth control knowledge to be obscene, particularly for women. As already indicated, Margaret Sanger and her supporters were jailed and stigmatized for bringing information and services to women.

The churches were never helpful in the struggle. While some at least remained neutral, the Catholic Church and many fundamental Protestant churches protected the power of men over women by stigmatizing women and threatening them with punishment after death for using any method of birth control except abstinence. It is only in the last twenty years that most Catholic women have been able to stand up to the power of the church and declare their private birth control practices their own territory. Many fundamentalist Protestant women continue to adhere to the preaching of their churches.

Another conclusion that can be drawn from this history is that contraceptives for men are still an underdeveloped field. Condoms are the only male contraceptive that has become popular, and as a matter of fact they are not easy to sell even in these times of peril from AIDS and other sexually transmitted diseases. Men simply do not have the same stake in contraception as women; indeed, for some men the freedom that contraception gives to women is most unwelcome.

The remarkable changes that have occurred in the roles and status of women since 1960, when the first oral contraceptives were marketed, suggest that the possibility of birth control led to basic challenges to the traditional place and role of women in society. Long-held assumptions have been questioned, and that most basic myth of all—that men were inherently superior—has been shattered. Once women could control their own bodies relative to reproduction, they became more autonomous. This new freedom allowed women in general, not just a select few, to seek opportunities in the formerly male-dominated professions, such as medicine, law, police work, and administration. The fruits of this revolution are just beginning to appear, although it will take much longer for them to be fully realized. Old myths, even when exposed, die hard.

The traditional mechanisms of religious repression based on a belief in male superiority continue to handicap many women; but even when they cannot confront the male power structure openly, some women are finding other ways to cope, including the secretive use of three-month Depo-Provera® injections. The braver women are simply ignoring the negative sanctions placed on them by the clergy. In the less developed countries, the traditional bastions of male power remain relatively untouched. Still, as birth control technology becomes widely disseminated, major changes will take place as the old myths about the necessity for female subordination continue to be challenged.

NOTES

1. Donald McFarlan, ed., *Guinness Books of Records, 1989* (New York: Sterling Publishing, 1988).

2. Ibid.

3. L. M. Laing, "Declining Fertility in a Religious Isolate: The Hutterite Population of Alberta, Canada, 1951–1971," *Human Biology* 52 (1980): 289–310; K. A. Peter, "The Decline of Hutterite Population Growth," *Canadian Ethnic Studies* 12 (1980): 97–110.

4. Clive Wood and Beryl Suitters, *The Fight for Acceptance* (Aylesbury, England: Medical and Technical Publishing Co., 1970), p. 10.

5. Richard Harrison Shyrock, *The Development of Modern Medicine,* 2d ed., rev. (New York: Alfred A. Knopf, 1947), p. 102.

6. Alfred E. Kinsey, Wardell B. Pomeroy, and Clyde E. Martin, *Sexual Behavior in the Human Male* (Philadelphia: W. B. Saunders, 1948), pp. 336, 356, Tables 81 and 88.

7. John T. Noonan, Jr., *Contraception: History of Its Treatment by Catholic Theologians and Canonists* (Cambridge, Mass.: Harvard University Press 1966), p. 332.

8. H. V. Muhsam, "Fertility of Polygamous Marriages," *Population Studies* 10 (1956–57): 3–16.

9. Norman E. Himes, *Medical History of Contraception* (New York: Schocken Books, 1970).

10. Ibid.

11. Ibid., pp. 59–88.

12. Thomas Robert Malthus, *An Essay on the Principle of Population,* 2d ed. (London, 1803).

13. Thomas McKeown, *The Modern Rise of Population* (New York: Academic Press).

14. Peter Fryer, *The Birth Controllers* (London: Secker and Warburg, 1965), pp. 43–57, 72–74.

15. Himes, *Medical History of Contraception,* pp. 216–217.

16. Fryer, *Birth Controllers* pp. 92–93.

17. Charles Knowlton, *Fruits of Philosophy,* edited by Norman Himes and Robert Latou Dickinson (Mount Vernon, N.Y.: Peter Pauper Press, 1937) p. 60

18. Himes, *Medical History of Contraception,* pp. 233–34; Fryer, *Birth Controllers,* pp. 110–11.

19. Vern L. Bullough, *Sexual Variance in Society and History* (Chicago: University of Chicago Press, 1976), pp. 652–53.

20. Angus McLaren, *Birth Control in Nineteenth-Century England* (New York: Holmes & Meier Publishers, 1978).

21. Paul S. Boyer, *Purity in Print* (New York: Charles Scribner's Sons, 1968).

22. Edward Bliss Foote, *Medical Common Sense Applied in the Causes, Prevention and Cure of Chronic Diseases and Unhappiness in Marriage,* revised and enlarged (New York: Published by the Author, 1866), pp. 378–81.

23. Margaret Sanger, *My Fight for Birth Control* (New York: 1931); Fryer, *The Birth Controllers,* pp. 201–19.

24. Fryer, *Birth Controllers,* pp. 223–34.

25. Himes, *Medical History of Contraception,* pp. 186–206.

26. Vern L. Bullough, "A Brief Note on Rubber Technology and Contraception: The Diaphragm and the Condom," *Technology and Culture* 22 (January 1981): 104–11.

27. R. Cautley, G. W. Beebe, and R. L. Dickinson, "Rubber Sheaths as Venereal Disease Prophylactics: The Relation of Quality and Technique to Their Effectiveness," *American Journal of Medical Sciences* 195 (February 1938): 155–83.

28. H. E. Butts, "Legal Requirements for Condoms under the Federal Food Drug and Cosmetic Act," in M. H. Redford, G. W. Duncan, and D. J. Prager. eds., *The Condom: Increasing Utilization in the United States* (San Francisco: San Francisco Press, 1974).

29. "Condoms—Now More than Ever," *Population Reports,* series H, number 8, September 1990.

30. "You Can Rely on Condoms," *Consumer Reports* 54 (March 1989): 135–42.

31. Rosemary Mastrangelo, "New Choices on the Contraceptive Front," *Advance for Nurse Practitioners,* May 1993, pp. 6–8, 20.

32. Vern L. Bullough and Bonnie Bullough, *Contraception: A Guide to Birth Control Methods* (Amherst, N.Y.: Prometheus Books, 1990), pp. 41–44.

33. W. P. A. Mensigna, *Über facultative Sterilitat. I. Beleuchet vom prophylactischen und hygenischen Standpunkte für praktische Ärzte II. Das Pessarium Occlusum und dessen Applikation* (Neuwald und Leipzig, 1885). The second part discusses the diaphram. For the United States the first clinical report was by James F. Cooper, *Techniques of Contraception* (New York: Day-Nichols, 1928), pp. 134–35.

34. Elizabeth B. Connell, "Barrier Methods of Contraception," in *Principles and Practice of Clinical Gynecology,* edited by Nathan G. Kase, Allan B. Weingold and David M. Gershenson, 2d ed. (Ann Arbor, Mich.: Books on Demand, 1990), pp. 981–91.

35. Robert A. Hatcher, Felicia Stewart, James Trussell, Deborah Kowal, Felicia Guest, Gary K. Stewart, and Williard Cates, *Contraceptive Technology, 1990–1992* (New York: Irvington Publishers, Inc., 1990), pp. 200–202.

36. Ibid., pp. 193–225; A. A. Shihata and Erica Gollub, "Acceptability of a New Intravaginal Barrier Contraceptive Device (Femcap)," *Contraception* 46 (December 1992): 511–19.

37. "Spermicides—Simplicity and Safety Are Major Assets," *Population Reports* 7, no. 5 (September 1979).

38. B. Voeller, "Mineral Oil Lubricants Cause Rapid Deterioration of Latex Condoms," *Contraception* 39 (January 1989): 95–102.

39. Hatcher et al., *Contraceptive Technology,* pp. 193–225.

40. J. Bennett, *Chemical Contraception* (New York: Columbia University Press, 1974).

41. Vern L. Bullough, *Science in the Bedroom: A History of Sex Research* (New York: Basic Books, 1994), pp. 193–94.

42. G. Pincus, *The Control of Fertility* (New York: Academic Press, 1965); G. Pincus, J. Rock, C-R. Garcia, E. Rice-Wray, M. Paniagua, and J. Rodriquez, "Fertility Control with Oral Medication," reprinted by L. L. Langley (Stroudsburg, Pa.: Dowden Hutchinson & Ross), pp. 413–26.

43. Hatcher et. al., *Contraceptive Technology,* pp. 227–300.

44. T. Luukkainen, "Contraception after Thirty-Five," *Acta Obstetrica et Gynecologia Scandanavica* 71 (1992): 169–74.

45. A. Rosenfield, D. Maine, D. Rochat, J. Shelton, and R. A. Hatcher, "The Food and Drug Administration and Medroxyprogesterone Acetate, What are the Issues?" *JAMA* 249 (June 3, 1983): 2922–28.

46. Andrew M. Kaunitz, "DMPA: A New Contraceptive Option," *Contemporary OB/GYN* 38 (1993): 19–34.

47. Ernst Graffenberg, "An Intrauterine Contraceptive Method," in *The Practice*

of Contraception: An International Symposium and Survey, edited by M. Sanger and H. H. Stone: Proceedings of the 7th international Birth Control Conference, Zurich, Switzerland, September 1930 (Baltimore, Md.: Williams and Wilkins, 1931), pp. 33–47.

48. T. Ota, "A Study on Birth Control with Intrauterine Devices," *Japanese Journal of Obstetrics and Gynecology* 17 (1934): 210–14.

49. Jack Lippes, "PID and IUD," paper presented at the World Congress of Gynecology and Obstetrics, Tokyo, October 1978.

50. Goran Ryboi, Kerstin Anderson, and Viveca Odlind, "Hormonal Intrauterine Devices," *Annals of Medicine* 25 (1993): 143–47.

51. Morton Mintz, *At Any Cost: Corporate Greed, Women and the Dalcon Shield* (New York: Pantheon Books, 1985).

52. Hatcher et al., *Contraceptive Technology,* pp. 355–85.

53. J. Billings, *Natural Family Planning Method: The Ovulation Method* (Collegeville, Minn.: Liturgical Press, 1973); E. Billings, and A. Westmore, *The Billings Method: Controlling Fertility without Drugs or Device* (New York: Random House, 1980).

54. J. B. Brown, L. F. Blackwell, J. J. Billings, et al., "Natural Family Planning," *American Journal of Obstetricis and Gynecology* 157 (1987): 1082–89.

55. Hatcher et al., *Contraceptive Technology,* p. 387.

56. Leon Speroff and Philip D. Darney, *A Clinical Guide for Contraception* (Baltimore, Md.: Williams and Wilkins, 1992), pp. 263–96.

57. G. P. Talwar, Om Singh, Rahul Pal, Nirjhar Chattergee, S. N. Upadhyay, et al., "A Birth Control Vaccine Is on the Horizon for Family Planning," *Annals of Medicine* 25 (1993): 207–12.

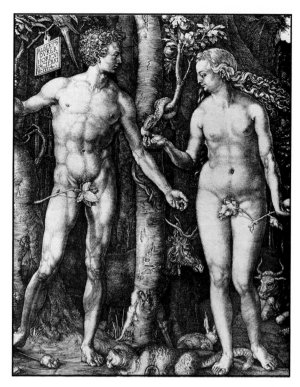

Figure 1. Albrecht Dürer, *Adam and Eve* (1504). This painting depicts a common theme in Western civilization: woman as a powerful and seductive sexual temptress. Bibliothèque Nationale, Paris. Giraudon / Art Resource, New York.

Figure 2. Prostitutes advertising their wares as a parade passes by. This cartoon was made for James Garfield, elected U.S. President in 1880.

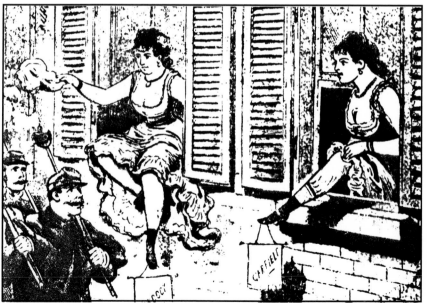

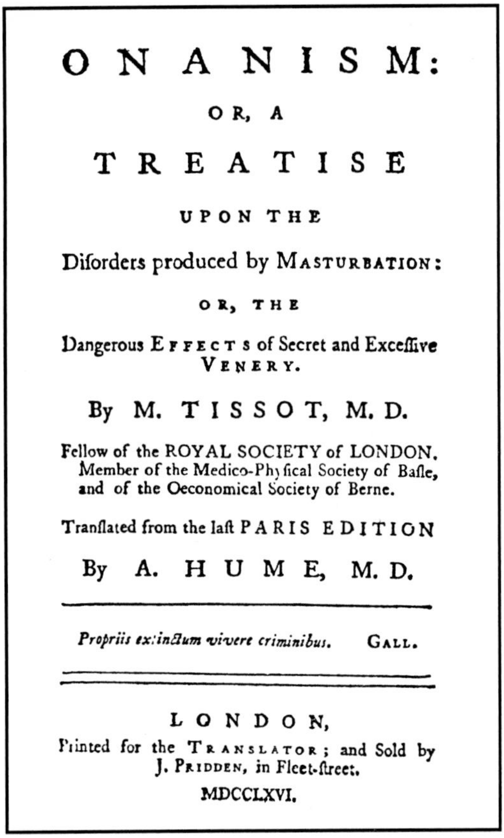

O N A N I S M:

OR, A

T R E A T I S E

UPON THE

Diſorders produced by MASTURBATION:

OR, THE

Dangerous E F F E C T s of Secret and Exceſſive
VENERY.

By M. TISSOT, M.D.

Fellow of the ROYAL SOCIETY of LONDON,
Member of the Medico-Phyſical Society of Baſle,
and of the Oeconomical Society of Berne.

Tranſlated from the laſt PARIS EDITION

By A. HUME, M.D.

Propriis ex:inĉum vivere criminibus. GALL.

LONDON,
Printed for the TRANSLATOR; and Sold by
J. PRIDDEN, in Fleet-ſtreet.
MDCCLXVI.

Figure 3. A treatise on "onanism," or masturbation, by the eighteenth-century physician S. A. D. Tissot, whose ideas were widely accepted.

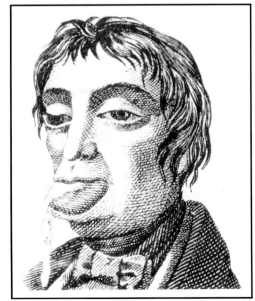

Figure 4. This nineteenth-century drawing illustrated the supposed effects of masturbation, including insanity, epilepsy, poor eyesight, and loss of memory.

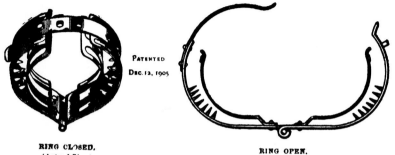

THE TIMELY WARNING

PATENTED
Dec. 12, 1905

RING CLOSED.
(Actual Size.)

RING OPEN.
(Actual Size.)

PREVENTS NIGHT EMISSIONS BY AROUSING THE WEARER

*Made of aluminum---weighs but two drams
and saves pounds of drugs and worry. . . .*

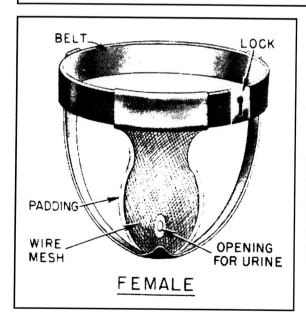

BELT   LOCK

PADDING

WIRE
MESH

OPENING
FOR URINE

FEMALE

To prevent the evil of masturbation, several devices were patented in the nineteenth century. Figure 5, above. Dr. E. B. Foote, proprietor of a New York clinic, invented "The Timely Warning," a ring of sharp metal spikes worn around the penis to prevent nocturnal emissions. Figure 6, left. A female harness had perforated wire-type meshing, so girls could urinate through it without touching themselves.

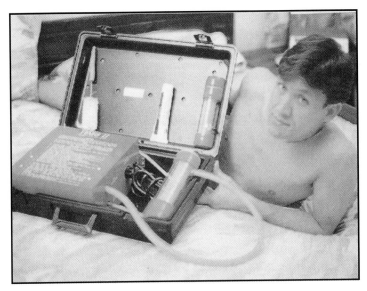

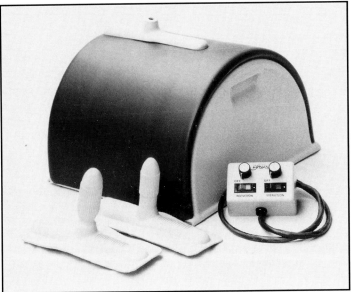

Modern aids to sexual stimulation. Figure 7, upper picture. The "Venus II" ™ masturbation machine for men. Figure 8, lower picture. The SYBIAN ™ stimulator for women. Courtesy Abco Research Associates, P.O. Box 354, Monticello, Ill. 61856.

8

Abortion

Abortion is an ancient practice, evidence of which can be found in the writings of many ancient cultures. An Egyptian papyrus medical of 1550 B.C.E. describes several mixtures of herbs that can be placed in the vagina to cause abortions.[1] Plato advised that any pregnant woman over forty abort. Aristotle argued that excess population should be controlled by means of abortions before sense and life had entered into the embryo.[2]

The second-century C.E. Greek physician Soranus of Ephesus specialized in what would now be called gynecology.[3] His writings include prescriptions (recipes) for antifertility drugs, some of which would be now be classified as contraceptives and others as abortifacients.[4] Soranus did not, however, divide them according to these categories; rather he classified them as substances that could be placed in the vagina as suppositories, and drugs that were to be taken orally. Several of the suppositories featured the use of pomegranate peel. Soranus's four major oral prescriptions each included a variety of herbs such as silphium (fennel), wallflower, rue, Queen Anne's lace, and myrtle. Modern testing of these herbs has shown the majority to have either contraceptive or abortifacient qualities.[5] Some of these herbs are also used in contemporary folk medicine as abortifacients.

Other ancient practices have survived until modern times as folk remedies. In addition to taking herbal preparations that date back to antiquity, Egyptian women insert mullohaya, a stiff grass, into the uterus to cause abortions.[6] The women of Thailand use a deep massage technique that dates back to ancient times. Ergot, a fungus that grows on rye, was widely used as an abortifacient wherever rye was grown. Because ergot can cause severe poisoning and even death, the practice was not without danger. Ergotamine, a modern drug used to stimulate uterine contractions, is an alkaloid of ergot.

While there were significant variations in the positive or negative sanctions for abortion from one culture to another, most societies had some type of abortion practices. Five major types of procedures were used: (1) the ingestion of herbs and other abortifacients; (2) the insertion of objects through the vagina and into the uterus; (3) the insertion of irritating substances into the vagina; (4) external injury with heavy massage or pounding, or violent physical exertion; and (5) magic.[7] Clearly the most effective means were also the most dangerous. Significant injuries and infection were likely with the insertion of objects into the uterus and heavy pounding of the abdomen was dangerous to the woman. Most of the oral remedies were less dangerous but less effective, and magic the least dangerous and least effective remedy of all. Abortion procedures were usually carried out by the woman herself or by midwives. Throughout most of the historical past, laws and rules, which tended to be the business of men, did not extend to women's matters.

The early Christian writers were an exception to this rule: they came out against both contraception and abortion although they did not consider the early expulsion of the fetus an abortion. This belief was based upon the teachings of Aristotle, who held that the rational soul entered the body of the male fetus forty days after conception and eighty days after conception for females. Some medieval theologians argued for different time frames, including Thomas Aquinas, who believed that the rational soul entered the fetus at the time of quickening (when the mother feels movement), making this the point in time that marked the prohibition against abortion.[8] In 1869, Pope Pius IX eliminated the distinction between the early, nonviable fetus and the later, viable fetus by declaring that abortion at any point after conception would be considered murder.[9]

There were also other moves made against abortion in the nineteenth century. English common law, which had accepted abortions as legal until quickening, was changed in 1803 when a law was passed outlawing abortion by poisoning. Later revisions strengthened the law by outlawing surgical procedures, and dropping the distinction between abortions before or after quickening. In the United States, abortions were caught up in the struggle between physicians and midwives, which occurred as physicians moved into the field of obstetrics and gynecology. Physicians argued that midwives were unsavory characters who performed abortions, so midwives and their skills should be eliminated to save the lives of women. Laws were therefore passed in the late nineteenth and early twentieth centuries outlawing midwives in most states. Laws were also passed against abortions, with the first such statute enacted in Connecticut in 1821 outlawing abortions after quickening. A revision in 1860 made all abortions illegal. Other states quickly followed; as a result, abortion was outlawed in all the states by the beginning of the twentieth century, although there was some state-to-state variation in what precisely was prohibited. One of the exceptions in most states was the right of physicians to perform therapeutic abortions if they were essential to save the life of the mother.

The anti-abortion statutes were written in an era of increasing labor markets fueled by industrial expansion. However, in spite of the nation's need for a large work force, the pay for laborers was meager, and the number of children who could be fed with a worker's salary limited, so the working-class was trapped in an impossible situation. Options for limiting births were relatively few, with celibacy, *coitus interruptus,* anal intercourse, vaginal sponges, and condoms being the choices other than abortion. Since only the wealthy could afford condoms before the 1920s, unwanted pregnancies were common, and desperate women turned to illegal abortionists.

The Kinsey study of the late 1940s included questions to 7,074 female participants about their past experience with abortions. The study found that in spite of their illegality, abortions were a common event, with one-fourth to one-third of the women reporting a past abortion. Most of these were not done as therapeutic abortions (to save the mother's life). Consequently they were illegal. Methods used for the illegal abortions were described as surgical procedures performed by a doctor or someone else with some medical knowledge. Only 9 percent of the white women successfully induced the abortion themselves, and this was usually with drugs rather than self-surgery. More black women, particularly among the very poor, reported abortions using the old folk remedies, such as drinking turpentine, tansy tea, rusty nail water, horseradish, bluing, aloes, ergot of rye, bitters and whiskey, or ginger tea.[10]

In spite of the fact that illegal abortions were common procedures, only 116 persons were convicted as abortionists in the year 1944, for example. This suggests that the laws against illegal abortions were not being enforced with much rigor.[11] Illegal abortions were not without danger, however. Even if the abortionist was a licensed physician, he might not have the hospital facilities available for emergencies, such as hemorrhaging. Nonphysicians were further cut off from mainstream medical care and had even fewer options for dealing with untoward events. When antibiotics became available in the 1940s, the illegal abortionists had difficulty obtaining them for their patients because they were available only with a physician's prescription. Statistics related to mortality rates for illegal abortions are difficult to obtain. However, studies done in 1929 and 1944 estimated that between 20 and 35 percent of the maternal deaths related to pregnancy and delivery were caused by illegal abortions.[12]

Despite some concern over these deaths, the United States held back on changing its abortion laws. The first country to legalize abortion in the twentieth century was the newly formed Soviet Union in 1920. Thereupon abortions quickly became the major method of birth control. However, in 1936, Joseph Stalin banned abortions and the prohibition remained until his death in 1953. When abortion was legalized again in 1955, most of the countries then in the Soviet bloc also legalized it.[13]

The Scandinavian countries were progressive in studying abortion as an option and in passing laws to permit it. Iceland in 1934 was the first to pass a modern abortion law. Denmark had established a study commission in 1932 to consider the matter and passed a liberal abortion law in 1939. In 1938 Sweden passed a law allowing pregnancies to be interrupted if the mother was ill, if she had been impregnated under circumstances contrary to law, or if a there was the possibility of a hereditary disease. The Swedish law was amended in 1946 to allow abortion if it could be assumed that the mother's physical or mental strength would be seriously impaired by the birth and care of the child.[14]

In 1948 Japan made history by becoming the first country to legalize abortions with the conscious aim of regulating population growth. The original 1948 law had legalized abortion only for women whose health might be impaired from the physical or economic standpoint but within a few years it was broadened to allow abortion on request. The Japanese birthrate quickly dropped from 34.3 per thousand women in 1947 to 16.0 per thousand by 1961. In recent years the number of abortions have decreased somewhat with the improvements in contraceptive technology and the growing wealth of the country, but abortions are still available and selected by many women as the method of choice for controlling pregnancies. The birthrate in Japan remains low with a virtually stable level of population growth.[15]

Although the leadership of the Chinese revolution in 1949 opposed birth control measures of any kind, within a few years it became apparent that the rapidly increasing population in that country was wiping out all efforts to increase the standard of living. Various measures were tried, but none were particularly successful given the degree of political upheaval marking those times. By 1981, when the population had reached 1.2 billion, China became the first country in the world to embark on a deliberate and comprehensive course to reach zero population growth by the year 2000 or as soon after that as possible. To achieve this goal the Chinese government called on the people to limit their families to one child. The limitations are enforced by the Danwei, collectives which are used to organize the factories, farms, and even the city blocks. In addition to facilitating abortions, birth control, and sterilizations, the Danwei arranges rewards at work and better schooling for the child if the couple has complied with the one-child norm.[16]

Though the Chinese government has allowed many more exceptions in recent years, the family planning policy was further emphasized in 1993 when the Party Congress approved a bill to forbid marriages of persons with hepatitis, venereal disease, or mental illness. The goal is to reduce the number of congenitally disabled persons as well as to limit population growth.

American policy toward abortion started changing in the 1960s. Relatively insulated from concerns about world population growth, Americans were primarily influenced by the growing women's movement. Improved methods of contraception, including oral contraceptives, had given women a growing sense of control over their biological destiny; with this power over the reproductive cycle they wanted more. Betty Friedan's *The Feminine Mystique,* published in 1963, raised the consciousness of many women, and made the concept of choice over whether or not to reproduce a respected goal.[17] The Model Penal Code adopted by the American Law Institute proposed that state laws be changed to allow termination of pregnancy when the physical or mental health of the mother was greatly impaired; when the child might be born with a grave physical or mental defect; or when the pregnancy resulted from rape, incest, or other felonious intercourse, including illicit intercourse with a girl under sixteen.[18]

Public interest focused on abortion laws in 1962 with the case of Sherri Finkbine, a Phoenix, Arizona, mother of four, who had taken the tranquilizer thalidomide during the first few months of her fifth pregnancy. Since the drug had not been approved by the American Food and Drug Administration (FDA), it was not marketed in the United States; however, Sherri's husband had returned from Europe with a bottle of thalidomide which she had then taken. Two months later the news of the deformities that the pill was causing in European children—notably stunted or missing arms and legs—was made public. Sherri consulted her physician, who estimated that the chances of her infant being born deformed were at least 50 percent. He then arranged to admit her to the hospital for a therapeutic abortion. Sherri told a friend about her planned surgery and the story reached the newspapers. Fearful of further publicity, the hospital canceled the abortion. The Finkbines flew to Los Angeles, planning to travel to Japan for the abortion, but the Japanese consulate, also afraid of negative publicity, refused them a visa. The couple then flew to Sweden where Sherri had the abortion. The fetus was deformed.[19]

This incident brought the discussion of American anti-abortion laws and practices out in the open and helped crystallize a movement for abortion law reform. In California, the Committee for Therapeutic Abortion was established in 1965, representing a coalition of civil libertarians, women's organizations, physicians, and liberal religious groups. That same year the National Organization for Women (NOW) was established, with reproductive rights as one of its major concerns. The National Association for the Repeal of Abortion Laws was established in 1968.[20]

Beginning in 1967, several states repealed their restrictive abortion laws, using all or part of the proposals of the American Law Institute. By 1970, thirteen states had passed such legislation and others were considering it. The advocates for legal reform also worked through the courts, so that by 1972 state court decisions had liberalized abortion privileges in three jurisdictions.[21] In 1973 the United States Supreme Court heard the case of *Roe* v. *Wade*; in a landmark decision the Court struck down state prohibitions against first-trimester abortions, ruling that during the first three months of pregnancy the decision to abort could be made by the woman and her physician. During the next three months the states could regulate abortion to ensure reasonable standards of care. Only in the last trimester could abortions be outlawed and not even then if they were necessary to preserve the life of the mother. This decision nullified more restrictive legislation by states.[22]

This decision brought strong reactions from opponents of abortion on moral and religious grounds, including the leadership of the Catholic Church and fundamentalist Protestantism, as well as individuals who felt moral repugnance to the idea of abortion. A strong backlash followed. Some of the anti-abortion activity was sponsored directly by churches, but most of it was coordinated by several different organizations under the collective title "Right to Life." The radical fringe of these groups bombed abortion clinics or chained themselves to clinic doors to block entrances.[23] More mainstream members worked through the political process to weaken the right to abortion by passing restrictive state laws. Some of these laws required the husband's consent; others added parental consent for minors, cut off public funding, or added procedural requirements such as waiting periods. When these state laws were tested in the courts, many of them were struck down because they were not congruent with *Roe* v. *Wade*. However, the political and ideological makeup of the Supreme Court changed during the administration of Ronald Reagan (1981–1989). Reagan made an anti-abortion stance the most important selection criterion for federal judges and supreme court justices. It took time for his policy to be felt in the judicial decisionmaking process, but by 1986 there had been enough turnover to affect the decisions on this matter. President George Bush (1989–1993) pursued the same policy, making an anti-abortion stance the litmus test for judicial selection. Consequently the Supreme Court became more reluctant to defend *Roe* v. *Wade* against the various state restrictions. The 1989 decision in *Webster* v. *Reproductive Health Services* tested a Missouri law that included a preamble arguing that life begins at conception. Although the Supreme Court refused to uphold it, the right-to-life advocates perceived the Court's sharp division as the next to the last step before the dismantling of *Roe* v. *Wade.*[24]

The election to the presidency of William Clinton in 1992 marked a change in justice selection policy with judicial criteria and other political agendas being used. The decision in *Roe* v. *Wade* still stands, although there are continuing attempts being made to overturn it. The political climate has undoubtedly been influenced by a countermovement using the slogan "Pro-Choice." The most clearly defined organizations within this camp are the National Abortion Rights Action League (NARAL), Planned Parenthood Federation, and the American Civil Liberties Union (ACLU). These groups have been active in preserving what they call "reproductive freedom."

Abortion procedures are now performed primarily in ambulatory free-standing clinics, with only second-trimester abortions being done in hospitals. "Morning-after" pills are prescribed in doctor's offices. When successful, these medications take effect before the fertilized ovum reaches the uterus and attaches to its wall. They are sometimes called postcoital methods, or menstrual regulation, and are often used for rape victims. Various hormones have been used for this purpose, including diethylstilbestrol (DES) and the oral contraceptives that contain estrogen and progesterone combinations, or either of these hormones alone.[25] The doses of these hormones used for postcoital contraception are large enough to cause unpleasant side effects, including nausea and vomiting, so their use should be medically supervised. Since the oral contraceptives have not been approved for this purpose by the FDA, federally funded clinics are not allowed to used this method.

It is anticipated that the French compound, RU-486, developed by Étienne-Émile Baulie and marketed in France since 1985, will be a more effective postcoital drug. It is one of a family of antiprogestins which prevents implantation of the egg in the uterus; if used at a later date, it causes an abortion at any time during the first nine weeks of pregnancy.[26] American testing by the FDA was held up for nine years because the pharmaceutical house Roussel-Uclaf considered the drug too controversial to market in the

United States. In 1994 they turned the American rights over to the non-profit Population Council for Marketing. As a result RU-486 is currently being tested by the FDA. It is anticipated that when the drug is marketed, abortions, or at least early abortions, will be a much more private matter. Drugs can be prescribed by a personal physician, so patients will not have to run the gauntlet of the right-to-lifers currently picketing the abortion clinics.

Postcoital insertion of a copper IUD has also proven effective in preventing implantation of the fertilized ovum in the uterus. The IUD is inserted one to seven days following unprotected intercourse, and can be left in place to prevent future pregnancies.

Most first-trimester abortions utilize a suction procedure developed in Asia, used in the former USSR, and brought to the United States in the 1960s. It is the most common abortion procedure, although American physicians often combine it with curettage to make sure the uterine lining is completely removed. A dilation and curettage (or D and C) is used if the pregnancy is in the late first trimester, or if the physician feels there is some problem requiring the procedure. The cervix is dilated and a curette is used to scrape the uterine walls. Various techniques can be used to facilitate the dilation of the cervix, including the insertion of laminaria, i.e, cervical tampons that swell from three to five times their original diameter when placed in a moist environment.

Second-trimester abortions usually involve the insertion of hypertonic saline solution into the amniotic sac. In addition, prostaglandin, which stimulates uterine contractions, is sometimes used, followed by the dilation and curettage. Sometimes a hysterotomy, i.e., a surgical opening of the uterus, is done. Many second-trimester abortions are undertaken because of fetal abnormalities discovered through amniocentesis. However, recent improvements in the technique of amniocentesis make it possible to do the procedure as early as the tenth week, so there will probably be fewer second-trimester abortions in the future.

The basic ethical issue marking the abortion debate focuses on the rights of the fetus.[27] Conservatives argue that the minute the sperm enters the ovum, the ovum has exactly the same moral status as a person, and its rights should not be terminated by abortion. Some adherents to this argument would hold that this is true even if the fetus is grossly deformed, or if several eggs have been removed from the mother for purposes of in vitro fertilization. Since this procedure involves the use of fertility drugs that produce multiple eggs, and since an unlimited number of multiple births can threaten the viability of all of the fetuses, the judgment about how many eggs to reintroduce then becomes difficult.

Liberals take a view nearly opposite to that of conservatives, claiming that fetuses are not persons and have no rights, or whatever rights the fetus may have are superseded by the privacy rights of the mother. Liberals argue that abortion on request should be legal and without punishment by moral sanctions. The intermediate or moderate view would hold that fetuses may have rights after they reach viability, but moderates do not worry about the rights of fertilized eggs. Moderates would allow abortions for a variety of reasons, including anything that would harm the fetus, as well as rape, incest, teen-age pregnancy, and poor maternal health. Most moderates in the United States do not accept economic deprivation as a criterion for abortion, although this is probably the major reason for both legal and illegal abortions in most of the Third World, where food is scarce.

This broad spectrum of views can be identified in the national surveys of public opinion. Repeated Gallup polls on abortion indicate that the overwhelming majority of Americans favor abortion under certain circumstances, including rape, incest, pregnancy of unmarried minor children, genetic or intrauterine problems, or illness of the mother; but they oppose granting women the right to abortion under all circumstances. A small group of extreme conservatives favors outlawing abortions altogether while a small group at the other end of the political spectrum advocates a free choice for women. Although earlier polls showed Catholics significantly more opposed to abortion than Protestants, the major religious groups now hold a similar range of opinions.[28]

Given the fact that a substantial number of Americans oppose abortion, at least in some cases, it is noteworthy that the United States has a high abortion rate, with approximately one-third of pregnancies (29.7 percent) ending in an abortion. Among the industrialized countries only Italy, Japan, and the states making up the former Soviet Union have abortion rates higher than or comparable to that in the United States. This high rate of American abortions is related to the fact that half of the pregnancies are unplanned or unwanted, a rate higher than most other industrialized countries. Most unintended pregnancies in the United States occur among women from disadvantaged backgrounds and who are under the age of twenty-five. A study published in 1989 compared those countries with low rates of unplanned pregnancies with the United States in order to identify the factors that might explain this situation. Two such factors emerge: (1) the United States does not do a good job reaching young men and women with contraceptive information and services, and (2) it does not have a comprehensive health-care plan to pay for birth control for all its young people. Those countries in the study with low rates of unintended pregnancies had comprehensive national health plans which made family planning services readily available to all women regardless of their income and age, and the community supported their quest for contraception.[29] The high rate of unplanned pregnancies also suggests that group norms in the United States have not yet fully changed to fit the belief in an overpopulated world. The fact that not all states allowed the dissemination of contraception until 1965 emphasizes the difficulty family planning has had in being accepted. Until it is fully accepted and financed, unplanned pregnancies will continue, and abortions will still be sought by large numbers of young women.

Most anti-abortion activists do not accept the link between abortions and an inadequate health-care delivery system that fails to provide sufficient contraceptive services for poor young women. Rather, they continue to espouse the myth that women who seek abortions are depraved sinners. Other myths are believed by the general public, including the one that abortion is something new that has appeared on the scene only in the twentieth century. As indicated in this chapter, abortion is clearly an ancient practice and one that has been employed in all parts of the world. While the men in some of these societies decried the practice, women knew that abortion was sometimes called for, and since the spheres of men and women were separate women could sometimes participate in a world closed off to men. Perhaps the greatest myth of all is that the Christian church has always opposed early abortions. It is important to remember that even in the Catholic Church life was supposed to begin at quickening. Only in 1869 did Pope Pius IX proclaim that this was no longer the case, thus making early abortions a sin.

NOTES

1. John M. Riddle, *Contraception and Abortion from the Ancient World to the Renaissance* (Cambridge, Mass.: Harvard University Press, 1992), pp. 71–72; B. Ebbell, editor and translator, *The Papyrus Ebers: The Greatest Egyptian Medical Document* (London: Humphrey Milford, 1937), pp. 109–110.

2. Aristotle, *The Politics,* translated by H. Rackham (London: Heineman; New York: Putnam, 1832).

3. Soranus, *Gynecology,* translated by Oswei Temkin (Baltimore: Johns Hopkins University Press, 1956), 1. 19, pp. 60–68.

4. John M. Riddle, J. Worth Estes, and Josiah C. Russell, "Ever Since Eve . . . Birth Control in the Ancient World," *Archaeology* 47 (March/April 1994): 29-35.

5. Riddle, *Contraception and Abortion,* pp. 25-30.

6. Bonnie Bullough, Personal conversations with Egyptian nurses, 1966-67; See also Riddle, *Contraception and Abortion,* p. 70.

7. Paul H. Gebhard, Wardell B. Pomeroy, Clyde E. Martin, and Cornelia Christenson, *Pregnancy, Birth Control and Abortion* (New York: Harper Brothers and Paul B. Hoeber, Inc., Medical Books, 1958), p. 191.

8. Lawrence Lader, *Abortion* (Indianapolis: Bobbs Merrill Inc., 1966), pp. 77-78; Vern L. Bullough, *Sexual Variance in Society and History* (Chicago: The University of Chicago Press, 1976), p. 325.

9. John T. Noonan, Jr., *Contraception* (Cambridge, Mass.: Harvard University Press, 1966), p. 405.

10. Gebhard et al., *Pregnancy, Birth Control and Abortion,* pp. 189-214.

11. United States Census, 1945-46, *Judicial Criminal Statistics, 1944,* cited in Gebhard et. al., *Pregnancy, Birth Control and Abortion,* p. 192.

12. R. W. Holmes et. al., "Factors and Causes of Maternal Mortality," *Journal of the American Medical Association* 93 (1929): 1440-46; C. Newberger, "An Analysis of the Obstetric Activities in Hospitals of Cook County during 1944," *American Journal of Obstetrics and Gynecology* 51 (1946): 372-86.

13. Lawrence Lader, *Abortion,* pp. 120-23.

14. Ibid., pp. 117-18.

15. Ibid., pp. 132-43; "Japan, a Crowded Nation Wants to Increase Its Birthrate," *Science* 167 (February 13, 1970): 960-62.

16. Vern and Bonnie Bullough, "Population Control vs. Freedom in China," *Free Inquiry* (Winter 1983-84): 12-15.

17. Betty Friedan, *The Feminine Mystique* (New York: Norton, 1963).

18. Lader, *Abortion,* p. 145.

19. Ibid., pp. 10-16.

20. Lawrence Lader, *Abortion II: Making the Revolution* (Boston: Beacon Press, 1973), pp. 73-86.

21. Ruth Roemer, "Abortion Law, Reform and Repeal: Legislative and Judicial Developments," in *Abortion and the Unwanted Child,* edited by Carl Reiterman (New York: Springer Publishing Co., 1971), pp. 39-58.

22. *Roe* v. *Wade,* 410 U.S. 174-177 (1973).

23. Lawrence H. Tribe, *Abortion: The Clash of Absolutes* (New York: W. W. Norton, 1990), pp. 161-96.

24. Ibid., pp. 172-76.

25. "Ovral as a Morning-After Contraceptive," *The Medical Letter on Drugs and Therapeutics,* October 20, 1989, p. 93; Albert Yuzpe, "Postcoital Contraception," *International Journal of Gynecology and Obstetrics* 16 (1979): 497-501.

26. Étienne-Émile Baulieu with Mort Rosenblum, *The "Abortion Pill": RU-486: A Woman's Choice* (New York: Simon and Schuster, 1990).

27. Robert M. Baird and Stuart E. Rosenbaum, *The Ethics of Abortion* (Amherst, N.Y.: Prometheus Books, 1989).

28. Noonan, *Contraception,* pp. 143–300; Lawrence Lader, *Abortion* (Indianapolis: Bobbs-Merill, 1966), pp. 79, 185.

29. Elise F. Jones, Jacqueline Darroch Forrest, Stanley K. Henshaw, Jane Silverman, and Aida Torres, *Pregnancy, Contraception and Family Planning Services in Industrialized Countries.* A Study of the Alan Guttmacher Institute (New Haven: Yale University Press, 1989).

9

Infertility, Impotence, and Artificial Insemination

Infertility may be loosely defined as the inability to conceive a child. This is not a new diagnosis but one that dates from ancient times. Through much of history the inability to conceive has been regarded not only as a misfortune but a disgrace, even a curse from some demon or displeased god needing to be propitiated with prayers, religious rites, and magic incantations. Most often in the past the failure to conceive was blamed upon the woman unless the man was impotent or his penis had been damaged. Infertile women were called barren or sterile while men who were unable to achieve an erection—one of the recognized reasons for failure to get a woman pregnant—were described as impotent. In cases where sterility resulted either from a physical injury or from an obvious penile deficiency, society's treatment of males who were not regarded as fully "male" was even harsher than for barren women. In the Jewish Scriptures, for example, a man whose testicles had been crushed or whose penis had been cut off was forbidden to enter the house of worship.[1]

In the last few decades of the twentieth century we have tried to lessen the judgmental aspect of such statements by calling the inability to conceive infertility, and shifting the total burden of infertility from the female by emphasizing that the male can also be infertile, even though he may be able to achieve an erection. One of the major reasons for this change in attitude is our better understanding of the physiology of reproduction; much of this understanding has only come in the twentieth century.

HISTORICAL BACKGROUND

The emotional problems of infertility are poignantly portrayed in one of first stories in the Jewish Scriptures and the Christian Bible. Sarah, the wife of Abraham, unable after years of marriage to bear a child, brought Hagar, her maid, to Abraham, encouraging him to take her to bed that he might have a son. Though the ancient Israelites were polygamous, it was still an emotional blow to Sarah when Hagar did become pregnant. Beside herself with jealousy, she drove Hagar away although, as Sarah's fury lessened, Hagar was allowed to return. Finally Sarah, after numerous prayers, found that Jehovah had answered her prayer and that she was pregnant even though ninety years old.[2] Similarly, one of the miracles performed by Peter and John, following the death of Jesus, was the restoration of potency to a man over forty years of age, an action, the scriptures emphasize, that impressed many.[3]

Fertility and potency remedies, incantations, and prayers were a mainstay of ancient medical literature. The inhabitants of the Tigris-Euphrates valley, for example, have left us many potency incantations. These formulas, ostensibly recited by a woman, are directed toward stimulating the man to get a sufficient enough erection to engage in sexual intercourse. They include such statements as "Let a horse (make love to me)," or "Let his penis be a stick of martu-wood."[4] By the same token, so important was the reproductive potential of a woman that would-be brides were examined carefully by the female relatives of the groom or by midwives for any obvious physiological or anatomical defects which would prevent them from becoming pregnant. Obese women were not regarded as good wife material, nor were those whose genitalia were in any way unusual or whose menses seemed sparse or irregular.

One particularly graphic test is described in the Hippocratic corpus, a series of writings associated with the name of the Greek physician Hippocrates (fifth century B.C.E.):

> If a woman does not conceive, and you wish to know if she will conceive, cover her round with wraps and burn perfumes underneath. If the smell seems to pass through the body to the mouth and nostrils, be assured that the woman is not barren through her own physical fault.[5]

Behind such practices was the belief that the inside of the female body was hollow and that the uterus had an almost independent existence within it, traveling up and down. A uterus long deprived of being pregnant would move upward in the body, constricting the windpipe; this, it was claimed, not only complicated breathing but caused hysteria,[6] a term derived from the Greek term for womb. If vapors passed through, the uterus was not functional.

Various explanations were offered for male impotence, many of them the same as for female infertility. Impotent or infertile people might be overweight or underweight, their humoral composition too hot or too cold.[7] Age obviously was recognized as a factor, and it was known that a woman who did not menstruate could not conceive. Treatments for impotency, besides incantations, involved eating lentils or other foods considered aphrodisiacs, massaging both the body and the penis, and surrounding the impotent male with beautiful nubile boys and girls, or reading love stores that included graphic sex scenes. The very word pornography, meaning literally writing about prostitutes, indicates this ancient tradition.

The Hippocratic corpus, unlike some other medical writings of the ancient world, held that sometimes males, too, could be infertile even though they were not impotent. This condition may arise,

> either because of the rarity of the body the breath is borne outward so as not to force along the [male] seed; or because the density of the body liquid does not pass out; or through the coldness it is not heated so as to collect at this place; or through the heat this same thing happens.[8]

This concern with male infertility reflects the belief of the Hippocratic corpus in general, which held that both the male and female contributed semen to bring about pregnancy.[9] Most Greek medical writers followed Aristotle in emphasizing the greater significance of the male seed in reproduction. It was the male's semen which supplied the form, while the female, who lacked semen, only supplied the matter fit for shaping.

> If then, the male stands for the effective and active, and the female, considered as female, for the passive, it follows that what the female would contribute to the semen of the male would not be semen but material for the semen to work upon.[10]

Thus if the male was able to produce semen, a visible enough demonstration of his fertility even though there might be a variation in its viscosity, and he could implant this in the female, the failure to conceive must be hers because the seed found only a barren field and could not grow. Since Galen, the most influential medical writers of the ancient world, adopted Aristotelian gynecological ideas, the emphasis on the female as the major factor in infertility has become dominant.[11]

This left impotency as the real problem for the male to face, which meant that his failure to produce children was a threat to his very maleness. This perhaps explains why so many male writers tried to blame the female. Still, it was believed that even an impotent male might father a child since it was held possible for a woman to conceive without being penetrated provided semen came in contact with her vagina. One of the earliest mentions of this possibility is found in the Babylonian Talmud dating from the sixth century C.E. A Talmudic student, concerned with the question of when a woman might be considered to have committed adultery, submitted to his rabbi-teacher the hypothetical case of a woman who became pregnant after bathing in water that, unknown to her, contained seminal fluid excreted by a man who had bathed in the same water before her. The rabbi ruled that the woman was innocent and was not an adulteress because no intercourse had taken place; insemination was accidental or, in modern terms, artificial.[12]

Theoretically then, artificial fertilization was considered a possibility even in ancient times, although we have no evidence that it was ever done deliberately in humans. Part of the problem is that the human female differs from almost all other animals in that she has no obvious fertile period; moreover, it was not until well into the twentieth century that the process of ovulation was fully understood. Even when a fertile couple is intent upon the female partner becoming pregnant and engages in regular intercourse, there is only a 3 percent chance that pregnancy will occur, and only if the couple engages in intercourse with considerable frequency.

This is not true of animals (primates being an exception) where the female has an estrous cycle, known in popular parlance as "being in heat." In some mammals (mares, cows, ewes, and sows) the estrous cycle occurs at rhythmic intervals during the year or during one limited breeding season; it is often stimulated by the lengthening or shortening of daylight so that the pregnancy will terminate in the spring. In other mammals the estrous cycle occurs periodically so that there can be several cycles during the year, as happens in dogs or cats. This cycle is obvious and would make artificial insemination much more predictable. It is from an Arab tale dating back to 1322 that the first mention of deliberate artificial insemination occurs. The story describes how hostile tribes secretly inseminated their enemies' stock of thoroughbred horses with sperm from inferior stallions.[13] The matter-of-fact recounting of such an incident seems to emphasize that the possibility of artificial insemination, at least in some animals, was accepted as a reality.

Arab medical writers led the challenge to some of the assumptions of Aristotle about reproduction. Avicenna (987–1037) compared conception to the process of making cheese, equating the male sperm with the clotting agent in milk, while the female element served as the coagulum.[14] This, however, did not explain why some embryos developed into males and others into females. It was Albertus Magnus, or Albert the Great (1206–1280), who held that the female fetus came about from a weaker seed than that which produced a male.[15] This was popularly interpreted to mean that the most potent of males would have more sons than daughters and gave further emphasis to worries about male potency.

The worry was real, not only in terms of self-image but because impotency was also a cause for divorce. To make certain, however, that claims of impotency were not just being used by a couple who wanted to separate for other reasons, the male's inability to get an erection had to be tested in front of witnesses, who could offer various enticements (including nude young women) to make certain that the man could not become erect.[16]

Inevitably impotency and infertility were blamed on witchcraft and sorcery. A witch, for example, could make the penis disappear by casting a "glamour," or spell, over it. Once this occurred only the witch herself could make it reappear. Though the disappearance of a penis might seem to be something that could be easily documented (it was often a claim used by women who were impersonating males), less subject to proof was the charge that witches could cause a male to fail to achieve an erection or cause a woman to miscarry. Impotence, for example, was believed to be the result of a ligature; that is, the witch, by tying knots in threads or hanks of leather, could cause impotence in the person over whom she had cast her spell. Impotence would last until the hidden knot was discovered or the witch removed the spell. Generally, however, believers in witchcraft held that the Devil and his allies, the witches, preferred to encourage, not discourage, fornication, and so ligature was believed to be less common than the other forms of *malefica,* or "evils," that a witch might impose. Miscarriages or female sterility were also widely believed to be due to witches,[17] and were accepted as something the witches were more likely to do since it did not prevent sexual activity.

CHALLENGES TO TRADITIONAL IDEAS

The popular belief that witches might be involved in female sterility did not, however, prevent the physicians of the time from trying various experiments to increase the possibility of pregnancy in an apparently infertile woman. For example, the anatomist Bartolomeo Eustachio (1520–1574), who lived during the heyday of belief in witchcraft, advised a fellow physician's wife, who was having difficulty getting pregnant, to have her husband insert his finger into the vagina after intercourse in order to move the semen closer to the os of the cervix. Eustachio reported that when this was done the women conceived, although today we would hold that success by this method was accidental.[18]

Improved understanding of human anatomy made rapid progress after the work of Andreas Vesalius (1514–1564), the founder of modern anatomy. Particularly important in furthering anatomical study of the reproductive organs was Gabriele Fallopio (1523–1562), who described the clitoris (which had long been known but not in anatomical detail), reported the existence of the fallopian tubes (to which he gave his name), coined the word "vagina," and demonstrated the existence of the hymen in virgins, a matter long under dispute. He also disproved the popular notion that the penis entered the uterus during coition, and described the *arteria profunda* of the penis which fills with blood to support penile erection.[19]

With a better understanding of anatomy came further exploration in the physiology of conception. A major challenge to traditional ideas came from physician and anatomist William Harvey (1578–1657), best known for demonstrating the circulation of the blood. Later in his life, Harvey became interested in the question of how generation came about; his work in this area entitles him to be regarded as one of the major founders of embryology. He made a wide variety of observations on reproduction in all types of animals, but primarily his attention was centered on the day-to-day development of the chick embryo and on his dissection of the uteri of deer at various stages during mating and pregnancy. Harvey emphasized the importance of the egg and the female contribution to reproduction, and though he could not actually see an egg in the deer he postulated the existence of a mammalian egg. Similarly, while Harvey could not find the existence of a seminal mass in the chicken egg, he felt that it had to have some influence anyway. To prove this he demonstrated that though a hen could lay fertile eggs for a brief time after the rooster had been removed from the pen, later eggs would be infertile. To Harvey this meant that the contribution of the rooster's semen was indirect and incorporeal; it simply conferred a certain fecundity on the hen and then played no further role in the actual generation of the egg or chick. This was a total reversal of what Aristotle and Galen had hypothesized. Harvey went on to hold that the same thing happened in deer since in his dissection he observed that it was some time after the male semen had disappeared from the body of the female that the first evidence of conception appeared.[20] Other researchers after Harvey came up with similar conclusions, including Marcello Malpighi (1628–1694), whose study of the embryo in hens' eggs was published in 1672. Regnier de Graaf (1641–1673) speculated that the same thing that happened in animals happened also in humans; he adopted the term "ovary" to describe the female mammalian gonad. De Graaf also described what we now call the Graafian follicle, the capsule-like structure in the ovary that nurtures the development of the ovum, although he mistook it for the ovum itself.[21]

Challenging the growing tide of the ovists were the studies of Anton van Leeuwenhoeck (1632–1723), which were made possible by the invention of the microscope. Johan Ham, a medical student, brought van Leeuwenhoek a bottle containing the semen of a man who suffered from nocturnal emission. Ham put the semen under a microscope and saw little creatures (animalcules) in it. He then sought to confirm his findings. Leeuwenhoeck supported this finding but went on with further experiments. He at first noticed that there were thousands of little round animalcula with tails five or six times as long as their bodies swimming around in ejaculate which had been collected from the patient. After finding the same creatures in the semen of healthy males, he called them *spermatozoa* and concluded that they were important in fertilizing the female egg.[22]

The proof of this hypothesis was confirmed by Lazzaro Spallanzani (1729–1799) in 1780,[23] but the female mammalian ovum remained elusive. The first real breakthrough was by Karl Ernst von Baer (1792–1876), who initially observed them in a female dog he dissected; spurred on by this discovery von Baer soon reported them in other animals. He summarized his findings by stating that "every animal which springs from the coition of male and female is developed from an ovum, and none from a simple formative liquid."[24] To explain how this happened, Oscar Hertwig (1849–1933), after discovering that fertilized eggs had two nuclei while unfertilized eggs only had one, hypothesized that there was a joining together of the male and female elements to bring about the two nuclei.[25] It was not, however, until 1877 that the Swiss biologist Hermann Fol (1845–1892) observed the actual entry of the sperm into the ova of a sea urchin, thereby finally demonstrating how pregnancy did occur.[26]

This, however, did not answer the question why some women were infertile, although it certainly indicated that the male might be a contributing factor. Still the major effort in terms of sexual research on males focused on impotence rather than infertility. Like so much in the history of sexuality, various tantalizing leads into the problem of impotence appeared but they usually turned out to be dead ends or became the subject of the pseudosciences.

Perhaps because the aging male has more difficulty getting an erection than the young male, initial studies aimed to solve the problems of men who, either through age or vascular problems, were no longer able to achieve an erection. This effort had been given new impetus by a reputable scientist, a professor of experimental medicine at the Sorbonne, Charles Édouard Brown-Séquard (1817–1894) who, when in his seventies, recognized the importance that newly discovered internal secretions (now called hormones) had on sexual functions, and sought to use an extract made of pulverized animal testicles to inject himself in order to restore his youthful vigor. He reported astonishing results,[27] although others who tried to replicate the experiment failed to get the same satisfaction.

Taking a somewhat different approach was the Viennese physician Eugen Steinach (1861–1944). Steinach had grafted genital glands from younger animals onto older ones and found restored vigor. Since he could not do the same with humans, he hit upon the idea of restoring potency by the ligature of the vas, the ducts through which the sperm is transported to the prostate, performing what we now call a vasectomy. Steinach believed, as did the ancient Chinese (and many of his own contemporaries), that seminal discharges involved the loss of vital elements which, if retained in the body, would not only maintain potency but could help restore it to those who had lost it. This was because the energy normally lost through ejaculation of sperm could be maintained in the body.[28] Though vasectomies are now a common form of sterilization, belief in the vital secretion theory of Steinach is no longer held. Nevertheless, we who advocate vasectomies for sterilization, sometimes regret the disappearance of the belief that vasectomies would restore potency since such a belief would undoubtedly increase the number of vasectomies, particularly in Third World countries where female sterilization is common but male sterilization is not, in large part because of male fears about damage to their potency.

Other researchers got into the act of finding new remedies for male impotency, including Serge Voronoff, a Russian living in France, who grafted monkey testicles into the human scrotum. He claimed that rejuvenation took place even if the transplanted testicle shriveled up and disappeared.[29] Brown-Séquard, Steinach, and Voronoff all achieved reputations for major contributions to medicine before they seemed to get carried away with their experiments on male "rejuvenation." This was not the case with John J. Brinkley, popularly known as "Goat-Gland Brinkley," the ultimate salesman of rejuvenation promises. Brinkley promised to restore virility in the male by implanting goat glands into the scrotum while he claimed to be able to rejuvenate a female's sagging erotic desire by using the "royal jelly" of the honey bee. Brinkley, an American, carried news of his operation and elixirs on the newly developed medium of radio; he even owned his own radio station in Kansas with which he blanketed much of the Midwest. Using his popularity, Brinkley ran for governor of Kansas in 1932 and received 244,607 votes, running third to Alfred M. Landon (with 278,581 votes) who later ran for president against Franklin D. Roosevelt in 1936. When the Kansas government later revoked Brinkley's medical license and attempted to close his radio station, Brinkley moved to Mexico where he established a clear channel radio station said to be more powerful than any in America. For a time his broadcasts reached one-third of all potential American radio listeners. From his new base Brinkley continued to pitch his cures until the Mexican government finally closed him down.[30]

ARTIFICIAL INSEMINATION

The attempts to treat infertility were not quite so outrageous as those dealing with male potency, although the concentration remained on the female. Spallanzani, mentioned above, had managed to inseminate a female dog artificially, but the first experiment on humans might have been conducted by his contemporary, John Hunter (1728–1793), one of the major founders of modern medicine. Hunter himself never reported the experiment but it was written up by a colleague, Everard Home, in 1799, nearly twenty years after Spallanzani had published his experiments and after Hunter was dead. Home reported that Hunter had been consulted by a man with a hypospadias who found that he could not eject semen into his wife's vagina.

> The late Mr. Hunter was consulted, to remedy, if possible, this inconvenience, and enable the person to beget children. After the failure of several modes of treatment which were adopted, Mr. Hunter suggested the following

experiment. He advised that the husband should be prepared with a syringe, and . . . [inject the ejaculate] into the vagina, while the female organs were still under the influence of coitus, and in the proper state for receiving the semen.

The patient followed through on the recommendation, and the wife did become pregnant.[31] If this account is to be believed, it marks the first actual recorded instance of what might be called artificial insemination in humans.[32]

Hunter's patient, however, was simply lucky and it was difficult for others to replicate this success. The American physician Marion Sims (1813–1883), the founding father of experiments into artificial insemination in humans, performed a series of fifty-five intrauterine inseminations utilizing the sperm of the husband; however, he had only one success, and this took place on the tenth try. Unfortunately the woman aborted. Since Sims attributed over 50 percent of his failures to faulty technique, he estimated that his true success rate should be one in twenty-seven instead of one in fifty-five.[33] While this would have given him a success rate approaching the statistical average of pregnancy as one in every thirty-three acts of intercourse, it still emphasized the haphazard nature of the whole process.

In spite of the low success rate, a number of individuals, including the American gynecologist and pioneer sex researcher Robert L. Dickinson (1861-1950), continued to experiment with artificial insemination in humans, sometimes successfully. Much more widespread was the use of artificial insemination in animal husbandry where the fertility cycle was easier to observe. In 1907 the Russian physiologist Ilyra Ivanovich Ivanov (1870–1932) published a book on artificial insemination in animals.[34] The method Ivanov advocated, insemination by injection, was gradually adopted for breeding horses, cattle, and other farm animals. Beginning in 1940, the practice spread rapidly throughout the United States, particularly among dairy farmers, since it cut down the necessity of having a bull in the herd. It could also be utilized to gradually upgrade the quality of the herd by using the semen of prized bulls. One bull, through artificial insemination, could serve more than 400 cows. Originally semen was obtained from a cow in estrus that had just been "serviced" by a bull. This proved difficult and so an artificial vagina was developed for wear either by a real cow or a dummy. Semen can also be secured from the bull (or other males) by other means, including electrical stimulation or massage of the male penis (masturbation). Electrical stimulation is also now used in humans, particularly in the case of paraplegics.

THE HUMAN FEMALE REPRODUCTIVE CYCLE

Before artificial insemination could be done with a high probability of success in humans, it was necessary to understand the female reproductive cycle. Unfortunately the animals on which experiments were performed did not menstruate, and so researchers tried to compare the menstrual cycle to the estrus phase of the animal cycle. This simply did not work. Other researchers who concentrated on human ovaries failed to find any evidence of ovulation at or near the time of menstruation. Obviously factors were at work which they did not yet know about. Still researchers persisted. The first breakthrough came between 1909 and 1915, when a number of researchers, mostly from Germany, especially Robert Meyer and Robert Shroeder, demonstrated that menstruation was the result of the breakdown of the progestational endometrium due to the degeneration of the *corpus luteum,* the sack that is left after expulsion of the ovum.

Although the lack of communication among scientists during World War I briefly held up the dissemination of such knowledge, by 1920 it was widely accepted that ovulation took place at about the middle of the intermenstrual stage, although the reasons why were not so clear. However, even this finding led to a better success rate for those experimenting with artificial insemination in humans.

An era of concentrated research on the unsolved problems of reproduction began in 1921, when the Rockefeller Foundation set up its Committee for Research in the Problems of Sex, which operated under the auspices of the National Research Council.[35] Among the researchers sponsored were Edgar Allen and Edward Doisy, who discovered the hormone that would eventually be called estrogen. Other researchers discovered progesterone, and still others elaborated upon the male hormones. By 1936, C. G. Hartman summarized the current state of knowledge, namely, that in the standard twenty-eight-day menstrual cycle, ovulation could occur on any day from day 8 to day 22, counting from the first day of menstrual flow but with a sharp peak of frequency on days 11 to 14.[36]

One of the first results of the new findings was not so much to aid fertility as to use the research to further contraception. Two researchers working independently of each other, H. Knaus and K. Ogino, plotted what initially came to be called the rhythm method.[37] With further refinements, including the use of basal body temperature and observations of cervical mucus, the term "Natural Family Planning" came to be adopted, as was discussed earlier.[38] Since timing of ovulation was necessary to calculate the safe period when pregnancy was least likely, the exact same techniques could be used to calculate the fertile period. This led to a higher success rate for artificial insemination, which led in turn to more people turning to this method of begetting children, until by 1941, over ten thousand pregnancies had taken place by artificial insemination, over two thirds of them with semen donated by the husband, known by the acronym AIH (Artificial Insemination Husband). The number was estimated to have doubled to 20,000 by 1950, and more than doubled again to 50,000 by 1955.[39]

By the 1970s, the methods for artificial insemination had become so much a part of general public information that many women who wanted to have a baby but did not desire to marry or to have intercourse could impregnate themselves by using a turkey baster, a long syringe-type instrument. One woman whom we know has had two pregnancies through this method. She carefully chose the man she wanted to father her children, and persuaded him to give blood to a local blood bank which resulted in an automatic testing for the common blood-borne sexually transmitted diseases. Once she found the sperm donor to be disease-free, she then had him masturbate, depositing his semen in a container, near the time she anticipated she would ovulate, and stored the semen in her freezer. Then, as her fertile period approached, with the cooperation of a woman friend, she defrosted the semen. Using sterile technique she inserted a speculum in order to visualize the entrance to the cervix, aspirated the semen in the turkey baster, and injected it into the mouth of the uterus.

The large majority of individuals, however, turn to physicians for help; in most cases the semen is donated by the husband although it can also be given by a donor, usually anonymous (originally known by the acronym AID [Anonymous Insemination Donor], which, in view of the development of AIDS, has been changed to DI, i.e., donor insemination).

LEGAL, SOCIAL, AND RELIGIOUS RAMIFICATIONS

It is this kind of artificial insemination that has raised the most legal questions. One of the first legal cases on the issue was tried early on in the development of artificial insemination. This was a 1921 Ontario, Canada, case known as *Orford* v. *Orford*. The wife allegedly had been artificially inseminated with semen other than her husband's without sexual intercourse, although it is not clear how. Since she had not received her husband's permission to do so, the court decided that she had committed adultery.[40] Similarly a 1922 case in England, *Russell* v. *Russell,* in which a woman had conceived a child without penetration by a man other than her husband, also resulted in the woman's being found of guilty of adultery.[41]

The legal opinions reflected the ambivalence of the medical profession as well as its uncertainty on how to proceed in the case of DI. The conservatism of the profession was most evident in an editorial in the *Journal of the American Medical Association*:

> The fact that conception is effected not by adultery nor fornication but by a method not involving sexual intercourse does not in principle seem to alter the concept of legitimacy. This concept seems to demand that the child be the actual offspring of the husband of the mother of the child. If the semen of some other male is utilized, the resulting child would seem to be illegitimate. The fact that the husband has freely consented to the artificial insemination does not have a bearing on the question of the child's legitimacy. If it did, by similar reasoning it might be urged that the fact that a husband had consented to the commission of adultery by his wife would legitimatize the issue resulting from the adulterous connection.[42]

Eventually in the United States most states enacted legislation to specifically legitimatize children born through DI provided the women receiving the donated sperm had the written consent of their husbands.[43] In other states where such legislation was lacking, a child conceived through DI was illegitimate. The consensus of legal opinion on the matter has been, however, that even though the child technically might be illegitimate it is almost impossible to prove that it is. This is because of the legal concept known as "the presumptions of legitimacy," which holds that any child born to a couple during a legally valid marriage is assumed to be legitimate unless it can be conclusively proven otherwise.[44]

Not only the legitimacy of offspring but also selection of donors was an issue. As early as 1945, two contributors to a British medical journal expressed their concern:

> The principles which govern the choice of donors are designed to reduce obvious biological dangers. There must be no history of transmissible disease; the family history of the donor must be free of adverse characteristics as possible genetical significance, such as alcoholism, criminality, or tuberculosis. Excessively pronounced physical features are undesirable not only because they might be objectionable themselves but also because they might facilitate identification of the donor.

> Positive considerations concerning the eugenic quality of the donor's stock will largely be governed by the scientific views and perhaps the individual preferences of the physician concerned. Our choice has favored men of intellectual attainment whose family history indicated that the members of at least two proceeding generations were not only intelligent but also endowed with good capacity for social adjustment. Others might prefer donors characterized less by mental than physical characteristics or achievements. . . .[45]

The two physician authors did not indicate that they followed the desires of the parents on selection of a donor, but simply emphasized that the selection of donors was a wide and complex problem. One of the interesting aspects of the discussion of donors is the biases inherent in the writers about what exactly constituted genetic problems.

Perhaps influenced by the article in the *British Medical Journal,* the then Archbishop of Canterbury set up a commission to investigate the problems associated with donors of semen for artificial insemination. The commission quickly concluded that the practice raised difficult moral problems and recommended that the whole practice be made illegal.[46] Fortunately the Anglican Church eventually changed its position, and rather than condemning the process, it emphasized the need for protection of the child.

The Catholic Church for its part initially used an 1897 statement of the pope to justify its opposition to artificial insemination by donors; this opposition was specifically restated to condemn such practices in 1949 by Pope Pius XII, in 1968 by Pope Paul VI, and again in 1987 by Pope John Paul II. The Vatican position has been summed up and criticized by Elizabeth Noble:

> The majority of Catholic theological opinion opposes not only DI but also artificial insemination with the husband's sperm. The Church's position is based on an unwillingness to tamper with God's universe, but this view, of course, does not take into account man's creativity in solving his earthly problems, including many life-saving procedures. The Church views DI as immoral because it combines both the evils of masturbation and adultery (despite the mutual agreement of all parties involved). All of the medically practical means of obtaining semen are considered "pollution." Any separation of the germ cells from the generative organs is "intrinsically sinful" and therefore wrong, no matter what it seeks to accomplish.[47]

Similarly, Orthodox Judaism has opposed DI as an evil without reservation because of the possibility of later incestuous marriages, an increase in promiscuity, and the possibility of women "satisfying their craving for children" without husband or home.[48] Both Conservative and Reformed Judaism have accepted DI; Israel, for example, has several operating sperm banks. Most mainline Protestant groups have come out for DI. Some evangelical Christians, however, have reservations which were expressed by D. Gareth Jones, who held that donor insemination

> should not be regarded as a medical procedure devoid of moral overtones. While it is true it appears to be widely accepted within many communities, its acceptance has occurred surreptitiously and at a time when there was little ethical debate about medical matters. Such acceptance should not be used as an argument in favor of the wholesale acceptance of gamete donation, regardless of the circumstances and of whether sperm or ovum donation is involved.
>
> AID [the old term] should only be carried out by registered medical practitioners, in authorized clinics. Only in this way can the procedure be adequately monitored.[49]

A more hostile view has been advanced by Oliver O'Donovan, a professor of theology at the University of Oxford. He argued not only against artificial insemination by a donor but against all artificial insemination on the grounds that any child not conceived through a natural act of sexual intercourse between a man and a woman is not begotten but made, and that such a child therefore is alien to us. Although O'Donovan realizes that DI can deal with infertility, he holds it is not a curative accomplishment but a compensatory one since the person remains infertile.[50]

Even the most liberal religious groups, however, have found it difficult to accept the fact that a pregnancy can be created with the use of the turkey baster. Most want to insist on rigid rules and safeguards. Undoubtedly most physicians who do DI do so with great care and caution, but some have not. Some have apparently used their own semen at times. In 1992 an Alexandria, Virginia, physician, Cecil B. Jacobson, was found guilty of fifty-two counts of fraud and perjury for misleading his female clients as to the anonymity of the sperm donor. The prosecutors charged that Jacobson may have fathered as many as seventy-five children by using his own semen to artificially inseminate patients, although he claimed to have matched the donor with the women's husband as to physical and even religious characteristics.

So seriously have the legal implications been regarded that the European Parliament, the legislative body for the growing European Community, called upon its member states to adopt legislation in order to safeguard individuals and protect the interests of society at large.[51] Obviously artificial insemination is one of the by-products of our new understanding of human physiology but it is not the only one.

The next logical step was *in vitro* (literally, in glass) fertilization of the ova by the sperm in a test tube or petri dish outside the human body. The breakthrough on this technique came in 1978 when the world's first in vitro fertilized baby was born in England. Her birth resulted from the work of Robert Edwards and Patrick Steptoe. In vitro fertilization involves the removal of the ovum as the women ovulates. Current methods utilize several ova which the ovaries are stimulated to produce through fertility drugs. Though these were originally removed by surgery, they now are removed through a needle inserted into the follicle, placed in a dish, and fertilized with the male sperm. After mitosis has taken place and two to four cells have appeared, the ova (usually more than one) are again implanted in the woman. The pregnancy rate for in vitro fertilization, as of this writing, is between 15 and 20 percent although about one-fourth of these result in spontaneous abortion and another 5 percent become ectopic pregnancies (i.e., outside the uterus). In vitro fertilization represents a last desperate step for infertile couples: it helps the male with a low sperm count as well as the female who has been unable to get pregnant by other means.[52]

In vitro fertilization has made it possible also to utilize a surrogate mother, in which the fertilized egg of one woman and her male partner is transferred into the uterus of another. Through this method a sister has borne a child for her sister, and a mother for her daughter, making her the grandmother of her own child. Many of the surrogates, however, have been paid to bear someone else's child, and this, though often successful, has also led to legal controversy.[53] These controversies, however, lie beyond the scope of this chapter.

IMPOTENCY

Although potency is no longer a necessary impediment to fertility since it is often possible to overcome this by placing sperm in the woman's vagina, it still remains a major emotional problem for the male. One important step forward has been to drop the emotionally loaded word "impotent" and to replace it by the term "erectile dysfunction." This implies something that can be overcome. With the new diagnosis came a new precision in categories, distinguishing three different causal factors: (1) organic, due to anatomical defects in the reproductive organ or in the brain or spinal cord; (2) functional, caused by a circulatory or inflammatory condition, an interference with nerve tracts, subnormal levels of male hormones, or simple exhaustion, many of which result from a disease such as diabetes; (3) psychogenic or inhibitory, due to psychological factors.

William Masters and Virginia Johnson were particularly successful in dealing with this last factor, although they went much too far in asserting that anxiety about sexual performance was the most important immediate cause of erectile dysfunction. They held that once a man has experienced an inability to have or maintain an erection (or, in the case of a woman, to have vaginal lubrication), he or she may become obsessed with failing again. The majority of men who experience problems with erection after having had a period of normal responsiveness respond well to treatment, but the prognosis is not so good for men who have never been able to attain or maintain an erection with a partner. Masters and Johnson reported a 60 percent success rate with primary erectile function, although 11 percent of their clients had suffered relapses within five years.[54] Their rate was much higher with secondary impotence, including premature ejaculation which Masters and Johnson dealt with far more successfully through training in the use of the squeeze technique and through attempts to remove extraneous pressures on performance. Unfortunately, later investigators failed to achieve the success rate of Masters and Johnson, perhaps because their clientele was more rigidly selected and excluded many with severe medical problems.

The result was a renewed emphasis on organic factors in erectile dysfunction. Treatment varies with the diagnosis. Many causes of erectile dysfunction such as anemia, vitamin deficiency, hypothyroidism, fatigue, and exhaustion, can be treated by correcting the physical deficiency itself. In other cases of asthenia where the debility might be due to insufficient stimulation, drugs are used to stimulate the parasympathetic nervous system and sedation of the sympathetic nervous system. Where an endocrine imbalance is noted, male hormones might be given, and where a vascular deficiency is involved, surgery might resolve the problem if it is not due to a disease. Many cases of sexual dysfunction involve excessive intake of alcohol or the use of drugs, either for recreational purposes or for treatment. Drugs to treat hypertension, for example, often lead to erectile dysfunctions.

Often if the cause is not apparent, surgical implants are utilized. Early bone implants resulted in a state of constant or semirigid erection and proved embarrassing to most patients. Another alternative was called the Coitus Training Apparatus, which was mounted over the penis with a ring at the base to hold it in and another to fit behind the head of the penis. The retractable arms were then stretched out and the contraption was covered by a condom.[55] Supposedly it worked, although we have no record of what the women involved with a man using such a device said. Since the 1970s there have been silicone implants, one a semirigid rod that can be bent for concealment under clothing. Another kind of silicone implant is an inflatable device developed for implanting under the skin of the penis. Erection is achieved by pressing a pump implanted in the scrotum which injects fluid into the penis. While such implants are costly, most users are able to experience ejaculation and orgasm.[56] In some cases, surgery to increase blood flow to the penis is indicated, and in a growing number of cases has proved successful.

SUMMARY

Obviously the problem of infertility remains even though modern science has given us many more ways of overcoming it. Coinciding with efforts to deal with infertility have been attempts to examine its multiple causes. One of the major causes is as a result of sexually transmitted diseases (particularly gonorrhea, syphilis, and chlamydia) or other infections (such as tuberculosis) that cause a scarring and blockage of the fallopian tubes in women or the vas deferens in men, thereby preventing the passage of ova or sperm. Sometimes an intrauterine device is implicated in the spread of infection to the pelvis, causing pelvic inflammatory disease (PID). Certain viruses, such as herpes simplex or venereal warts, can also lead to problems by damaging the cervical mucus. The rate of infertility following infections tends to increase with age, in part because the likelihood of contracting a sexually transmitted disease increases with the number of sexual partners. This only emphasizes the importance of early diagnosis and treatment of sexually transmitted diseases.

Another causal factor in male infertility is low sperm count. Men need to produce approximately 60 million sperm per ejaculate to be considered fertile. Most healthy young men produce at least 300 million sperm per ejaculate. However, because sperm count decreases with age, the chances of becoming infertile increase accordingly. In addition, stress, diet, radiation, excess heat (lengthy periods in hot tubs), mumps after puberty, a varicocele (a varicose vein in the scrotum that raises the temperature of the testicles), an undescended testicle, and drug use can interfere with production of sperm. One of the more common sources of fertility problems is wearing jockey shorts or athletic supporters which raise the temperature of the testicles above the desired maximum. Any problem that interferes with sperm placement during intercourse is also a cause of infertility. Glandular difficulties which cause lowered levels of testosterone, follicle-stimulating hormone (FSH), and luteinizing hormone (LH) can also cause sterility. Obviously many of the difficulties can be overcome by medical intervention or by alternative strategies.

In females, age is a factor in infertility since aging women may fail to ovulate. They are also likely to carry genetic abnormalities. The risk of miscarriage likewise increases with age. Other conditions contributing to infertility in women include endometriosis (in which part of the endometrial lining of the uterus migrates into the abdominal cavity), acidity of the vagina (which interferes with sperm motility), thick cervical mucus, cervical polyps, amenorrhea, uterine abnormalities, vaginismus (in which the muscles at the entry of the vagina squeeze so tightly that penetration by the penis is impossible), lack of ovulation (sometimes a result of low levels of body fat necessary to metabolize sex hormones), smoking, and drug use. There is also the possibility of structural disorders in the fallopian tubes or uterus or hormonal imbalances. Again many of these problems can be overcome by medical or surgical intervention.

It should be obvious that both males and females can be infertile, and infertility can exist in either or both partners. The problems of infertility, moreover, become even more complicated by what has come to be called the "crisis of infertility" characterized by couples' excessive anxiety, damaged self-esteem, grief, uncertainty about the future, and strained relationships both with each other and with family and friends.

The trauma of being diagnosed as infertile is heavily influenced by social and cultural norms. Most people, long before they become sexually active, assume fertility. Their initial questions are really about whether they want children, when they will have them, and how many. If they tend to have some initial difficulty in getting pregnant, the emotional crisis not only adds to the problem of infertility, but can itself be a causal factor. Isolation of the infertility factor often results in resentment against the partner so diagnosed, and the strain on the relationship increases. Each failure to get pregnant through the various methods outlined above, adds to the feelings of anxiety, hurt, and desperation. Since many of the methods, such as in vitro fertilization, are very costly, the emotional burden is complicated by an economic one. Unfortunately, science has as yet offered no easy solution to the problem. Perhaps the simplest is the old-fashioned solution of adoption, but even this in today's world is not as easy as it once was.

Recent research has solved many of the problems associated with infertility and impotence; but in spite of the change in terminology to erectile dysfunction or sexual dysfunction, many problems still remain. Not all problems of infertility have been solved, and there are still men who have difficulty getting an erection, and women who are nonorgasmic or who experience pain upon penetration. We do know that not all these problems are psychological, as was claimed for a brief time. There are real organic problems present in many cases of sexual dysfunction and infertility. We have not yet really isolated them all, and even many of those we know about we have not been able to treat successfully. Moreover, the treatment available often does not prove satisfactory to those seeking it.

NOTES

1. Deut. 23:1.

2. Gen. 16:1–16, 17:1–27.

3. Acts 4:9, 14, 22.

4. Robert D. Biggs, *SA.ZI.GA: Ancient Mesopotamian Potency Incantations,* in *Texts in Cuneiform Sources,* II (1967), p. 25, No. 8, lines 14–15.

5. Hippocrates, *Aphorism,* V, lix, in *Hippocrates,* ed. and trans. by W. H. S. Jones, 4 vols. (London: William Heinemann, 1968), vol. 4.

6. See Ilza Veith, *Hysteria: The History of a Disease* (Chicago: University of Chicago Press, 1965), p. 7, and Vern L. Bullough, *Sexual Variance in Society and History* (Chicago: University of Chicago Press, 1976), p. 61.

7. Hippocrates, *Aphorism,* V, lxii. This particular passage applies to a woman but similar scattered passages throughout the Greek medical corpus deal with men.

8. Ibid., V, lxiii.

9. T. U. H. Ellinger, *Hippocrates on Intercourse and Pregnancy* (New York: Abelard Schuman, 1952), and Joseph Needham, *A History of Embryology,* 2d ed., rev. (New York: Abelard Schuman, 1959), pp. 31–37.

10. Aristotle, *Historia animalium,* translated by D'Arcy W. Thompson, in *The Works of Aristotle* (Oxford: Clarendon Press, 1910), 4. 608B. See also Aristotle, *Politics,* edited and translated by H. Rackham (London: Heinemann, 1944), 1. 2 (1252 B). 7.

11. Needham, *History of Embryology,* pp. 69–74.

12. Haggadoth, 14B–15A, *Babylonian Talmud,* edited by Isidore Epstein (reprint London: Soncino Press, 1952).

13. For a discussion of animal insemination see Enos J. Perry, *The Artificial Insemination of Farm Animals*, 4th ed. (New Brunswick, N.J.: Rutgers University Press, 1968).

14. Avicenna, *Canon of Medicine*, I, 196, translated by O. Cameron Grunner (London: Luzac and Company, 1930), p. 230.

15. Albertus Magnus, *De animalibus libri XXVI*, edited by Herman Studler, 2 vols. (Munster: *Bietrage sur Geschichte des Mittelaters*, vols. 15–16, 1916–20), lib. IX, tract 2, cap. 3, pp. 714ff;, lib. XV, tract. 2, caps. 4–11, pp. 1026ff.

16. For an account of this in France see Pierre Darmon, *Trial by Impotence*, translated by Paul Keegan (London: Hogarth Press, 1985).

17. For example, see H. C. Lea, *Materials toward A History of Witchcraft*, edited by Arthur Howland, 3 vols. (reprint New York: Thomas Yoseloff, 1957), 1: 162–70.

18. Harvey Graham, *Eternal Eve: The History of Gynecology and Obstetrics* (New York: Doubleday and Company, 1951), p. 639.

19. See C. D. O'Malley, "Fallopio," in *Dictionary of Scientific Biography* (New York: Charles Scribner's Sons, 1971), 4: 519–21.

20. Harvey's work on the topic, *Anatomical Exercitations concerning the Generation of Living Creatures*, was published in Latin in 1651 and translated into English under the above title in 1653. For a discussion see Arthur W. Meyer, *An Analysis of the De generatione animalium of William Harvey* (Palo Alto: Stanford University Press, 1936), and Elizabeth B. Gasking, *Investigations into Generation, 1651–1828* (Baltimore: Johns Hopkins University Press, 1967), pp. 16–36.

21. F. J. Cole, *Early Theories of Sexual Generation* (Oxford: Clarendon Press, 1930).

22. See Clifford Dobell, *Antony van Leeuwenhoek and His "Little Animals"* (reprint New York: Russell and Russell, 1958), and Cole, *Early Theories of Sexual Generation*.

23. Lazaro Spallanzani, *Expériences pour servir à l'histoire de la génération des animaux et des plantes* (Geneva: Chirol, 1785, 1786). See also Perry, *Artificial Insemination*, p. 3.

24. Karl Ernst von Baer, *De ovi mammalium et hominis genesi epistola* (Leipzig, 1827), reprinted in George Sarton, "The Discovery of the Mammalian Egg and the Foundation of Modern Embryology," *Isis* 16 (1931): 325–78, and translated into English by Charles Donald O'Malley, *Isis* 47 (1956): 117–53. The quote is from p. 139 of this last citation.

25. Robert Olby, "Wilhelm August Oscar Hertwig," in *Dictionary of Scientific Biography*, edited Charles Coulton Gillespie (New York: Charles Scribner's Sons, 1972), 6: 337–40.

26. Garland E. Allen, "Hermann Fol," in *Dictionary of Scientific Biography*, 5: 51–53.

27. Charles-Édouard Brown-Séquard, "Expérience démonstrant la puissance

dynamogénique chez l'homme d'un liquid extrait de testicules d'animaux," *Archives de Physiologie Normale et Pathologique,* ser. 1, 5 (1889): 651–58.

28. Eugen Steinach, *Sex and Forty Years of Biological and Medical Experiments* (New York: Viking, 1930), pp. 239–40.

29. Serge Voronoff, "Rejuvenation," in *Encyclopedia Sexualis,* edited by Victor Robinson (New York: Dingwall-Rock, 1936), pp. 707–15.

30. Gerald Carson, *The Roguish World of Doctor Brinkley* (New York: Holt, Rinehart and Winston, 1960).

31. Everard Home, "The Dissection of an Hermaphrodite Dog. With Observations on Hermaphrodites in General," *Philosophical Transactions of the Royal Society of London* 18 (1799): 162.

32. See William Cary, "Experiences with Artificial Impregnations in Treating Sterility," *Journal of the American Medical Association* 14 (1930): 2184.

33. J. Marion Sims, *Clinical Notes on Uterine Surgery* (New York: William Wood & Co., 1873), p. 369.

34. P. N. Skatkin, "Ilya Ivanovich Ivanov," in *Dictionary of Scientific Biography,* 7: 13–33.

35. See Vern L. Bullough, "Katherine Bement Davis, Sex Research, and the Rockefeller Foundation" *Bulletin of the History of Medicine* 62 (1988): 74–89.

36. G. D. Hartman, *Time of Ovulation in Women* (Baltimore: Williams & Wilkins, 1936).

37. See K. Ogino, "Ovulationstermin und Konzeptionstermin," *Zentralblatt für Gynäkologie* 54 (February 1930): 464–79, and H. Knaus, "Die periodische Frucht- und Unfruchtbarkeit des Weibes," *Zentralblatt für Gynäkologie* 57 (June 1933): 1393.

38. See Vern L. Bullough and Bonnie Bullough, *Contraception: A Guide to Birth Control Methods* (Amherst, N.Y.: Prometheus Books, 1990), pp. 95–106.

39. Frances L. Seymour and Alfred Koerner, "Artificial Insemination: Present Status in the United States as Shown by a Recent Survey," *JAMA* 116 (1941): 2747–51.

40. Sidney B. Schatkin, *Disputed Paternity Proceedings,* 2d ed. (Albany, N.Y.: Banks and Co., 1947), pp. 16–17.

41. Ibid., pp. 17–18.

42. Ibid., pp. 18–19. I am indepted to my student Martin Pollack for the citations on the legal issues.

43. R. Snowden and C. D. Mitchell, *The Artificial Family* (London: George Allen and Unwin, 1981), pp. 18–19.

44. Albert E. Wilkerson, ed., *The Rights of Children* (Philadelphia: Temple University Press, 1974), p. 74.

45. Mary Martin and Kenneth Walker, "Artificial Insemination," *British Medical Journal,* January 13, 1945, p. 41.

46. Snowden and Mitchell, *The Artificial Family,* p. 13.

47. Elizabeth Noble, *Having Your Baby by Donor Insemination* (Boston: Houghton Mifflin, 1987), p. 210.

48. Ibid., p. 211.

49. D. Gareth Jones, *Manufacturing Humans: The Challenge of the New Reproductive Technologies* (Leicester, England: Inter-Varsity Press, 1987), p. 249.

50. Oliver O'Donovan, *Begotten or Made?* (New York: Oxford University Press, 1983), pp. 1, 32.

51. European Parliament, *Ethical and Legal Problems of Genetic Engineering and Human Artificial Insemination* (Luxembourg: European Parliament, 1990), p. 5.

52. See the discussion by Sarah Freeman and Vern L. Bullough, *The Complete Guide to Fertility* (Amherst: N.Y.: Prometheus Books, 1993), *passim,* for further and more detailed information.

53. For a discussion of this see Freeman and Bullough, *The Complete Guide to Fertility,* pp. 100–11.

54. William Masters and Virginia Johnson, *Human Sexual Inadequacy* (Boston: Little Brown, 1970), pp. 137–56.

55. This device is described in G. Lombard Kelly, "Impotence," in Albert Ellis and Albert Abarbanel, *The Encyclopedia of Sexual Behavior,* 2 vols. (New York: Hawthorne Books, 1961), p. 525.

56. R. J. Krane, "Surgical Implants for Impotence: Indications and Procedures," in *Male Reproductive Dysfunction,* edited by R. J. Santen and K. S. Swerdloff (New York: Marcel Dekker, 1986), pp. 563–76, and F. B. Scott, I. J. Fishman, and J. K. Light, "A Decade of Experience with Inflatable Penile Prosthesis, *World Journal of Urology* 1 (1983): 244.

10

Pornography and Obscenity

One of the keys to examining past attitudes toward sex is the place pornography or obscenity held in a society. Etymologically the two words differ, although in practical usage they have often become synonymous. Technically the term "pornography" is derived from the Greek *pornographe,* literally, "writing about prostitutes," and it carries the suggestion of erotic imagery which results in sexual arousal. It is a kind of psychological aphrodisiac, and for this reason there has been in recent years an attempt to replace the term pornography with the word erotica, in part because it seems to enjoy a more positive public reception. In theory, obscenity has a quite different meaning, but because of the psychological factors involved in the definition, the two can be synonymous. "Obscenity" is a Latin word, probably derived from the base word *caenum,* meaning "dirt" or "filth or excrement," but which also meant "penis"; in its plural form it could refer either to the genitals or the buttocks. Scatology (derived from the Greek word *skatos,* or dung) has some of the same overtones. It is also possible that the word is derived from the Latin *scaena,* meaning "stage," and thus could mean something that took place offstage (*ob-scaena*) because it was inappropriate to depict onstage. The difficulty in distinguishing obscenity from pornography stems from the fact that what is sexually suggestive—erotic if you will—to one person, is sexually repulsive or filthy to another. The portrayal of an adult urinating or defecating would probably be regarded as crude or even obscene by most observers, but to the individual who enjoys watching others urinate or defecate, such a portrayal might prove to be sexually arousing. Sometimes an illustration might be both pornographic and obscene to the same individual since, though he or she might be sexually aroused, the guilt and shame that the individual feels through such arousal could lead to revulsion. Thus Supreme Court Justice Potter Stewart, who wrote that, while he could not define what constituted hard-core pornography (meaning obscenity), he recognized it when he saw it, would simply be revealing his own sexual predilections whenever he ruled on a case.[1]

When we look at the past, however, it is not always clear that what we think of as either pornographic or obscene was regarded in the same way by the people of the time. In some societies, where the copulation of animals was accepted as an everyday part of life, the inclusion of such acts in an illustration might be regarded simply as a portrayal of reality. Pictures relating to sexual reproduction might be regarded as pornographic, obscene, or simply an illustration of the process, depending not only on the culture but the particular group within that culture for whom the pictures are intended. Medical texts, for example, often include graphic portrayals of anatomy or physiology that some would fine obscene. Still, even with this qualification, it seems that most societies have had some sort of pornography, that is, materials consciously designed to be sexually arousing. The forms these materials have taken have varied from culture to culture, although obviously, literary materials did not appear until the invention of writing. Simply because a culture is not literate, however, does not mean that it lacks pornographic materials. One of the largest surviving collections of sexually illustrative materials in pre-Columbian America has been excavated in Peru, and it seemingly had erotic connotations. The materials are made of pottery and show exaggerated phalluses and vaginas and various positions and forms in sexual intercourse, including anal intercourse and bestiality.[2] Hindu temples are full of sexual representations, either erotic or obscene (depending on the eye of the beholder), but there to be seen by all whether child or adult, literate or illiterate.[3] We have erotic and/or obscene sculpture and painting portraying all forms of sexual activity from ancient China,[4] as well as from Japan.[5] We also have quantities of sexually oriented material from ancient Persia,[6] from ancient Greece,[7] and from ancient Italy,[8] as well as from medieval Europe. Sometimes the imagery is symbolic and perhaps unconscious, as in the case of the medieval cathedral, where the phallus-like bell tower standing next to the vagina-like rose window has provided a field day for Freudian image-seekers.

From the very beginning some literature contained sexual or sensual overtones which some held to be pornographic. The *Song of Songs* in the Jewish Scriptures and Christian Bible has been banned as pornographic and was once printed separately from the Bible. When we turn to the world of Greece and Rome, we have, considering the amount of material that has been preserved, a surprisingly large corpus of erotic or pornographic materials. The Greeks in particular left us several surviving works about the life and works of prostitutes which are almost pornographic fantasies. Any list of such works would include *The Dialogues of the Courtesans* by Lucian, the *Deipnosophists* of Athenaeus, and the oration *Against Naera* by Demosthenes. Anyone interested in pursuing Greek or Roman ideas about masturbation, homosexuality, bestiality, flagellation, or almost any other aspect of sexual behavior will find a goldmine of information.[9] Ovid's *Ars amatoria,* or *The Art of Love,* has often been regarded as pornographic, and it has served as an example for hundreds of imitators. In addition, there is the *Satyricon* of Petronius, as well as the writings of Apuleius, Juvenal, Suetonius, and numerous others.

Christianity, being a sex-negative if not sexually repressive religion, had for that very reason a prurient obsession with sex. Inevitably there are vast quantities of materials dealing with sex, some so graphic that they have been left untranslated from the Latin until the last few years because of their erotic or obscene connotations. The most detailed accounts of sexual activity exist in the penitential literature and in canon law, but there are also erotic poems and stories that by the time of Chaucer had become quite bawdy. It should also be emphasized that those classical erotic works which have survived did so because they were preserved, read, and recopied in the Christian monasteries.

Literary erotic materials, as distinct from pictorial representations of sex, had a rather restricted audience until the last two hundred years. Few people could read, and books were expensive. Though we possess numerous surviving pornographic stories and poems from antiquity and beyond, it is not until the development of printing that literary pornography became an industry. Almost immediately there were collections of "dirty" jokes and epigrams, usually called jest books. One of the earliest of such collections was by the humanist scholar Poggio Bracciolini (1380–1459), which was published in Latin in 1450. As Poggio himself puts it, his work soon "flooded all Italy, overflowed into France, Spain, Germany, England, and every other country where Latin was understood." The stories were full of double entendres, accounts of cuckoldry and lust, and there are a large number dealing with bowel movements. Perhaps typical, and it is printed here because it is short, is the story concerning a noblewoman whose inkwell was empty:

> A messenger once asked a high-born lady of my acquaintance whether she desired him to take any letters from her to her husband, who was long away from home, as ambassador of the republic.

"How can I write him?" she said, "when he has taken his pen away with him and left my inkwell empty?"

Which is a clever and honorable retort.[10]

These jests were used to demonstrate literary skills as well as one's use of double entendres, and were composed and repeated for the amusement of members of the "academies" or eating clubs. They became a favorite of the educated elite, who tried to think up new and different terms for sexual intercourse or for the human reproductive organs.

In addition, there was a less literary, far more earthy kind of erotic or scatological writing. The earliest surviving example of this is the work of the sixteenth-century satirist Pietro Aretino and his various secretaries. He has a character in one of his dialogues say to another:

Oh, I meant to tell you and I forgot. Speak plainly and say "fuck," "price," "cunt," and "ass" [*cu, ca, po,* and *fo*] if you want anyone except the scholars at the university in Rome to understand you. You with your "rope in the ring," your "obelisk in the Colosseum," your "leek in the garden," your "key in the lock," your "bolt in the door," your "pestle in the mortary," your "nightingale in the nest," your "tree in the ditch," your "syringe in the valve," your "sword in the scabbard," not to mention your "stake," your "crozier," your "parsnip," your "little monkey," your "this," your "that," your "him" and your "her," your "apples," "leaves of the missals," "fact," verbigratia," "job," "affair," "big news," "handle," "arrow," "carrot," "root" and all shit there is—why don't you say yes when you mean yes and no when you mean no—or else keep it to yourself.[11]

Attributed to Aretino but probably written by his secretary Niccolo Franco is the classic *La putana errante* (*The Wandering Whore*), a fictional autobiography of a prostitute which includes a discussion of some thirty-five sexual positions. Various other ways of achieving sexual satisfaction are also mentioned since the courtesan heroine, Madalene, spied on her masturbating cousin when she was eleven, had a lesbian affair with an aunt, and so forth. The work is more famous for its illustrations than for its contents, although the originals have since been destroyed. The artist Giulio Romano did a surreptitious series of sixteen cartoons showing various positions of sexual intercourse on the walls of the Vatican and then painted over them. Before they were obliterated, however, Marcantonio Raimondi made a series of plates with designs taken from the cartoons, and Aretino supposedly composed a sonnet for each plate which formed the basis of his story. When the news of Romano's activities came out, Romano and Aretino had to flee Rome, while Raimondi was sent to jail. The story just recounted would put the number of plates at sixteen, but these were later expanded to twenty or to thirty-six (a frontispiece plus one illustration for each posture) either by Romano or Raimondi or some later imitator, only copies of which have survived.[12]

Authors and artists all over Europe turned to erotic writing and illustration. Probably the leading English writer of erotica was Thomas Nashe (1567-1601) who called himself an English Aretino. Nashe argued that if Italian models served as the mode for literary and courtly endeavors, they should also serve for erotic verse. His *Choise of Valentines* has been called the "most overtly pornographic poem" in English, at least in the sixteenth century. Nashe's purpose in writing it was to arouse his readers. It had no moral and Nashe refused to claim, as many other writers of pornography did, that he was trying to teach by negative example.[13]

One of the earliest descriptions of how a "pornographic" book affected a reader comes from the diary of Samuel Pepys in the seventeenth century. He recorded that on January 13, 1668, he

> stopped at Martin's my bookseller, where I saw the French book which I did think to have had for my wife to translate, called *L'escholle des filles,* but when I come to look in it, it is the most bawdy, lewd book that ever I saw, rather worse than *Putana errante,* so that I was ashamed of reading it, and so away home.[14]

This ought to have ended the matter, but Pepys's shock was not so great as he recorded it, because on February 8 he reported that he went to his bookseller and stayed there an hour before buying "the idle, roguish book *L'escholle des filles,*" in plain binding, avoiding the purchase of a better-bound edition, "because I resolve, as soon as I have read it, to burn it, that it may not stand in the list of books nor among them to disgrace them if [it] should be found."[15] Putting an erotic or pornographic work in a plain wrapper to disguise its contents is obviously an old practice. Actually the book that Pepys refers to is similar to the one by Aretino but with a simple plot. First published in 1655, it was finally printed in English in 1688 under the title of the *School of Venus.*[16]

The ambivalence that Pepys expresses about his "lewd" book helps explain why pornography has periodically come under attack, even by those who have enjoyed reading or looking at it. Initially, however, erotic materials were free from formal censorship. The first *Index librorum prohibitorum* (*Index of Prohibited Books*) drawn up in the sixteenth century by the Catholic Church was not concerned with erotic literature or pornography, but rather with the suppression of heresy and maintaining the prestige of the clergy. Aretino had found it wise to leave Rome for a time, but he was not prosecuted. The *Decameron* of Giovanni Boccaccio (1313–1375) was initially placed on the *Index,* but only because it included a number of stories of clerical sinners and erring nuns. When these were changed into lay people in new editions, the book was then removed. The Puritans in seventeenth-century England tried to impose censorship on the stage, and finally in 1642 abolished play-houses altogether, but left literary pornography more or less untouched. After 1660, when the theaters were reopened under the Restoration, censorship of the stage was imposed by the provisions of the Licensing Act passed in 1662, expired in 1679, revived in 1685, and allowed to die again in 1695. In general, however, the censors did not concern themselves with chap or jest books or amorous literature, some rather crude specimens of which were published.[17]

Although Great Britain had no specific legislation providing for censorship, there were occasional prosecutions for publishing or circulating salacious or scandalous books. A certain James Read was indicted in 1708 for printing a book titled *The Fifteen Plagues of Maidenhead.* He was acquitted on the grounds that it was a matter for the spiritual court. The justice who ruled on the case wrote that if "there is no [effective] remedy in the Spiritual court, it does not follow there must be a remedy here."[18] Penalties in religious court were for religious crimes, and the most extreme penalty was excommunication. By the eighteenth century, however, this was not necessarily a deterrent to large segments of the population, hence the attempt to use secular or civil courts. But the civil courts initially proved reluctant to enter the field without government legislation to do so. When Parliament refused to enact such legislation, some judges were persuaded to "make law" on the grounds that destroying the peace of the government was destroying public order, and then they proceeded to define public order as public morality. This rather farfetched interpretation of common law was first applied to Edmund Curll, a well-known printer and bookseller who got into trouble in 1725 for printing *Venus in the Cloister,* also known as *The Nun in Her Smock.* The judges in the case accepted the argument of the attorney general which was that publication of such a work constituted an offense to common law:

I do not insist that every immoral act is indictable, such as telling a lie, or the like. But if it is destructive of morality in general; if it does or may, affect all the King's subjects, it then is an offence of a public nature.[19]

Curll was sentenced to the pillory for his action, but this case did not clearly establish obscenity or pornography as a common law crime since probably only matters that discredited the official religion or religion in general were regarded as punishable.[20] Evidence for this conclusion is the scarcity of prosecutions during the eighteenth century.

Illustrative of the legal ambiguity is the case of John Cleland (1709–1789), whose *Fanny Hill,* or *Memoirs of a Woman of Pleasure,* is regarded as an erotic classic. Published in 1748, it went through several printings before Cleland was arraigned before the Privy Council. Cleland justified writing the novel by his need for money, and the case was settled by the president of the council, the Earl of Granville, a relative of Cleland, by granting Cleland a pension of a hundred pounds a year on condition that he not repeat the offense. Cleland agreed but then proceeded to issue anonymously the erotic classic *The Memoirs of a Coxcomb* (1751), after which he devoted himself to political and philological writing.[21]

Usually when writers of "obscene" materials were prosecuted in the eighteenth century, it was more for their political stands than their erotic writings. This was certainly true in the case of John Wilkes (1725–1797), whose radical agitations were extremely distasteful to King George III and his government. When Wilkes's *An Essay on Woman,* a rather clever parody of Alexander Pope's *Essay on Man,* appeared, Wilkes was in trouble. Dedicated to a popular prostitute, Fanny Murray, the poem was brought to the attention of Wilkes's political opponents in the House of Lords where it was read aloud to the assembled body. At the end of the reading, the House resolved that the poem was "a most scandalous, obscene, and impious libel," whereupon Wilkes was convicted *in absentia,* fined five hundred pounds, and outlawed.[22]

Still, there was also a real and growing concern with pornography in the last part of the eighteenth century. One motivating factor in this was the increase in literacy, which led to concern about preserving the morals of the newly literate groups. A second factor was the growing power of the middle class, which had a different set of moral standards than that of the more "dissolute" nobility. At the beginning of the eighteenth century, England can be said to have been composed of an illiterate mass of people governed by an educated, cultured, and sexually licentious upper class opposed to the Puritan strictures of an earlier period. Increasingly, however, this ruling class was being challenged for power by a rising, work-oriented middle class who were much more abstemious in their tastes, and whose moral attitudes were becoming increasingly influential. A third factor was the changing attitude toward sex, marked by the appearance of Tissot's work on masturbation, and a renewed fear of the dangers of sex. Still another factor was the growth of privacy, at least among the bourgeoisie, made possible by the new kind of house that separated the bedroom from the living room, and children from adults.

The most important factor, however, was the changing concept of women and family, especially in the middle class. Declining infant mortality rates saw a gradual shift in the treatment of children, which by the nineteenth century had begun to effect the nature of child-rearing. As children came to be treated as special creatures rather than as little adults, there was greater emphasis placed on the role of the mother and wife as the key to the family. Since the child had to be isolated from society, it seemed obvious, at least to some, that women, the children's natural guardians, should also be isolated. Motherhood became a special calling, demanding equal time with other occupations, and the tendency was to put woman on a pedestal. Although this concept of women had medieval precedents, it reached a new height in the nineteenth century. This was especially true of middle-class women, whose lives were far more restricted than those of the women at either the working-class or aristocratic level. The new mark of these middle-class women was gentility, which came to be associated with inactivity. Proper ladies simply did not do many of the things that women had always done in the past. Moreover, women, in a legal and economic sense, were the property of their husbands; as such, they could be conspicuously displayed as part of their husband's wealth and power. To compensate for their new gentility there was an even greater tendency to set middle- and upper-class women apart from the rest of humankind; they were a special species who had reached a higher moral level, and whose unique function was motherhood. The new elevation of women is evident in the instructions of a Presbyterian minister to his daughters:

> Though the duties of religion, strictly speaking, are equally binding on both sexes, yet certain differences in their natural character and education, render some vices in your sex particularly odious. . . . Your superior delicacy, your modesty, and the usual severity of your education, preserve you, in a great measure, from any temptation to those vices to which

we are most subjected. The natural softness and sensibility of your dispositions particularly fit you for the practice of those duties where the heart is chiefly concerned. And this, along with the natural warmth of your imagination, renders you particularly susceptible to the feelings of devotion. . . . One of the chief beauties in a female character is that modest reserve, that retiring delicacy, which avoids the public eye and is disconcerted even at the gaze of admiration.[23]

The capstone of gentility was the attainment of a higher moral susceptibility and delicacy in feeling. The genteel woman was to be a model of self-control, to attenuate sexual attraction as the mode of relation between the sexes, and to favor discreet withdrawal and even retreat in the face of vulgarity.

While the prudery associated with the new gentility has often been labeled Victorianism, it actually predated the accession of Queen Victoria, and remained a dominant theme after her death. The new mystique of motherhood granted women special status but at the same time guaranteed them inferiority. The female sex came to be made up of "good girls" and "bad girls." In a sense this was no different from the past except that it was more difficult to be a good girl, since one not only had to act properly but to think correctly and to demonstrate a purity of mind and spirit unclouded by any shadows of gross or vulgar thoughts. Although not all women bought into the system, they still had to give the illusion that they did or else be ostracized. Proper conduct was more important than real thought. The literature of the time, particularly the novels, tended to represent sexuality as dangerous and evil, thereby reinforcing the stereotypes of respectable young women and anxious wives adhering to their moral code of chastity and virtue.

Since women, in spite of their "delicate sensibilities," were becoming better educated—essential if they were to raise their children properly— one of the socially approved pastimes was reading, particularly reading aloud in a family group. By the beginning of the nineteenth century, it was assumed that most existing fiction was much too salacious for women, who had to be shielded from the grosser facts of life. Even Aphra Behn (1640–1689), usually regarded as the first professional woman of letters, became suspect for the new generation of women readers. Sir Walter Scott recorded the change in attitudes. He wrote that while he was visiting with one of his grand-aunts, she asked him if he had ever seen Mrs. Aphra Behn's novels. When Scott confessed that he had, she then asked him whether he could get some for her which, after he returned home, he mailed to her. The next time he saw his great-aunt, Scott wrote:

she gave me back Aphra, properly wrapped up, with nearly these words: "Take back your bonny Mrs. Behn; and if you will take my advice, put her in the fire, for I found it impossible to get through the very first novel. But is it not," she said, "a very odd thing that I, an old woman of eighty and upwards, sitting alone, feel myself ashamed to read a book which sixty years ago, I have heard read aloud for the amusement of large circles, consisting of the first and most creditable society in London."[24]

It was this change of attitude that led to the success of Dr. Thomas Bowdler, mentioned earlier, who expurgated Shakespeare so that it might be more suitable for women.[25]

The cleansing process of literature symbolized by Bowdler cut two ways. Coinciding with official literary prudery was the growth of a vast literary underground producing ever more pornographic work. Not a few prominent authors, such as Algernon Charles Swinburne (1837–1909), wrote pseudonymously for this audience. What was true in England also held true in the United States, although until 1846, when an enterprising Irishman, William Haynes, began to publish such materials in New York, all the American materials had to be imported. By 1870 Haynes was reputed to be selling about 100,000 books annually. Some famous American authors also turned their hand to underground literature. Probably the most famous was Mark Twain, whose short story "1601" recounts a "learned" discussion between Queen Elizabeth I and her courtiers on flatulence. Inevitably there was growing opposition to what was regarded as obscene literature, but little was done until the passage of the Obscene Publications Act in 1857 by the British Parliament. The bill, introduced by Lord Chief Justice Campbell of England, was designed, he said, to eliminate a "sale of poison more deadly than prussic acid, strychnine, or arsenic." Though the bill met with considerable opposition in the House of Lords, and was amended in the House of Commons, it became law in 1857. In spite of Campbell's protest that it was not designed to harm literature, this act has proved to have a baneful effect. It provided that a search warrant could be issued on sworn information that obscene publications were kept for sale or distribution on any premises, even though no sale of such publications had actually been made. Any obscene matter then found during such a search was to be brought into court, and the proprietor of the premises where it was displayed called upon to show cause why it should not be destroyed. Technically the law did not alter existing obscenity legislation, but it provided for effective enforcement.

Based upon the Obscene Publications Act prosecution was first brought against a militant Protestant named Henry Scott for publishing an anti-Catholic pamphlet, *The Confessional Unmasked: shewing the depravity of the Roman Priesthood, the iniquity of the Confessional and the questions put to females in confession.* Included in the pamphlet, supposedly based on Catholic confessional manuals, were examples of what a priest should get a penitent to confess, including a discussion of sexual intercourse and fellatio. Scott sold his pamphlets at cost so that he could not be accused of profiting from pornography, and argued that he was just doing his Christian duty. Nevertheless, Justice Benjamin Hicklin, a Wolverhampton magistrate, ordered the pamphlets seized and destroyed. After Scott appealed this decision to the local magistrate, who held that since Scott's purpose had been not to corrupt public morals but to expose the evils of the Church of Rome, the destruction order should be revoked. This decision was finally appealed to the Court of the Queen's Bench presided over by Chief Justice Cockburn, who in 1868 supported the original Hicklin ruling and held that in his mind the test for obscenity should be "whether the tendency of the matter charged as obscenity is to deprave and corrupt those whose minds are open to such immoral influences and into whose hands a publication of this sort may fall."[26]

Obviously any pious missionary tract such as Scott's, even though it depicted graphic sexual scenes, could not be termed pornography. This standard, however, served to determine obscenity in England until 1959. In the United States, which then frequently followed English court decisions in its own courts, there were some modifications of the original decision, but the basic standard of judgment stood until 1957. The difficulty with the Hicklin decision was indicated by Judge Learned Hand in 1913, when he wondered whether adult Americans would

> long remain content to reduce our treatment of sex to the standard of a child's library in the supposed interest of a salacious few, or that shame will for long prevent us from adequate portrayal of some of the most serious and beautiful sides of human nature.

He added that perhaps there would come a time when the word "obscene" would indicate the critical point at which any community might arrive in the compromise between candor and shame. Later, in a side remark, Hand indicated that the appropriate test for obscenity was to determine whether the disputed matter physically aroused the judge—not just any judge, but an exceedingly old one.[27]

It was under the Hicklin decision that dissemination of contraceptive information was suppressed in England. This suppression in 1877 led two atheists, Charles Bradlaught (1833–1891) and Annie Besant (1847–1933) to openly challenge the law by publishing Knowlton's *Fruits of Philosophy*, the American book on contraception discussed in chapter 7. Though the jury found the book was "calculated to corrupt public morals," it exonerated the defendants "from any corrupt action in publishing it." The judge regarded this as a verdict of guilty, and sentenced the two to six months' imprisonment plus a fine of 200 pounds each. On appeal, however, the conviction was quashed on the grounds that the indictment was erroneous.[28] The case nonetheless is an excellent illustration of the political uses which any anti-pornographic law can serve.

Such laws, however, did not stop the dissemination of pornography, which continued to flood the English and even the American markets. Many erotic works were published in Paris by Charles Carrington, who was not bothered by French censors since his books were in English and were sent under closed cover to England to selected customers. Sir Richard Burton found another way to avoid the censorship by privately publishing his unexpurgated translation of the *Thousand Nights and a Night* and selling it by subscription, a practice also followed by other English authors. The effect of all this was to put most erotic writing out of the reach of the ordinary reader while allowing the wealthy to buy what they wanted either in Paris or through private solicitation. And not only Paris published erotic and pornographic books in English, but Brussels and several other continental cities did as well. It is worth commenting that social class still remains an issue in censorship: books and materials most likely to be censored are those that seem most able to reach a mass audience: softcover books over hardcover, movies over the legitimate theater, and television over movies.

Those individuals who did not resort to some form of pretense often got into trouble, and this was particularly true of the English sexologist Havelock Ellis. His pioneering study, *Sexual Inversion*, which he had co-authored with John Addington Symonds, and which composed the first of what came to be seven volumes in the *Psychology of Sex*, was prosecuted in 1898 in England and successfully suppressed. Ellis and Symonds originally had issued the work in German without a problem, but by the time the English edition appeared, Symonds was dead and his executor insisted that his name be removed from the book. This led to the first printing being destroyed. When the book was finally reprinted, the publisher who issued it also brought out material for the Legitimation League, a group trying to obtain legal status for illegitimate children. This seemingly innocuous effort was seen by some government officials as an effort to put good and virtuous women on the same level as prostitutes and of increasing the likelihood of pandering. Since the league's bookstore also displayed Ellis's book, it and other materials were seized by a Scotland Yard detective. The owner of the bookstore was held for trial and pleaded guilty to selling material of the Legitimation League as well as *Sexual Inversion.* The result was the dissolution of the league and the withdrawal of Ellis's book on homosexuality. As a result Ellis turned to the United States which, in spite of the efforts of Anthony Comstock, was far more tolerant, particularly if the book did not enter the country through New York or was posted from a city other than where Comstock was in power. The American edition was published by F. A. Davis, a medical publisher in Philadelphia, who officially limited the book to the medical profession, a practice that applied to most books about sex in this country until almost the time of the Second World War.[29] While this was also a practice that could not be practically enforced, again it was easier for the well-to-do to purchase such a book than the ordinary citizen; moreover, libraries that purchased such books did restrict their distribution.[30]

Publication of books on sexual themes became somewhat easier with the death of Anthony Comstock in 1915, although it took a whole series of legal cases finally to end censorship. Many of the early challenges were over the dissemination of information on contraception for the general reader, but increasingly the challenges extended into other areas. One of the major breakthroughs came with the so-called *Ulysses* case: federal judge John M. Woolsey ruled that though the James Joyce classic contained obscene passages, the book, taken in its entirety, was a sincere and serious attempt to devise a new literary method for the observation and description of humankind. When the federal government appealed, the New York Federal Court of Appeals upheld Woolsey in a two-to-one decision. The government decided not to appeal any further, fearful perhaps that the Supreme Court would agree.[31]

Gradually, however, other cases did work their way to the Supreme Court. In the 1957 case *Roth* v. *U.S.,* the Court held that though obscenity per se was not protected by the Constitution, a work could only be considered obscene if to the average person, applying contemporary community standards, the dominant theme of the material taken as a whole appeals to prurient interests.[32]

The Court retreated from this stand somewhat when the justices in 1973 abandoned a national standard for what constituted obscenity and instead allowed the communities to establish their own guidelines. However, this has had little effect in the long run since through the efforts of television and other media, explicit sexual material has been increasingly integrated into mainstream culture. Although pornography still remains controversial and antipornography forces continue to claim a high moral ground, contemporary community standards are generally accepting of sexual expression, including explicit sexual material.

The changes taking place in the United States were being replicated in much of the rest of the Western world, thus leading to government efforts to find new answers to what constituted legal obscenity. Three important governmental commissions were established in English-speaking countries to this end, two in the United States and one in Britain. A separate Canadian commission, which included in its inquiries the topic of prostitution, was not so important to the question of pornography. President Lyndon B. Johnson appointed the first such American commission in 1968, which came to be known as the President's Commission on Obscenity and Pornography. In July 1977, the British Home Secretary appointed a Committee on Obscenity and Film Censorship, usually referred to as the Williams Committee, after its chairman. In May 1985, Attorney General Edwin Meese established a Commission on Pornography. One of the questions all the commissions were to resolve was whether pornography was harmful. Each answered differently.

The president's commission sponsored direct research on pornography and its effect, probably the first large-scale study. The commission liked neither the terms "obscenity" nor "pornography," both of which they thought had pejorative connotations, preferring the neutral phrase "explicit sexual materials." The Williams Committee thought the word "obscene" connoted disgust or repulsion while "pornography" served both to arouse its audience sexually and to contain explicit sexual representation. Similarly the Canadian commission decided that the words "pornography" and "obscenity" were impossible to define and preferred to use the more neutral term of "sexually explicit materials." The Meese commission, recognizing the difficulty, tried in general to avoid the word "pornography." It pointed out the obvious, namely, that individuals used "pornography" to designate the depiction of sex in a disapproved way, while "erotica" connoted a depiction of sex in a way that the user approved. "Obscenity" was used when the material appealed only to prurient interests, but it, too, was a loaded word.[33]

Part of the difficulty is that pornography, whether obscenity, erotica, or sexually explicit material, remains a divisive area no matter how we label or define it, and difficult, if not impossible, to discuss without revealing an ideological stance. One stance might be called *sexual naturalism,* the view that sexual expression is positive and natural. Its adherents defend pornography on First Amendment grounds, turning to scientific evidence to demonstrate the lack of serious and likely harm. A second view, which might be labeled *traditional morality,* sees sexual expression as undermining the family by allowing portrayals of nonprocreative sexual expression. It argues that pornography corrupts and depraves, leading to sexual addiction and perversion. In recent years, another ideological stance has emerged, pushed by Women Against Pornography, which sees the compulsive hetero-sexuality of men as violent in nature. It argues that pornography degrades women and promotes violence against them. At this writing the moralists and the feminists have melded into a single antipornography position.[34]

For example, Susan Brownmiller, a militant feminist, has said that pornography was a male invention designed to dehumanize women and to reduce the female to an object of sexual access, not to free sensuality from moralistic or parental inhibitions. "Pornography is the undiluted essence of antifemale propaganda."[35] Andrea Dworkin writes that pornography appropriates a woman's sex, possesses her body, uses her, and despises her.[36]

One result of such ideology was the formation in New York City of Women Against Pornography and an outburst of publications and articles on the topic and a reinvigoration of the censorship movement.[37] Prominent leaders of the movement, Catherine MacKinnon and Andrea Dworkin, together drafted an antipornography ordinance for the Minneapolis City Council, which argued that pornography was a form of sex discrimination against women and legally actionable as such.[38] Though the Minneapolis ordinance was defeated, a similar version passed in Indianapolis in 1984 but was ruled unconstitutional by both a district court and by the seventh circuit court of appeals, a ruling which the U.S. Supreme Court let stand. The justices accepted that pornography might well be an aspect of domination and might influence people's worldview, but it was, nonetheless, speech, and as such was protected by the First Amendment.[39]

Anyone who has read some of the feminist writing on the topic has been sensitized to the misogynistic qualities in much of pornography which traditionally was written by men for men. The question here, however, is not whether this is the case, but how far censorship should go. If women's civil rights are violated by pornography, doesn't Hitler's *Mein Kampf* violate Jews, and Ku Klux Klan literature violate blacks, and militant Protestant denigration of Catholics violate Catholics—which, after all, is where the whole censorship issue started? Ultimately, is not the writing of Catherine MacKinnon, Andrea Dworkin, and Susan Brownmiller degrading to men and deserving of censorship as much as the literature they accuse of being antiwomen? In sum, the issue, no matter how it is put, is quite clearly one of censorship.

It is a mistake to lump all feminists, or all women for that matter, into the same category where MacKinnon would put them. She herself is on the extreme edge and most feminists do not agree with her. In fact, it is quite possible to interpret MacKinnon's effort as a last-ditch attempt to unite the ever diverging feminist movement into a kind of "I hate males" crusade. The censorship effort failed for a variety of reasons, not the least of which was the refusal of most women to go along. Moreover, ignored in the discussion was the fact that women have always read erotic material and increasingly have written it, and created erotic paintings, statuary, and other forms of what traditionally has been classed as pornography. One of the fastest-growing literary markets is erotic fantasy literature for women. Joanni Blank, for example, and a collective of women established the Good Vibrations Bookstore in San Francisco as a nationwide mail-order service designed to reach women who desire erotic literature and sexual self-help devices, but who are unwilling to enter the traditional pornographic bookstores.

The movement had difficulties because the fundamental premise of the Women Against Pornography movement was the essential difference between femininity and masculinity, a difference which we, the authors of this book, would argue, cannot be an either/or situation. The movement, however, is not dead; the argument will continue to rage as long as society hunts for simple causal explanations to complex behavior. To say that rape results from pornography is to ignore the seriousness of the crime. Violence, sexism, and sexuality comprise three different realities: many acts of violence have nothing to do with sexism; sexism itself is not limited to matters of sex nor is it necessarily violent, and it is possible to show sex without violence or sexism.

Bernard Arcand used the Sherente myth of the jaguar and the anteater to summarize the issues over pornography. The Sherente, a Brazilian tribe, visualize life as a contest between two equally strong animals: the jaguar (symbol of sex and reproduction but also of mortality and danger), and the anteater, an asocial creature who, in the myth, also represents immortality. The Sherente ultimately picked the jaguar as their model, choosing to accept uncertainty, to live well and die. They came to believe that a long or prolonged life, or perhaps even an eternal life, the way of the anteater, is possible only in the form of a minimal existence. The only alternative for the anteater is to overcome death through reproduction, which is why the anteater is obsessed with sex. This does not mean that the Sherente repress their longing for the model of the anteater: to live comfortably in a protected and cozy isolation allows an individual to escape from traditional social constraint, but they realize this is not possible. The way of the anteater is seen by Arcand to be symbolic of pornography. He emphasizes that while the only real choice in life is to follow the path of the jaguar, the anteater allows some of us to escape into the closed universe of pornographic fantasy. However, we must also accept the fact that such an escape is one of lies and limitation, and also recognize that real life exists outside the fantasy. It is not wrong to indulge in one's fantasy; the danger is to live in fantasy as a retreat from life itself.[40]

Perhaps the concern that society today has over pornography is due as much to our own failure as a society to deal with sexuality as it is to anything else. While obvious pornographic fantasy has some effect on those who seek it out, it has always existed without as yet destroying civilization, and there is no historical evidence that it ever will. Moreover, the anti-pornography people seem to be retreating further from real life than those who escape to pornographic fantasies. In the past, sexually explicit writing has often served as a major source of sex information, misleading as it might have been. We hope this function can be served through modern sex education, but even when this happens erotic writing will probably serve as fantasy fiction for many.

NOTES

1. Commission on Obscenity and Pornography, William B. Lockhart, chairman, *Technical Report No. 2* (Washington, D.C.: U.S. Government Printing Office, 1970), p. 15.

2. Some of this has been illustrated in Rafael Larco Hoyle, *Checan: Essay*

on Erotic Elements in Peruvian Art (Geneva: Nagel Publishers, 1965). We have our own collection of some of these.

3. There are numerous collections of these, including Francis Leeson, *Kama Shilpa: A Study of Indian Sculptures Depicting Love in Action* (Bombay: D. B. Taraporevala Sons & Company, 1962); P. Thomas, *Kama Kalpa* (Bombay: D. B. Taraporevala Sons & Company, 1959); Mulk Raj Anand, *Kama Kala* (Geneva: Nagel Publishers, 1963); and *Kama Sutra: Ancient India in Vatsyayana's Time,* ed. Mulk Raj Anand (Atlantic Highlands, N.J.: Humanities Press, 1982), illustrated.

4. R. H. Van Gulik, *Sexual Life in Ancient China* (Leiden: E. J. Brill, 1961); also his *Erotic Colour Prints of the Ming Period,* 3 vols. (Tokyo: Privately printed, 1951); Marc de Smedt, *Chinese Erotism* (New York: Crescent Books, 1981); Abraham N. Franzblau, *Erotic Art of China* (New York: Crown Publishers, 1977); Étiemble, *Yun Yu* (Geneva: Nagel Publishers, 1970). There are many more.

5. See, for example, Charles Grosbois. *Shunga: Images of Spring* (Geneva: Nagel Publishers, 1965), and Tom and Mary Anne Evans, *Shunga: The Art of Love in Japan* (New York: Bookthrift, 1975).

6. Robert Surieu, *Sarv-E-Naz,* translated by James Hogarth (Geneva: Nagel Publishers, 1967).

7. Jean Marcadé, *Eros Kalos* (Geneva: Nagel Publishers, 1962).

8. Jean Marcadé, *Roma Amor* (Geneva: Nagel Publishers, 1965).

9. For a traditional summary of some of these see Friedrich Carl Forberg, *De Figuris Veneris: Manual of Classical Erotology* (reprint New York: Medical Press, 1964). In recent years there has been an outpouring of works on Greek as well as Roman erotic and sexual thinking.

10. Poggio Bracciolini, *Facetiae* (reprint New York: Valhalla Books, 1964), p. 100. There are numerous editions of this work.

11. *Aretino's Dialogues,* translated by Raymond Rosenthal (New York: Stein and Day, 1971), pp. 43–44.

12. For a discussion of this see David Foxon, *Libertine Literature in England 1660–1745* (New York: New Hyde Park, N.Y.: University Books 1965), pp. 19–30.

13. David O. Frantz, " 'Leud Priapians' and Renaissance Pornography," *Studies in English Literature* 12 (1972): 152–72, esp. 170.

14. *The Diary of Samuel Pepys,* edited by Henry B. Wheatley, 2 vols. (reprint New York: Random House, n.d.), 2: 768–69.

15. Ibid., 2: 790.

16. Foxon, *Libertine Literature,* p. 13.

17. Norman St. John-Stevas, *Obscenity and the Law* (London: Secker and Warburg, 1956), pp. 1–17.

18. *Queen* v. *Read,* 11 Mod. Rep. 142 (1708). See also Alec Craig, *Suppressed Books* (Cleveland: World Publishing Co., 1963), p. 25, and Foxon, *Libertine Literature,* p. 15.

19. *Rex* v. *Curll* in 2 Stra. 788 (1727); see also Craig, *Suppressed Books,* pp. 26–32, and Foxon, *Libertine Literature,* p. 15.

20. Theodore Schroeder, "Obscene Literature at Common Law," *Albany Law Journal* 146 (1907): 146.

21. H. Montgomery Hyde, *A History of Pornography* (London: Heinemann, 1964), pp. 97–100.

22. Ibid., pp. 160–64.

23. Quoted in Vern L. Bullough, Brenda Shelton, and Sarah Slavin, *The Subordinated Sex: A History of Attitudes toward Women* (Athens, Ga.: University of Georgia Press, 1988), p. 248.

24. Quoted in John Gibson Lockhart, *Memoirs of the Life of Sir Walter Scott,* 10 vols. (reprint Toronto: George N. Morant, 1901), 6: 303ff.

25. See also Milton Rugoff, *Prudery and Passion* (New York: G. P. Putnam's Sons, 1971).

26. *Queen* v. *Hicklin,* L.R. 3 Q.B. 360 (1868). See also St. John-Stevas, *Obscenity,* pp. 69–70.

27. Quoted in Richard H. Kuh, *Foolish Figleaves* (New York: Macmillan, 1967), p. 23.

28. See S. Chandrasekhar, *A Dirty Filthy Book* (Berkeley and Los Angeles: University of California Press, 1981).

29. St. John-Stevas, *Obscenity,* pp. 83–85, and Craig, *Suppressed Books,* pp. 54–70.

30. See *Libraries, Erotica, Pornography,* edited by Martha Cornog (Phoenix: Oryx Press, 1991), for a discussion of these kinds of issues.

31. *United States* v. *One Book Entitled* Ulysses, 5 F. Supp. 182 (S.D.N.Y. 1933), *affirmed* 72 F.2d 705 (2d Cir. 1934).

32. *Roth* v. *United States,* 354 U.S. 476 (1957).

33. See, William B. Lockhart, Chair, *The Report of the Commission on Obscenity and Pornography* (Washington, D.C.: U.S. Government Printing Office, 1970). Besides the report there are eight additional volumes of technical reports. Bernard Williams, Chair, *Report of the Home Office Committee on Obscenity and Film Censorship* (London: Her Majesty's Stationery Office, 1978); Henry Hudson, Chair, *Attorney General's Commission on Pornography: Final Report* (Washington, D.C.: U.S. Government Printing Office, 1986). There was also a special Canadian commission which looked at pornography and prostitution: Paul Fraser, Chair, *Report of the Special Committee on Pornography and Prostitution* (Ottawa, 1985) which precedes the Hudson Committee, and which decided that defining pornography was futile, opting instead for the term "sexually explicit material."

34. We are indebted to Donald Mosher, "Pornography," in *Human Sexuality: An Encyclopedia* (New York: Garland, 1994), p. 473, for this conceptualization.

35. Susan Brownmiller, *Against Our Will: Men, Women, and Rape* (New York: Simon and Schuster, 1975), p. 374.

36. Andrea Dworkin, *Pornography: Men Possessing Women* (New York: Perigree, 1981), p. 223.

37. See, for example, Betty-Carol Selles and Patricia Young, *Feminists, Pornography, and the Law: An Annotated Bibliography* (Hamden, Conn.: Library Professional publications, 1987).

38. Catherine MacKinnon and Andrea Dworkin, "Model Anti-Pornography Law," *Changing Men: Issues in Gender, Sex and Politics* 14 (Fall 1985): 23.

39. *Hudnut* v. *American Booksellers Association, Inc., et al.,* 1986. 106 S. Ct. 1172, 89 L.Ed.2d 29.

40. Bernard Arcand, *The Jaguar and the Anteater: Pornography Degree Zero,* translated from the French by Wayne Grady (New York: Verso [distributed by Routledge, Chapman and Hall], 1993).

11

Prostitution

Prostitution is often referred to as the oldest profession. The intention of such a statement is to indicate that it must always have existed, since by no stretch of the imagination could it be called a profession. Only a minority of women in the past have chosen to "profess" to being prostitutes, and none of the associated definitions of "professionalization" could be applied to prostitution.[1] Given Western Christian ambivalence toward sex, it would seem that prostitution should have been outlawed throughout much of Western history. In reality, however, prostitution has been not only tolerated but legalized. This contradiction between the celibate ideals and the reality of Western culture seem to be in large part due to the existence of a double standard, which holds that what is right for a man is wrong for a woman. Men have ever been conscious that women arouse sexual desires; but rather than regard this as a kind of natural attraction between the sexes in Western culture, they have often tended to feel guilty, putting the blame for this erotic desire on women themselves. Thus, according to myth and tradition, it was Eve who led Adam astray and Pandora who loosed evil upon humankind. Inevitably, the male lawmakers of the past attempted to control the erotic potential of the female by regulating the conduct of their daughters, wives, and sisters, thus making two distinct (and unequal) classes of women: those who were pure and those who were not. The latter were usually classed as prostitutes and were regarded as a necessary evil to protect the pure, who otherwise might unwittingly provoke the male to rape. The male in any case was not to blame. This double standard of morality has been deeply ingrained in Western culture and even has biblical backing.

One of the pertinent examples is the biblical case of Tamar whose story effectively illustrates the acceptance both of prostitution and of the double standard. Tamar's husband, Er, had been killed. Her father-in-law, Judah, following the Levirate law, then gave her as wife to his next son, Onan.

By custom it was Onan's duty to impregnate her so that she could continue the line of his dead brother. Onan (see Gen. 38:9) refused to do so by spilling his seed upon the ground, whereupon Jehovah struck him dead. By right, Tamar then should have been passed on to Judah's next son, Shelah, but Judah, fearing that Tamar was an evil influence, sent her back to her father's house childless and in disgrace. Unwilling to accept her childless condition, Tamar resolved to continue the line of her deceased husband by having intercourse with her father-in-law. To this end, she put on the heavy veils of a prostitute, then stationed herself at the side of a road on which Judah was accustomed to travel. When Judah saw the "prostitute" beckoning to him, he became sufficiently enamored to bargain for her services. Since he had not anticipated meeting with such a desirable interruption on his journey, he had neglected to bring sufficient money to pay the disguised Tamar for her services. Tamar eagerly agreed to take his signet, bracelets and staff as pledges, which he promised he would later redeem for cash. The two then engaged in intercourse. True to his word, Judah later tried to redeem his pledge but the prostitute was nowhere to be found. While this slight on his honor upset him, he had no qualms about his sexual relations with the prostitute. When word reached Judah, however, that his daughter-in-law had become pregnant, he ordered her to be brought before him to be punished for adulterous conduct. Tamar came willingly and showed Judah his own signet, bracelets, and staff, forcing him to recognize that she had been more righteous than he because she had gone to such lengths to continue the line of her husband, while he, righteous prophet that he was, had neglected to give her as wife to his third son.[2] The Jewish Scriptures contain numerous other stories of prostitutes. Rehab the harlot, for example, was instrumental in helping the Jews capture Jericho.[3] The point to emphasize, however, is that prostitution was accepted as a fact of life, and though the role of prostitute was not quite respectable, even prophets might seek them out.

The ambivalence about prostitutes and prostitution present in the Jewish Scriptures is heightened in Christianity by the importance of Mary Magdalene. According to Gospel tradition, Mary Magdalene had been a "woman of the city, which was a sinner," before she met Jesus.[4] This is usually interpreted to mean that she was a prostitute. In spite of this "sinful" past, however, Mary Magdalene played a significant role in the life of Jesus. She was among those who discovered that his grave was empty, and the first of Jesus' followers to whom he is said to have appeared after his resurrection. Jesus himself was also somewhat protective of prostitutes, telling the Pharisees, "Harlots go into the kingdom of God before you."[5]

With the words of Jesus as a guide, and with the life of Mary Magdalene as an example, the early Christian proselytizers made great efforts to convert prostitutes. Some are reported to have visited slave prostitutes, the lowest of the low, in a deliberate effort to convert them. If a prostitute received the gospel, the proselytizers changed garments with her on the spot so that she might escape. It was perhaps through just such zealous efforts at conversion that one courtesan was able to accuse Gregory Thaumaturgus (Wonder Worker) not only of having been her lover, but also of refusing to pay her the sum that had been promised. The man who would be saint immediately paid the woman what she asked, but his innocence was immediately demonstrated when the woman became possessed by a demon.[6]

Several prostitutes became saints. Their conversion stories early became part of the folk legend of the faithful, serving to emphasize that there was always the potential for salvation, even among the most fallen of women. Next to Mary Magdalene, the most famous of saintly prostitutes is the Mary known as the Harlot. According to the traditional story, she was the niece of a hermit ascetic by the name of Abraham, who had spent much of his adult life in a desert praying to God. When young Mary was seven, her parents died, and since her uncle was her only surviving relative, she was brought to him to be cared for. Conscious of his familial responsibilities, yet committed to his ascetic lifestyle, Abraham knocked out a window-like opening in his cell and built a small addition on to it in which he put Mary. She could observe him and he could see her, but otherwise contact was minimal. The youthful Mary quickly adapted to the ascetic life, content to spend her days in prayer and meditation, following the example of her uncle. The young girl grew to be an attractive, yet naive, adolescent, making her an easy victim for a lustful young man who laid careful plans to entrap her. He first asked her to pray for him to help him through a crisis. The dutiful Mary did as requested, and the young man continued to return seeking her intercession for his problem. Ultimately, he suggested that perhaps if they prayed together her prayers might be more effectively answered. Mary, ever willing to oblige, crawled out of her cell to help him, whereupon he fell upon her. When she came to her senses, she found she was no longer a virgin, and, unwilling to face her saintly uncle about her fall from grace, she fled to a nearby city where she ended up in a brothel.

Mary's uncle, who had been engaged in deep meditation all this time, remained blissfully unaware of what had happened. Eventually, however, he realized that Mary was no longer in her cell, and he began to ask his infrequent visitors if they knew of her whereabouts. Eventually he heard rumors that Mary had become a prostitute in the city. Determined to save his niece from herself, Abraham dressed in his old military uniform which he had somehow preserved, and set out for the city to find her. He soon saw her, and began propositioning her. Mary at first did not recognize her uncle, but gradually she became assailed by what was called "a certain odor of sanctity" (saints did not bathe) which reminded her of her uncle. As they reached her room, Abraham revealed himself to Mary, begging her to return with him and assuring her that God would accept her atonement if she did penance. Mary returned with him, whereupon her healing power was so enhanced by her experience that she was able to perform many miracles. Upon her death she was elevated to sainthood.[7] The devout fully believed such legendary stories, which undoubtedly made the Christian community somewhat more tolerant of prostitutes than they might otherwise have been.

A somewhat different story is told about Mary the Egyptian, who had worked as a harlot in Alexandria for some seventeen years before her conversion to Christianity. She then decided to spend an equal number of years in isolation purging herself of her sin. According to the legend, during this second seventeen years, she miraculously lived on only three loaves of bread plus the wild herbs she could gather. So holy did Mary become that when she made the sign of the cross, a monk by the name of Zosimus was able to walk on water. When Mary died, her body was placed in a cave frequented by a lion, but the lion willingly left the cave without touching her body.[8] There were many other prostitute saints,[9] with only slight variations of the story.

The more-or-less-official position of Christianity on prostitution was that put forth in the fifth century by Augustine, who held that even though there was nothing more sordid, more void of modesty, more full of shame than a prostitute, if they were removed entirely from human affairs everything would be polluted by lust.[10] In effect, Augustine justified the lust for prostitutes by his greater hostility to lust itself. Prostitutes, however, were to be excluded from the Church as long as they continued their profession,[11] but there was always the hope that they would eventually be converted to the true faith as were their saintly predecessors. Until that time they were to be tolerated because they served a useful function.

This attitude was reinforced in the Middle Ages by Thomas Aquinas, who argued that prostitution could not be disallowed entirely even though fornication itself was sinful. He compared prostitution to a sewer in the palace. If the sewer was removed, the palace would be filled with pollution;

similarly, if the prostitute were eliminated, the world would be filled with "sodomy."[12] Prostitution, in effect, was the lesser of two evils.

Similar attitudes appeared in the civil law codes as exemplified by the *Corpus juris civilis,* compiled under the direction of the emperor Justinian in the sixth century C.E. It was this compilation that served as the foundation for most later European civil and canon law. The compilers of the *Corpus* recognized the legality of prostitution, although they attempted to curtail it by banning procuresses and brothel keepers, keeping it, so to speak, as a free-enterprise occupation.[13] Earlier, there had been an attempt to abolish the tax on prostitutes on the assumption that the state should not have a vested interest in continuing prostitution,[14] but such a tax was not fully abolished until much later.

During the sixteenth century the reforming zeal of the Protestants originally led to a concentrated effort to eliminate prostitution. Some of the Protestant reformers, for example, urged that prostitutes be punished by excommunication and perpetual exile.[15] Probably the most extreme of the Protestants was Philip Stubbes, who, in his *The Anatomie of Abuses* (1582), recommended that all "whores" be cauterized with a red-hot iron on the cheeks, forehead, and other visible parts of the body.[16] Martin Luther, although he attempted to close the brothels in the cities adhering to his cause, recognized the difficulties that might ensue from such a ban. It was for this reason that Luther advised the city fathers of Halle to proceed with caution since premature eradication of the evil of prostitution might simply lead to greater evil.[17]

Luther's caution was undoubtedly justified, for there were few ways a woman not independently wealthy could survive without a husband except for prostitution. When the brothels of Strasbourg were closed, the prostitutes petitioned the authorities to reopen them or else give them honest work since they had become prostitutes not from desire but in order to earn a living. Some of the reformers attempted to find the prostitutes husbands or, failing that, some alternative means of work, but the abolition in general was only short-lived. In Zurich and some other cities, the brothels had never been closed, but rather were put under the supervision of an officer whose duty it was to see that no married men frequented them, a task that was not easy to perform. In London, the public houses were closed in 1546 and in Paris in 1560. In Rome, the pope ordered all prostitutes to leave the city in an edict of July 23, 1566, but this order was soon annulled, allegedly because some 25,000 persons, namely, the prostitutes and all their dependents, made preparations to leave.[18] Most other cities soon rescinded or ignored their prohibition of prostitution although prostitutes themselves increasingly came under greater government control because of a growing fear of sexually transmitted diseases (STDs). In fact, during the last four centuries it has been the association of prostitution with disease that has dominated most efforts to control it. Only in the last century have other factors entered in, primarily the rise of feminism.

SEXUALLY TRANSMITTED DISEASES

STDs, earlier called venereal diseases, have been around since recorded history; in fact, ancient skeletal evidence would indicate that they existed even before. The very term "venereal" implies an association of the disease with sex since it is derived from "venery," that is, the pursuit of Venus, goddess of love. Gonorrhea, from a Greek word meaning "a flow of seed," existed long before Galen coined the term in the second century C.E. Other forms of venereal disease that produce local genital ulcers or enlarged lymph nodes in the genital area have a venerable history although they appear often to have been confused with other diseases such as leprosy and elephantiasis. Syphilis, however, might have reached epidemic proportions only in the sixteenth century. The problem with looking at STDs in a historical context lies in diagnosing what diseases were described by ancient observers.

This is true of syphilis, which was the most feared of STDs until the appearance of the Acquired Immune Deficiency Syndrome (AIDS) in the late twentieth century. The first recorded reference to what has been diagnosed as syphilis occurred in the winter of 1494–1495 in Naples, when French soldiers garrisoned in the city reported the existence of tumors on their genitals. No sooner had these sores healed than they were followed by a series of eruptions such as sores inside their mouth or festering malignant ulcers on the legs or other parts of the body. Since the disease first occurred among soldiers of the French army, it inevitably was called *morbus gallicus* or the "French sickness." From Naples the disease spread over Europe with the virulence of a new plague. The name "syphilis" was ultimately given to the disease based on a poem by Girolamo Fracastoro, or Fracastorius (c. 1478–1553), a physician from Verona. The poem, *Syphilis sive morbus gallicus* (*Syphilis, or the French Disease*) (1530), recounted how a dreadful drought had afflicted the island of Hispaniola (Haiti), killing animals as well as humans. A shepherd, known as Syphilis, who felt that the drought constituted cruel and unusual punishment by the gods, rebelled against the sun god, Sirius, by switching allegiance to King Alcithous, an earthly mortal. Alcithous, intoxicated by this sudden allegiance, decreed that while the gods could have the heavens, he was king of the earth. In retaliation for this impiety, Sirius sent a new scourge to earth which claimed Syphilis as its first victim.[19] The poem not only gave the disease a name but also tied it directly to the Americas, an argument that is still debated.[20]

In recent years, the debate over whether syphilis was imported to Europe from the Americas or existed in Europe before the voyages of Columbus, has become of lesser importance, as other approaches to the subject of historical diseases have emerged. One such approach ignores ancient descriptions of disease, in this case syphilis, and instead studies the germ responsible for it within the broad biological and epidemiological context of the development of human treponematoses (the source of syphilis) and integrating these findings with paleopathological and historico-epidemiological studies.[21] Since there are a number of related infections caused by treponemal orgasms including yaws (a nonvenereal disease that produces ulcers and a fever), and pinta, a skin disease characterized by depigmented spots, as well as syphilis there is a variety of means of transmission depending upon the environment in which the treponema finds itself. It is quite possible that syphilis existed earlier in Europe in a nonvenereal form as bejel still does in the modern Middle East, where it thrives amid unhygienic living conditions.[22]

Still another approach is to look at the concept of syphilis rather than the history of the disease itself. That is, different diseases were considered by different generations to be syphilis, and the concept itself is a historical construct.[23] This has particular value in a study of syphilis, because it was not until the development of bacteriology and the isolation of the *Spirochaeta pallida* by Fritz Schaudin and Eric Hoffman in 1905 that it was clear what was meant by syphilis. In fact it was widely assumed in the eighteenth century that syphilis and gonorrhea were the same disease until Philippe Ricord (1799–1889) proved that syphilis and gonorrhea were indeed different, and hypothesized that syphilis had three stages. As indicated in chapter 6 on masturbation, there was also a widespread belief that many of the symptoms we now attribute to various STDs were believed to be simply a function of sexual activity itself.

Only in the last part of the nineteenth century, as some inkling of the real effects of STDs was gained, did prostitution come under attack not so much for moral reasons, but because of the disease spread by prostitutes and their clients to the innocent wives and children of those who were involved in prostitution. Massive campaigns were mounted against prostitution as a way of preventing disease; indeed, prostitution's link with STDs still dominates discussion of the topic today. Giving strength to the campaign was a growing feminist movement, which saw the elimination of prostitution as a way of challenging the sexual double standard.

STDS TODAY: A BRIEF OVERVIEW

Syphilis

Syphilis remains the most feared of the traditional STDs, although the early twentieth-century development of chemotherapy with salvarsan and related drugs made with arsenic and the mid-twentieth-century discovery and manufacture of antibiotics finally made it treatable. However, in past few decades new strains have appeared which are immune to many of the older antibiotics. The onset of syphilis is usually marked by the appearance of a chancre at the point where the spirochetes invade the body, usually on the genitals, but also on the lips, mouth, fingers, or breasts. Such chancres usually heal without treatment in a month or so and, though unsightly, are not particularly painful. The second phase of the disease appears from two to six months later in the form of lesions that appear in the mucous membranes of the mouth and anus, or in the body folds, and as rashes on the palms of the hand and soles of the feet. This secondary phase is usually marked by headaches, low-grade fever, and sore throat, as well as other aches and pains. Usually these symptoms also disappear within a few weeks or months, although they occasionally last longer. Syphilis then enters into a quiescent and noncontagious stage in which there are no clinical signs or symptoms directly attributable to it. Eventually, however, sometimes as long as twenty years after this benign stage has come to an end, the third stage of syphilis usually becomes manifest, although not everyone suffers the same degree of severity as occurred with the unwitting participants in the notorious Tuskegee experiments.[24] This lengthy period of incubation made it difficult in the past for physicians to link the later manifestation of what we know as syphilis with the syphilis that they thought they had cured. Moreover, not all the symptoms of the third stage are similar to those of the earlier stages, since the syphilis spirochete attacks a number of different organs. Probably the most noticeable symptom of the third stage are skin lesions, called gummata, which are ulcers that heal slowly with scarring. At the same time, a wide variety of organ systems may become painfully and chronically inflamed. It is the chronic inflammation which leaves the typical syphilitic mark on bones. When syphilis attacks the cardiovascular system, the aorta is often inflamed, resulting in a weakness of the artery wall and an outpocketing known as aneurysm. The result is an eventual rupture which causes death. Neurosyphilis affects the brain and spinal cord and can result in a deterioration of cerebral function or tabes dorsalis, i.e., an inability to coordinate muscular movement. The disease may also take the form of cerebral hemorrhage, brain tumor, deafness, blindness, mental disturbance, or epilepsy. The syphilis spirochete can cross the placental barrier, passing from the mother to the fetus. Children born with this disease usually enter the third stage before reaching their teens.

Gonorrhea

Gonorrhea can be easily identified because of its characteristic yellow discharge, and this symptom has a long history in the medical records. In men, gonorrheal urinary tract infections are acutely painful and disabling for up to a week. This led the military to pay particular attention to it because soldiers could be disabled during key battles. In women gonorrhea is often asymptomatic but can spread to the internal pelvic organs causing pelvic inflammatory disease and sterility. We believe it was a major factor in sterility of prostitutes in the past as well as of women whose husbands transmitted the disease to them. Although it does not cross the placental barrier, gonorrhea can spread to newborn infants in their passage through the birth canal and cause blindness. The realization of this infection resulted in one of the earliest twentieth-century breakthroughs in treatment, namely, the use of silver nitrate drops in the eyes of newborn infants, a treatment that has now been replaced by the use of antibiotics. The gonococcus causing it was isolated by Albert Neisser in 1879. It, too, can be treated by antibiotics although some strains are now resistant to some of the antibiotics currently being used.

Chlamydia

Chlamydia has been diagnosed only since the 1960s and, as of this writing, is the most common venereal disease in the United States, with more than four million cases a year. It is caused by a microorganism which for a time was believed to be a virus but which now appears to be a rickettsiaelike bacteria. Probably in the past many of the cases of chlamydia were diagnosed as gonorrhea, since it, too, can lead to pelvic inflammatory disease and sterility. Like gonorrhea, chlamydia is often asymptomatic in women while men may have a painful urethritis. A related disease, chlamydia trachomatous, is the most common cause of blindness throughout the world, although now both forms of chlamydia can be treated successfully with antibiotics.

Trichomoniasis

Trichomoniasis, though described in the nineteenth century, was confused with gonorrhea until almost the beginning of the twentieth century. It is marked by thick, frothy, yellow-green smelly discharges. Trichomoniasis, which is caused by a flagellate parasitic protozoon, is much more common in the female than the male. Treatment is by oral metronidazole, popularly known as Flagyl.

Herpes

Herpes is a viral disease with venereal and other forms, including herpes simplex, the common cold sore or fever blister. Genital herpes may start with flu-like symptoms and continue with painful blisters in the genital area and painful urination. Mild cases may go unnoticed, but anyone infected may in turn infect a sex partner. Herpes can be transmitted to newborn infants; indeed, until the development of intravenous acyclovir therapy, it was often fatal to the infant. While acyclovir treats the symptoms, it does not cure the disease which often reoccurs.

Venereal Warts

Venereal warts are caused by the papilloma viruses. Although some of them are relatively harmless, papilloma virus numbers 16 and 18 are particularly suspect and are now believed to be the cause of cervical cancer. Venereal warts can be removed with local application of chemicals or by surgery, but they can recur.

Gardnerella

Gardnerella, formerly called hemophilus vaginalis, is a bacterial infection that causes discomfort, a characteristic unpleasant odor, and may produce a pelvic inflammatory disease in women. There are a number of other sexually transmitted diseases including *molluscum contagiosum,* similar to venereal warts; *candida albicans,* a yeast infection more common in women than in men; and various parasitic infections such as scabies and lice.

AIDS

The disease dominating current thinking, however, is AIDS, which was discovered only in the 1980s. AIDS seems to be caused by a retrovirus that is constantly changing its characteristics. So far there is no cure or effective vaccine, which means that treatment is merely palliative. Moreover, many of the drugs used to treat AIDS are themselves toxic. AIDS compromises the immune system and leads to death through other diseases it facilitates, including pneumocystitis carinii (which attacks the lungs), Kaposi's sarcoma (cancer), yeast infections, and a particularly virulent form of tuberculosis. In fact, any opportunistic infection is made more difficult to treat because of the damage to the immune system that AIDS causes.

PROSTITUTION AND SEXUALLY TRANSMITTED DISEASES

As the dangers and extent of sexually transmitted diseases began to be better understood in the last part of the nineteenth century, there came a call for government-regulated and medically inspected prostitution—technically referred to as *réglementation.* Various cities in Germany and France already had established some sort of control, primarily in terms of public morals, but the fear of disease raised the need for greater medical and public health intervention.

Moreover, the rapid rise of urbanization and industrialization in the nineteenth century changed the nature of the demography of many Western countries. With people leaving the countryside in ever increasing numbers, particularly young men, to find their fortune in the cities, traditional village moral control was disappearing. Since there was a real shortage of women in the cities, prostitution flourished. Adding to the issue was the growing dissatisfaction of women with their traditional lifestyle; this led, both in

Europe and America, to the growth of feminism, which was marked by a demand for suffrage, for more attention to the needs of women and children, for greater opportunities for women, and for an end to the sexual double standard.

Many rich and powerful men, fearful of contracting a disease from a prostitute, attempted to avoid the problem by getting pure, i.e., virginal, uncontaminated, girls as bedmates. In London in the last part of the nineteenth century, the going price for a virgin girl from the working classes between fourteen and eighteen years of age was twenty pounds plus expenses for one night (supposedly the first night). Girls of higher social classes went for up to a hundred pounds, a small fortune for the ordinary person who earned less than a pound a week.

Undoubtedly many young girls who accidentally strayed into prostitution stayed there because they believed that once they had lost their virtue there was no hope for them except in a life of prostitution. Other girls found themselves involuntarily on the market. English girls, for example, were recruited for jobs on the Continent which, when they arrived more or less penniless, turned out to be in a brothel. If these young women refused to serve in the brothel, they found themselves stranded with no way of earning their way back to England. Newspapers connived in the illicit trafficking of girls by running advertisements designed to recruit them.[25] For example, many newspapers ran misleading advertisements requesting guardians or parents of "beautiful girls" from twelve to fifteen suitable for "adoption" to contact them: these were but thinly designed coverups for recruitment of young prostitutes.

Despite occasional protests about the "white slave" trade, a term coined at the end of the nineteenth century to describe the transfer of prostitutes from one area to another, there was no organized movement until Mrs. Josephine Butler (1828–1906) appeared on the scene. She had first become interested in the subject of prostitution in the 1860s when England had attempted to establish a regulated system of prostitution on the German model. Mrs. Butler's interest soon turned into a crusade. She made England the center of her battle against prostitution, although she herself always remained sympathetic to the women involved. Aiding her were a number of influential citizens and groups, most notably the Salvation Army, which had been started in 1865 in the East End of London by William Booth, better known under his title of General Booth. Almost from the first day the Christian Mission (the original name of the Salvation Army) in London opened its doors, Booth had been interested in the welfare of the prostitute.

In 1868 he opened his first shelter for prostitutes and vagrant girls. Also influential was "The London Committee for the Exposure and Suppression of the Traffic in English Girls for the Purposes of Continental Prostitution," organized in 1880.

Parliament, however, was reluctant to act, but this legislative impasse was broken largely through the efforts of W. T. Stead, editor of the *Pall Mall Gazette*. After determining the existence of "white slavery," Stead began to plan an exposé. To be successful, he felt it necessary to demonstrate that he himself could purchase a child in England for immoral purposes, then remove her to the Continent without any protest. Stead hired a "repentant" procuress to hunt for a "pure child" just over thirteen. The woman soon found a child who wanted to go into service in a "nice" house. Although the girl herself did not know why she was being selected, it was clear to her mother that her daughter was to have sexual relations with someone rich and powerful; the father also undoubtedly had a good idea of what it was all about. The child's mother was paid one pound for her daughter, an intermediary was given two pounds, and an additional two pounds were to be given to the mother after the child's virginity had been certified by a competent authority. Stead then took the girl to a hotel where he staged a "mock" seduction, then turned her over to the Salvation Army who whisked her off to the Continent. His series of articles on "The Maiden Tribute of Modern Babylon," which began to appear on July 4, 1885, caused a sensation and made Stead both a hero and a villain. He achieved his objective, however: by August 1885, Parliament had passed a bill raising the age of consent to sixteen and putting some teeth into the prohibition against trafficking in women and children. Stead's enemies, however (and there were many of them, including the London police), determined to punish him not only for the allegations he had made against them, but because of what they felt to be the unfavorable light he had thrown on British morals. Their opportunity came when the parents of the girl whom Stead had "purchased" sued to get her back, charging him with abduction. Stead was arrested, tried, and convicted, but this only served to give greater notoriety to his cause. Stead served three months in prison for his part in the abduction, the nominal basis for his conviction being that the girl's father had not been consulted on the sale (although it was later shown that he was not the biological father of the child and, in fact, had no legal rights over her disposal). One of the results of Stead's effort was the formation of the British Vigilance Society to curtail prostitution; another was the 1899 gathering of an international congress on the white slave traffic, which eventually led to an international agreement about the white slave trade. In the United States, passage of the Mann Act in 1910 made it a felony to transport or in any way aid, abet, or cause the transporting of a woman from one state to another for an immoral purpose.[26]

Many of the larger American cities tried to confine prostitutes to certain quarters, often known as "red-light" districts, although only St. Louis tried to follow the so-called *réglementation* system of Europe. At least seventy-seven cities and towns—in effect, all the larger cities—had established tolerated districts by the end of the nineteenth century. These districts came under attack in the twentieth century through the efforts of the American Social Hygiene Association, a combination of reformers, scientists, and feminists. One of the major successes of the reformers was to convince the U.S. Army during World War I to inspect soldiers rather than prostitutes, eliminating the military's need for *réglementation* and officially tolerated brothels. By the advent of women's suffrage in 1920, most of the tolerated red-light districts had been forced out of existence, and prostitution went underground. It continued to exist but now under the patronage of the criminal element, often in collusion with the police. In some all-male centers such as logging or mining camps, however, prostitution remained conspicuously open.

Despite its long history, prostitution has received little scholarly or scientific attention, although the libraries are full of moral tracts about it, and there is a vast bawdy literature which also exists outside the library. Perhaps the first real study of Parisian prostitutes was that done by A. J. B. Parent-Duchatelet in 1836. He found that the registered prostitutes as a rule were in their late teens or early twenties, illiterate, poor, probably illegitimate or from a broken family. Most also thought of themselves as temporary prostitutes, ready and willing to leave the field if something better turned up.[27] Parent-Duchatelet's great importance lies in his emphasis on the economic, educational, and sociological causes of prostitution, an almost radical change from the past, when the prostitute had been regarded as a "fallen" woman who had turned to prostitution because of some moral defect in her character—a defect that could be overcome only by religious conversion. Following Parent-Duchatelet's study, other investigators also emphasized the economic and sociological factors underlying prostitution. In 1855, Dr. William Sanger, with the assistance of the New York City police, had some 2,000 prostitutes fill out questionnaires giving information about their birth and parents, their age, economic background, and reasons for becoming a prostitute. The survey showed a correlation, which would seemingly hold today, between immigrant groups and prostitution. By far the largest number of prostitutes, some 706, were immigrants from Ireland. It was the Irish at the time who were fleeing poverty in their country, and who followed the black slaves and Native Americans as the most outcast and dislocated group. A large number of the native-born prostitutes came from New England, primarily from the declining textile towns that were centers of greater community disorganization.[28]

Fifty-seven years later, in 1912, George Kneeland made a similar study of 2,363 prostitutes in New York City based on police records. Russia, the home of a large number of Jewish immigrants, was the country of origin of the largest number of immigrant prostitutes while this time Ireland ranked a poor fourth, an indication of the changing status of the New York Irish. Blacks, a group totally ignored by Sanger,[29] were also becoming an increasing source of prostitution, which indicated the growing migration of African Americans from the South.

Both Sanger and Kneeland drew their information from police records or referrals; this meant that their statistics were heavily weighted toward the lower end of the social scale, since these were the women most likely to be arrested. Such studies concluded that prostitutes came from among the dislocated, dispossessed, and helpless; their finding led others to examine this aspect of prostitution. Because the economic causes were given so much stress in these statistical studies, serious attention began to be focused in the 1920s on the Soviet experience, since the Communists claimed that the chief cause of prostitution, capitalism, had been eliminated, and with it prostitution.[30] Despite such claims, however, prostitution continued to exist in the Union of Soviet Socialist Republics, albeit in a more covert form than it had in czarist Russia.[31] China, similarly, claimed for a time to have eliminated prostitution, but such claims could only be made by charging those arrested with other crimes.

Even though poor living conditions, unhealthy neighborhoods, neglected homes, inadequate education, low levels of intelligence, ignorance of sexual matters, or premature sexual experience are found in the backgrounds of a great many prostitutes,[32] these elements in themselves do not necessarily lead to prostitution. The remarkable thing is not that women with such backgrounds become prostitutes but that so many women with the same kind of background do not. This fact caused early twentieth-century investigators to look at the psychological factors related to prostitution.

Interestingly, perhaps because prostitution had so long been accepted by society as a "necessary evil," it did not attract the attention of the early pioneer researchers of human sexuality of the last part of the nineteenth century. Richard von Krafft-Ebing, for example, did not deal with the subject in his work on sexual pathology. Havelock Ellis was one of the first to do so although not in any detail. Still, Ellis rejected most of the popular ideas of his era about prostitutes, including the economic explanation, the theory of the Italian criminologist-physician Cesare Lombroso (1836–1909) that prostitutes had inherited criminal tendencies, and the folk wisdom which held that recruits were drawn into "the life" because they were extremely sensual women. Rather, Ellis looked for psychological explanations, maintaining that prostitutes selected their occupation because they were troubled women.[33]

While Sigmund Freud did little investigation into the topic himself, some of his disciples and followers carried Ellis's insight much further. They went so far as to erect a theoretical model conceptualizing the whole institution of prostitution as a psychopathology. Karl Abraham, for example, theorized that it was only when a woman could not enjoy the sex act with one partner that she felt compelled to change to another. The result was that the prostitute could avenge herself on every man by demonstrating that the sex act, which was so important to him, meant very little to her, allowing her unconsciously to humiliate all men.[34] Edward Glover interpreted prostitution as evidence of an unresolved Oedipal conflict: the woman still hated her mother and was disappointed with her father. Consequently she was hostile, frigid, and had homosexual tendencies. Glover further argued that prostitutes' customers were able to enjoy sex only with people they held in low esteem.[35]

The theme of latent or overt homosexuality was even more strongly advocated by Frank Caprio, who held that prostitution was a defense mechanism against homosexual desires; prostitutes turned to pseudo-heterosexuality rather than admit they were homosexual.[36] Similarly, Helene Deutsch identified a theme of hostility toward men which she felt was caused by an identification with a hostile mother and a rejection of paternal authority which even extended to rejection of the institutions built by men, such as law and morality.[37] Maryse Choisy, a French psychoanalyst, believed that the union of the prostitute with her client was one of debasement in which both partners expressed their aggression and hostility in a sadomasochistic relationship. The women were seeking revenge against their fathers and the men who sought them out wanted revenge against their mothers; the money that changed hands was a symbol of the mutual contempt they felt for each other.[38]

None of these writers used any kind of control group to test their generalizations, nor did they specify the samples they were using. Not surprisingly, some of the conceptualizations ran contrary to one another: Glover identified mother hatred as a basic mechanism while Deutsch saw father hatred as the motivating force. Considering the primitive state of psychoanalytic research methodology at the time, a 1958 study by Harold Greenwald stood out as a landmark. His initial sample included twenty "call girls," the term for the affluent prostitutes whose clients communicated with them by telephone. Greenwald identified rejection by both parents as a common element in the histories of his respondents, although he felt maternal rejection to be crucial.[39]

Yet even with the addition of Greenwald's empirical data, the psychoanalytic approach is questionable. Without any controlled analysis, we do not know whether prostitutes hate their clients more than married women hate their husbands, or whether there are more lesbians in the ranks of prostitutes than in any field dominated by women. However, the major problem of this approach is that it is too narrow, just as the economic explanation or any other prostitute-focused analysis is too narrow. Almost all the studies focused on one person in what is really a two-person relationship. To illustrate, while it may be true that used-car salesmen or surgeons have certain childhood traumas and personality traits in common with other members of their occupations, no responsible authority is willing to argue that cars are bought and sold or that operations are performed merely to satisfy the emotional needs of these workers. A market relationship that involves buying and selling of commodities or services must always be viewed within a broader context if it is to be understood. Nevertheless, a major theme in the literature for much of the twentieth century has been that prostitutes are mentally ill and should be treated in order to cause them to abandon their occupation. This has been advanced as a method for lessening the "evil" of commercialized sex and for cutting down sexually transmitted diseases. In practice, few prostitutes have actually been given any psychotherapy, although many have been jailed sporadically. These sanctions are enough to perpetuate the stigma of the prostitute as a sinful and sick woman, but insufficient to eradicate the institution.

Empirical research that was not psychoanalytical seems to be more valid. A 1955 English study titled *Women of the Streets* was based on a sample of 150 women. The author reported that there were social-class differences in the group. Those who worked in affluent neighborhoods seemed charming, educated, and sympathetic, while those who worked in poorer neighborhoods tended to be embittered and were more obviously out to get the best of their customers.[40] The Kinsey group gathered information on prostitutes which was never published, although some of it was finally reported in 1965 by Wardell Pomeroy. Using a sample of 175 prostitutes, most of whom were in prison, Pomeroy reported that contrary to the psychoanalytic assumptions, prostitutes were not necessarily frigid; they were in fact more sexually responsive than the other women interviewed for the major Kinsey study on sexual behavior. Ninety percent of the prostitute group reported having orgasms in their nonprofessional contacts, and 80 percent reported an occasional orgasm with a client. Nearly two-thirds indicated they felt no regrets about their choice of occupation, although the prison inmates did regret being in jail. Reasons for choosing prostitution included the income, the opportunity to meet interesting people, the fact that they regarded it as comparatively easy work, and sexual pleasures.[41]

Of course, it is difficult to generalize from a prison group to the rest of the population, but the hundreds of available personal and literary accounts suggest that a more variable and often more healthy personality among prostitutes seems reasonable. Some are troubled, but others are not. Some even fit the earlier stereotypes of the sensual woman, while others do not. Some are charming and cultured; other are malicious and dishonest. Some are affluent and live comfortably, while others are trapped in the life by poverty and drug addiction. A few see themselves as permanently in the life, but most feel that their occupation is a temporary one.

The earlier Kinsey study of the sex practices of American men brought out another important point. In 1947, Kinsey and his associates reported that 69 percent of the male sample had experienced some contact with prostitutes and 15 percent of the group visited them on a regular basis. The major users were single men. Significantly, older men had utilized the services of prostitutes more than had younger men.[42] This generational difference seems to be a significant, continuing trend: fewer men now turn to prostitute partners than formerly. The major factor in this change does not seem to be any personality change among American women, or any great growth in morality; rather it seems to reflect a decline in the double standard and more open acceptance of the sexuality of women made possible by modern contraceptives, abortion, and greater economic independence. Sexual intercourse has become less a salable commodity and more a shared, reciprocal activity.

This does not mean that the institution has disappeared completely. Rather the users are drawn from a narrower spectrum. Martha L. Stein did a study in the 1970s of 1,230 encounters between high-priced call girls and their clients. From her observations Stein drew up nine customer profiles which she labeled "the opportunist," "fraternizers," "promoters," "adventurers," "lovers," "friends," "slaves," "guardians," and "juveniles." Regardless of type, however, all seemed to want their sex needs met conveniently, professionally, and without further obligations other than monetary, although several of the types described by Stein enjoyed a temporary illusion of love or friendly involvement.[43] These men continue to patronize the higher-priced call girls because they do not want the involvement of a reciprocal relationship. Others turn to prostitutes for sadomasochistic or fetishistic desires because they do not want to confess these to a friend. Thus the market remains for specialized needs. It is, however, now a narrower market, which less often includes the so-called average man.

Prostitution is difficult to research, in part because it is a hierarchized occupation, and in part because it is a temporary occupation for many women who leave it if something better turns up, and who return to it if things do not work out. Some of them repeat this process several times. One of the more fascinating insights comes not from the research of professional scholars but from the biographies and autobiographies of the more literate prostitutes and ex-prostitutes. Many of these accounts report prostitutes suffering feelings of degradation that made them the willing victims of dope salesmen, pimps who beat them, and sadistic clients, and even of suicide. What comes through most strongly in these personalized accounts is that prostitution is hazardous work, and, though some women obtain extremely high fees, many find it difficult to hold on to the money they earn. The call girl has to see the same shows night after night and yet act enchanted and delighted with her sponsor, while the lowly streetwalker has to snag a customer in order to pay for food. The woman who works in a brothel has her life carefully circumscribed. Though most of the women who write about themselves are concerned with some sort of self-justification, and might not tell the truth even if they know it, a surprising number report that they have found satisfaction with their lifestyle.[44] The guilt they feel about what they do is less inherent than imposed on them by society.

One aspect of the changing picture of sex for compensation is the growing number of sexual surrogates who teach impotent, frightened, or handicapped clients how to enjoy sexual intercourse. Most of these surrogates are women, but there are also some men. Clients are referred to them by therapists who feel the surrogate can give them the loving, nurturing, and nondemanding help needed to make clients sexually more adequate. This unusual new occupation is undoubtedly one that was often performed by the prostitute in the past; her teaching and counseling and permission-giving functions have often been overlooked.

CONCLUSION

Obviously, in spite of everything prostitution still exists; however, there seems to be little reason for singling out the prostitute for punishment when her customers are allowed to go free. The disease factor, which once made it so fearful, has reemerged with AIDS, emphasizing the importance, both for the prostitute and her client, of using condoms with spermacides. The moral attitudes which condemned the prostitute but not her customer now seem like curiously dated relics of a double standard. The conceptualization of prostitution as a psychopathology also is increasingly viewed as an over-extension of the psychotherapeutic model. As society has finally begun to allow women some semblance of equality with men, it might be a logical next step to allow women to give or sell their sexual services as they see fit, without threat of arrest, although perhaps society has some right to demand discretion on the part of both the prostitute and her clients. It seems clear that no society, however repressive, has been able to eliminate prostitution.

We have thought long and hard about how to deal with prostitution. It might well be to examine the conflicting recommendations given by various individuals and groups and the difficulties inherent in them. Our conclusions can be grouped into five alternatives.

1. Perhaps the most extreme recommendation that could be made would be to outlaw prostitution entirely, to throw all the resources of the state into a legal campaign to eliminate it altogether. In our opinion such a policy would be doomed to failure, if only because it would be impossible to enforce unless police powers, using all the efforts of the state, were brought to bear on every act of sexual intercourse. This policy would be much worse than any problem it purports to solve; moreover, it would not only contravene all historical insights but would violate privacy and ignore the biological needs and drives of men and women.

2. A lesser solution would be to outlaw certain forms of behavior associated with prostitution, primarily zealous solicitation, but immediately difficulties appear in what constitutes solicitation. Almost every female has been solicited at least some time in her life, and though female solicitation of males is less blatant and less obvious, most women have to give signals that they

would like to know a man better for him to approach her.[45] The whole concept of romantic love is based upon the assumption that males and females have some kind of attraction for each other and that one of them has to make the approach to the other. If no power relationship exists, and it is simply a proposition in which either side can say no without endangering themselves or their economic well-being, then defining solicitation becomes a problem. The courts, in wrestling with this problem, have usually insisted that the solicitation be to commit a sexual act for money. This has led to further difficulties in enforcement because male vice officers then have to hold off arrest until such an offer is made, and a streetwise prostitute is reluctant to name money until the officer himself does. The end result is entrapment, and basic perversion of the law. But if we are going to arrest prostitutes for solicitation, should not her customers be arrested for propositioning her? Probably yes, but the same difficulty exists here, since in order to arrest soliciting customers, a vice officer has to act the part of a prostitute and encourage her would-be client to offer money, in effect entrapping him. Moreover, the difficulty with an arrest for solicitation is that only the more obvious prostitutes, primarily the streetwalkers, are arrested. This leaves more discreet call girls or high-class party girls untouched. The result is a class bias in law enforcement that mocks equal justice under the law.

3. A third alternative is to legalize and control, usually justified on the grounds of preventing the spread of STDs. The medical reason advanced in the nineteenth century turned out ultimately not to be a valid one. This is because to control venereal disease every prostitute's client would have to undergo examination before being given access to her (or him) and the examination would have to be more than superficial and involve laboratory workups as well. Indeed, the prostitute herself (or himself) would have to be examined daily.

Réglementation is not only a failure in controlling disease, it raises other problems. It makes prostitution a long-term career choice for many who might otherwise have been involved only temporarily. It fosters police fraud because they control the licensing and can also prevent women from leaving the field or blackmail them if they try to change careers.

4. Some jurisdictions have attempted to avoid some of these problems by setting aside certain districts for prostitution, since it was believed that by concentrating vice in one area, police could better control crime. Two factors are at work which tend to make this ineffective. One is the standard plea

of "Not in *my* neighborhood." Where should such a place be located? And even if that problem is solved by establishing a specific district, it does not lessen police problems but complicates them. Such districts demand heavy law enforcement because both the prostitutes and their customers are considered fair game by many of the criminal element, and unless the area is heavily policed so-called respectable clients will not come. On the other hand, if police enforcement is too overbearing, they will not come either.

Often cities do not overtly designate such an area but allow the business to develop as it will. As of this writing, New York City's Times Square has mounted a massive campaign to "clean up the area" so "respectable" tourists will feel safe visiting and, more important, tax-paying businesses will reestablish themselves there. Such areas cost more than they produce in revenue, and demand constant efforts to prevent their further deterioration. Though Times Square might well soon be abandoned by the prostitutes, the new area they adopt will soon face the same problems.

In the small Nevada towns where prostitution is legalized and ghettoized, one or two houses can be located in isolated areas and still attract customers; but if such a policy is followed in New York, Los Angeles, San Francisco, Chicago, or even in Las Vegas, one house of prostitution will not be enough. Massive districts are required. Moreover, the legalized district has to be set up in areas where tourists and transients are most likely to go; if the legal district is far from the focus of other activity, the prostitute will go to the location where the action is. This puts the police in the situation of arresting people for actions in one part of the city that would be legal in another. Again the problem is also that such districts deal with only the more blatant forms of prostitution, while less obvious or more discreet forms take place elsewhere.

5. The obvious solution, at least to us, is the decriminalization of sexual activities between consenting adults whether or not money changes hands. The merit of such a system is that it would free the majority of the members of the urban vice squads for other tasks, specifically for crimes involving victims. Prostitutes could be encouraged to be discreet, advertising their services in the so-called underground press; establishing telephone-answering services; recruiting customers in parlors emphasizing erotic massages, in adult bookstores, and through special escort services; and establishing erotic clubs. Those who want prostitutes could find them, and those who do not could avoid them.

We strongly believe that the law should protect young girls from being enticed into prostitution, but the laws on statutory rape and age of consent already deal with this. The strong prohibitions against involuntary prostitution should remain on the books. As we have emphasized, Western society, in spite of all its apparent condemnations, has actually condoned prostitution. It has indicated its ambivalence by making the prostitute subject to harassment, imprisonment, fines, and other penalties, but then enforcing these penalties only sporadically and mainly against the poorer and less fortunate of prostitutes. Although we think that prostitution will continue to decline as a percentage of the population's total sexual contacts, we can predict that there will be a demand for the foreseeable future. We need to deal with prostitution realistically and not brush aside the problems associated with it as we do today. Passed over in this chapter is any discussion of homosexual prostitution, which will be discussed under homosexuality.

NOTES

1. For an extensive treatment of the subject of professionalization, see Vern L. Bullough, *The Development of Medicine as a Profession* (New York: Science History, 1966).

2. Gen. 38.

3. Josh. 2:1ff.

4. Luke 7:37.

5. Matt. 21:31.

6. Vern L. Bullough and Bonnie Bullough, *Women and Prostitution: A Social History* (Amherst, N.Y.: Prometheus Books, 1987), p. 67.

7. The story of St. Mary the Harlot was exceedingly popular during the Middle Ages. A retelling of the story can be found in Helen Waddell, *The Desert Fathers* (reprint Ann Arbor: University of Michigan, 1957), pp. 190–201.

8. *Butler's Lives of the Saints,* edited and revised, and supplemented by Herbert Thurston and Donald Attwater, 4 vols. (London: Burns and Oates, 1956), 2: 14–15.

9. Bullough and Bullough, *Women and Prostitution,* pp. 68–69.

10. *De ordine,* II, iv, 22, in J. P. Migne, *Patrologiae Latina* (hereafter *PL*) (Paris: Garnier Fratres, 1877) XXXII.

11. *Constitutiones Apostolicae,* II, xxvi, in *PL* I.

12. Thomas Aquinas, *Summa Theologica* (New York: Benziger Brothers, 1947), II, Part II, x, II, and ix, 2 and 5.

13. *Corpus juris civilis* (Amsterdam, 1664), *Digest,* lib. XII, titulus v, and *Novella,* XIV, collatio, III, titulus i, "De lenonibus."

14. *The Theodosian Code,* translation and commentary by Clyde Pharr, in

collaboration with Theresa S. Davidson and Mary B. Pharr (Princeton: Princeton University Press, 1952), *Novellae*, "De lenonibus," titulus 18, p. 504.

15. Derrick Sherwin Bailey, *Sexual Relation in Christian Thought* (New York: Harper & Brothers, 1959), p. 206.

16. Nina Epton, *Love and the English* (London: Cassell, 1960), pp. 68, 91.

17. Bailey, *Sexual Relation,* p. 182.

18. Preserved Smith, *The Age of Reformation* (New York: Henry Holt and Company, 1920), pp. 506–507.

19. There are various translations of this. We used the one published as Hieronymus Fracastoro, *Syphilis* (St. Louis: The Philmar Company, 1911).

20. The controversy over syphilis's origins dates from at least the beginning of the sixteenth century, with some arguing for a New World origin and others for its existence in Europe before the discovery of America. Since syphilis often leaves lesions that are uniquely identifiable, the debate goes beyond traditional medical sources and looks at skeletal remains. Among discussions of it are Alfred W. Crosby, *The Columbia Exchange: Biological and Cultural Consequences of 1492* (Westport, Conn.: Greenwood Publishing Company, 1972), and Theodor Rosebury, *Microbes and Morals: The Strange Story of Venereal Disease* (New York: The Viking Press, 1971). Much of the debate centers around the Spanish writers of the time: Crosby is more inclined to credit them than is Rosebury. The person most responsible for the New World origin was Jean Astruc, *De morbis venereis* (Paris, 1756), who was determined to change the name from the French disease to syphilis or some other name less identifiable with the French. Karl Sudhoff, *Der Ursprung der Syphilis* (Leipzig: F. C. W. Vogel, 1913), argued against such an interpretation. Sudhoff's collection of tracts on the topic was reedited and in part translated by Charles Singer, *The Earliest Printed Literature on Syphilis* (Florence: R. Lier and Company, 1925). Disagreeing with Sudhoff was Iwan Bloch, *Der Ursprung der Syphilis*, 2 vols. (Jena: Gustav Fischer, 1901–1911).

21. C. J. Hacket, "On the Origin of the Human Treponematoses (Pinta, Yaws, Endemic Syphilis and Venereal Syphilis)," *Bulletin of the World Health Organization* 29 (1963): 7–41; Corinne Shear Wood, "Syphilis in Anthropological Perspective," *Social Sciences and Medicine* 12 (1978): 47–55.

22. E. H. Hudson, *Non-Venereal Syphilis* (Edinburgh: E. & S. Livingstone, 1958), and E. H. Hudson, *Treponematosis* (New York: Oxford University Press, 1946).

23. This is a concept first put forth by Ludwik Fleck in the 1930s but not widely adopted until after the translation of the work into English: Ludwik Fleck, *Genesis and Development of a Scientific Fact,* translated by Fred Bradley and Thaddeus J. Trenn, and edited by Trenn and Robert Merton (Chicago: University of Chicago Press, 1979).

24. This was a long-term project carried out on African Americans in Tuskegee, Alabama, by the United States Public Health Services from 1932 to 1972. Patients were under the illusion that they were receiving treatment, although they were not.

Even after the effectiveness of penicillin had been demonstrated, the experiment was carried on to determine the long-term effects of syphilis. See James H. Jones, *Bad Blood: The Scandalous Story of the Tuskegee Experiment* (New York: Free Press, 1981).

25. Charles Terrot, *Traffic in Innocents* (New York: E. P. Dutton, 1960), pp. 22–44.

26. See Josephine E. Butler, *Personal Reminiscence of a Great Crusade* (London: Horace Marshall and Sons, 1896); Adolph F. Niemoller, *Sexual Slavery in America* (New York: The Panurge Press, 1935); Howard B. Woolston, *Prostitution in the United States* (New York: The Century Company, 1921); and Michael Pearson, *The 15 Virgins* (New York: Saturday Review Press, 1973). See also Bullough and Bullough, *Women and Prostitution*, pp. 358–90.

27. A. J. B. Parent-Duchatelet, *De la prostitution dans la ville de Paris*, 2 vols. (Paris: J. B. Baillière, 1836), 1: 38–39.

28. William L. Sanger, *The History of Prostitution* (New York: Harper and Brothers, 1858), p. 460. The book has often been reprinted.

29. George J. Kneeland, *Commercialized Prostitution in New York City* (New York: The Century Company, 1913), p. 251.

30. See V. Bronner, *La lutte contre la prostitution en URSS* (Moscow, 1936), and Dyson Carter, *Sin and Science* (New York: Heck-Cattell, 1946), *passim*.

31. Various observers in the 1930s and afterwards reported the continued existence of prostitution. One of the problems, however, was finding a place to have sexual intercourse since housing until the dismemberment of the USSR remained a critical issue. This was no problem in the summer when the great outdoors furnished plenty of space, but in the winter it was difficult. This meant that a number of people had to be involved: an individual entrepreneur could not operate without the connivance of doormen, family members, or others. One of the favorite haunts was the Moscow-Leningrad train where many of the compartments were taken up by prostitutes and their clients. In the Russia of today, prostitution is practiced openly.

32. A whole host of such factors was given by Woolston, *Prostitution in the United States*, pp. 300–301. See also Maude E. Miner, *Slavery of Prostitution* (New York: Macmillan, 1916), pp. 53–87, and the League of Nations, *Prevention of Prostitution*, C.26.M.26 (1943), IV, pp. 25–32.

33. Havelock Ellis, *Studies in the Psychology of Sex*, 7 vols. in 2 (reprint New York: Random House, 1936), "Sex in Relation to Society," 2, part 3: 269–72, 277–80, 295–96. Freud had also recognized the psychological factors, although he did little work in the field himself.

34. Karl Abraham, *Selected Papers*, translated by Douglas Bryan and Alex Strachey (London: The Hogarth Press, 1942), chap. 22, "Manifestations of the Female Castration Complex," p. 361. The paper was originally written in 1920.

35. Edward Glover, *The Psycho-Pathology of Prostitution* (London: Institution

for the Scientific Treatment of Delinquency, 1945), p. 4. This paper was also reprinted in Glover, *The Roots of Crime* (New York: International University Press, 1960), pp. 244–67.

36. Frank Caprio and Donald Brenner, *Sexual Behavior: Psycho-Legal Aspects* (New York: Citadel Press, 1961), pp. 249–52.

37. Helen Deutsch, "The Genesis of Agoraphobia," *International Journal of Psychoanalysis* 10 (1929): 51–69, and vol. 1 of *The Psychology of Women* (New York: Grune and Stratton, 1944).

38. Maryse Choisy, *A Month among the Girls,* translated by C. Blochman (New York: Pyramid Books, 1960; first published in 1928).

39. Harold Greenwald, *The Call Girl: A Social and Psychoanalytic Study* (New York: Ballantine Books, 1958), *passim,* esp. pp. 91–98.

40. *Women of the Streets,* edited by C. H. Rolph (London: Secker and Warburg, 1955), pp. 46–50.

41. Wardell B. Pomeroy, "Some Aspects of Prostitution," *The Journal of Sex Research* 1 (November 1965): 177–87.

42. Alfred C. Kinsey, Wardell B. Pomeroy, and Clyde E. Martin, *Sexual Behavior in the Human Male* (Philadelphia: W. B. Saunders, 1948), pp. 596–609, esp. p. 603.

43. Martha L. Stein, *Lovers, Friends, Slaves: Nine Male Sexual Types: Their Psycho-Sexual Transactions with Call Girls* (New York: Berkley Publishing Corporation and G. P. Putnam's Sons, 1974).

44. For a list of biographies and autobiographies see Bullough and Bullough, *Women and Prostitution,* p. 363, n. 15, and for more comprehensive listing Vern L. Bullough, Barret Elcano, Margaret Deacon, and Bonnie Bullough, *A Bibliography of Prostitution* (New York: Garland, 1977), and Vern L. Bullough and Lilli Sentz, *Prostitution: A Guide to Sources, 1960–1990* (New York: Garland, 1992).

45. Timothy Perper, *Sex Signals: The Biology of Love* (Philadelphia: ISIS Press, 1985).

12

Homosexuality, Sex Labeling, and Stigmatized Behavior

In 1974, the American Psychiatric Association removed homosexuality from the category of pathological conditions. The final decision to do this was done by mail ballot. More people previously judged ill by the medical profession and by society were declared well and healthy in one stroke than had ever occurred before in history. Two other examples of rejected pathologies have already been mentioned, namely, masturbatory insanity and female menstrual cycles, although in neither case was there quite such a sudden reclassification. How many other forms of sexual behavior regarded as pathological today will be reinterpreted in the immediate future? How can a pattern of sexual behavior be pathological one day and classified as something else the next?

We have pointed out that many long-held attitudes about sex were based on erroneous if not fantastic assumptions which came to be incorporated into the medical model that emerged in the late nineteenth and early twentieth centuries. However, the major advantage of the medical model over previous conceptualizations of sex as sin, or as crime, was that calling socially disapproved sexual activities "illnesses" allowed them to be studied. Therefore, physicians, psychologists, and others could carry on a wide range of research in previously forbidden areas.

One of the first results of the new sex research was to define and name behaviors, distinguishing them from each other, and in the process determining entirely new categories in what had once been lumped together indiscriminately. We have already examined such recently defined terms as "transvestism" and "transsexualism," but there are many others coined from Greek and Latin roots, including coprophilia (arousal by feces), urophilia (arousal by urine), mysophilia (love of filth), and pyromania (a compulsive desire to set fires). Other examples are necrophilia (sexual use of corpses) and gerontophilia (sex with a considerably older person). Sometimes the names of individuals have been utilized to describe behaviors. Sadism, the need to inflict pain in order to achieve sexual satisfaction, was named for the Marquis de Sade (1740–1814), who had a reputation for enjoying cruelty. (We'll be discussing the Marquis de Sade at greater length in the following chapter.)

The one who most effectively put the imprimatur of science on the developing labeling system for sexual activities was Richard von Krafft-Ebing (1840–1902) His *Psychopathia Sexualis* included new labels for a wide variety of sexual activities, all of which he disapproved of. In the process he undoubtedly created abnormalities out of activities that had not been associated with illness before.[1]

John Money is the most well-known contemporary sexual scientist active in developing the nomenclature of sexuality. He has described and named over a hundred variations in sexual behavior.[2] Money, however, was preceded by Havelock Ellis, who summed up the variety of sexual diversity by stating there has been "no excretion or product of the body which has not been a source of ecstasy" to someone;[3] we may add that there is nothing that can be done either to the body or by the body that does not give someone erotic stimulation and sexual satisfaction.

One result of the passion for classification and description of the various forms of sexual impulse has been to give medical credence to stigmatizing behavior. The danger in this was summarized by the sociologist Howard Becker:

> Social groups create deviance by making the rules whose infraction constitutes deviance, and by applying those rules to particular people and labeling them as outsiders. From this point of view deviance is not a quality of the act the person commits, but rather a consequence of the application by others of rules and sanctions to an "offender." The deviant is one to whom the label has successfully been applied; deviant behavior is behavior that people so label.[4]

Defining behaviors as belonging to a certain category thus had implications not only for medicine but for society, since this was the necessary first step in establishing something as deviant. But classifying certain behaviors as deviant has other implications. It tends, if the category is broad enough, to create a special group of people, and those who recognize any part of such a description in themselves may conform or attempt to conform to the description. A classic past example of stigmatized behavior leading to the creation of a special class of deviants was witchcraft. Through much of the medieval period the Christian Church denied that witchcraft existed; it was not until the fifteenth century that the church gave its official recognition and defined what witchcraft was. The official definition was set forth in a handbook, *Malleus maleficarum* (*Hammer of the Witches*), written in 1484–1486 by Heinrich Kramer (Institoris) and Jakob Sprenger.[5] Once defined, not only could a witch be recognized by the public at large, but certain people whose slightly deviant behavior was stigmatized as being that of witches began increasingly to conform to the accepted definition of witchcraft. Even if they did not fully conform initially, they usually would do so when apprehended or taken into custody as witches because there was almost no defense against an accusation of witchcraft except confession, and the accused were carefully fed the charges to which they would confess. The result was a reinforcement of what it meant to be a witch. A similar response is noted in reference to stigmatized sexual behavior. Someone who feels that he or she is different or whom others say is different, or who is told that he or she is a masochist, a voyeur, or a homosexual, often begins to conform to the expected behavior of such a stigmatized group. Sometimes, however, individuals so labeled consciously turn away from the stigmatized behavior pattern because they are unhappy with such an identity, or else fearful of ostracism or other punishment.

Usually when enough individuals manifest behavior that has been stigmatized, there is a tendency for them to band together; when this happens, the particular stigmatized behavior is enhanced and made more visible. This is because the group helps to form a self-identity for the stigmatized individual, giving reinforcement to the kind of behavior for which society has ostracized him or her. If outside pressure is great enough, the stigmatized group often turns to religious or pseudoreligious concepts for reinforcement, embracing the principles of morality to emphasize their propriety, and portraying their own particular group as worthwhile while viewing others as immoral, sinful, or self-deceiving. Those who join the group but who do not follow what the group defines as norms are often ostracized. Not infrequently the stigmatized group develops its own pattern of conformity and the suppression of deviants. This is particularly true if the society at large is particularly hostile. If society is somewhat more tolerant, and those whose behavior has been labeled as abnormal or pathological are numerous enough, a number of diverse groups will form; for example, the organizational history of sadomasochists, transvestites, or homosexuals has been studied. Usually the group can effectively mask its key sexual identity from the larger public while privately seeking support of like-minded persons. Like other organizations these groups are subject to internal splits and intense rivalry. As cliques and more specialized groupings grow in number, the more varied are the individuals who engage in a particular form of stigmatized behavior.[6] Some forms of sexual behavior are so private or personal that they are not dependent upon others (masturbation might be an example), and individuals who practice such behavior hardly ever organize.

One of the results of medical classification was to focus greater attention on those sex activities which had previously not been regarded as sex crimes or even sins, although many of the acts so defined were often performed in houses of prostitution. The few prostitutes who have penned their memoirs have described clients who took erotic satisfaction from watching others defecate or urinate, or simply from looking at the sexual organs of the same or opposite sex. Many houses of prostitution had rooms where clients could achieve voyeuristic satisfaction by observing couples engaged in intercourse, or where others who enjoyed exhibiting themselves in public could put on a show. Such activities generally were not regarded as aberrant behavior until so described in medical journals. Exhibitionism, for example, was first described and categorized in 1877,[7] although we know it existed much earlier.

Other forms of sexual activity which varied from culture to culture and century to century remained ambiguous until codified by medical terminology. Incest, which some regard as a universal taboo, is derived from the Latin *incestus*, meaning "impure," "immodest," "lewd," and which in the early medieval period also meant "adulterous." Later with the development of canon law, incest was used to describe sexual intercourse between those for whom marriage was prohibited by law, although these prohibitions varied from area to area. For example, marriage between first cousins is defined as incest in a number of American states but not in all.[8] Even though incest has biological and psychological implications, it essentially has to remain a question of legal definitions since what constitutes incest varies considerably depending on the culture.

The interaction between stigmatized behavior and the medical community, and the development of a medical model of pathology, can perhaps best be seen in the case of homosexuality, and it is to this subject that much of the rest of this chapter is devoted. Originally the concern was almost entirely confined to men, with the early focus on the wasted semen in homosexual activities. As we described earlier, Western culture once defined all nonprocreative sex as a sin against nature; in the eighteenth century nonprocreative sex also became a medical pathology through the efforts of S. A. D. Tissot (1728–1787), whose work on masturbation has already been discussed (see chapter 5). With Tissot's advocacy of the belief that the loss of semen could eventually lead to madness, a number of other researchers rushed in to amplify, to categorize, and to point out the dire consequences. Among the nineteenth-century figures who might briefly be singled out is the American reformer Sylvester Graham (1794–1851), for whom the Graham cracker is named, since, in addition to his writing on sex, Graham was a great advocate of "natural" foods such as unbolted wheat flour. Graham taught that the loss of an ounce of semen was equivalent to the loss of several ounces of blood; thus every time a man ejaculated he lowered his life force, thereby exposing himself to diseases and premature death.[9]

Second, we may mention the nineteenth-century French physician, Claude-François Lallemand, who so worried about the loss of male semen that he felt even daydreaming was dangerous: if an erotic thought crossed a man's mind, he might lose a little semen.[10] William Acton (1814–1875), an Englishman, held that the emission of semen imposed such a great drain on the nervous system that the only way the male could avoid damaging himself and shortening his life or endangering his sanity was to engage in sex infrequently, and then without any effort to prolong the act. Acton believed that this was possible because God had created humanity in such a way as to make women indifferent to sex. Only out of the need for babies or out of fear that their husbands would desert them for courtesans or prostitutes (women with a distorted sexual sense), did good women waive their own sexual repugnance and submit to the ardent embraces of the male. So great was women's loathing of sex, however, that even under such circumstances, the husband was forced to perform his necessary biological function of impregnation as expeditiously as possible, and thus manage to avoid severe damage to his nervous system.[11]

The obvious loophole in these arguments was the evidence that people had engaged in sex since the beginning of time and somehow had managed to survive and reproduce. The critics of active sexuality, however, responded that though this might have been true in the past, it was no longer the case. They held that the growing complexities of modern civilization, and the higher evolutionary development that humans were attaining, had created greater problems for humanity's animal nature, and that now the only way men and women could continue to advance was by limiting their sexuality. One of the popularizers of this absurb idea was American physician George M. Beard, who maintained that "modern civilization" had put such increased stress upon humankind that ever larger numbers of people were suffering from nervous exhaustion, particularly those who worked with their brains. Since the use of the brain was believed to increase as civilization advanced, and the brain worker by implication was more advanced than the manual worker, it became more and more necessary for the brain worker to save his nervous energy. According to Beard, the human body was to be looked upon as a reservoir of "force constantly escaping, constantly being renewed," but always in danger of unbalance. One of the major causes of nervous exhaustion was sexual intercourse: unless the nervous energy that went into it was carefully regulated and guarded, nervous collapse would inevitably result.[12]

Since the only permissible activity in the minds of these and the many other advocates of diminished sexuality was procreative sex, by implication anyone who purposely engaged in nonprocreative sex was in danger of losing his or her mind; if such nonprocreative activity was engaged in with a person of the same sex then insanity almost inevitably resulted. There have always been homosexuals, however, and some attempted to justify homosexuality in medical terms. The inevitable result was the classification of homosexuality as a pathological illness.

The modern study of homosexuality began with Karl Heinrich Ulrichs (1825-1895), who publicly proclaimed his own homosexuality and set out to challenge traditional concepts. Under both the pseudonym Numa Numantius and then his own name, Ulrichs issued a series of polemical, analytical, and theoretical pamphlets between 1864 and 1870 defending homosexuality. His very defense, however, came to be used as an argument to prove that homosexuality was a pathological illness. What Ulrichs attempted to demonstrate was that the instincts causing men and women to turn to the same sex were inborn, and therefore natural to a significant percentage of human beings. Sex between such individuals was no more dangerous than procreative sex between married couples. Since homosexuality did not derive from bad habits, hereditary disease, or willful depravity, those who engaged in it could not be classed as physically or intellectually inferior to heterosexuals, who were superior merely by their number. He hypothesized that up to a certain stage of prenatal development all sexes were the same, after which a threefold division took place: male, female, and *Urning* (male homosexual)

or *Urningin* (female homosexual), with many gradations within the homosexual realm. This third group had the physical features of one sex but
their sexual instinct did not correspond to their sexual organs. It was natural,
therefore, for these individuals to prefer partners of their own sex.[13]

Similar ideas were expressed by Karoly Maria Benkert (later Kertbeny)
(1824–1882), who wrote a pamphlet defending homosexual orientation, and
who coined the word "homosexual," a hybrid form since it derives from
the Greek *homos,* meaning "same" (not the Latin *homo,* meaning "man"),
and the Latin *sexus,* or "sex." In spite of etymologists' horror over the coining
of such hybrids, homosexuality is the term most commonly accepted.
Kertbeny had ideas similar to Ulrichs's, although he did not focus on a
third sex so much as inborn urges.[14]

The advocates of homosexuality as a congenital anomaly won grudging
acceptance from the medical community, but instead of accepting this
inheritance as normal, they came to regard it as pathological. Karl Westphal
(1833–1890), the physician who coined the term *die konträre Sexualempfindung,* or "contrary sexual feeling," to describe a homosexual transvestite,
and whose work marked the real beginning of the medical community's
interest in homosexuality per se, held that homosexuality was a form of
moral insanity due to "congenital reversal of sexual feeling." Westphal later
went on to study other cases of homosexuality, which he claimed resulted
from psychopathological or neuropathological conditions.[15]

The nineteenth-century French physician Paul Moreau set out to explain
the pathological origins of such a congenital reversal of sexual feeling. He
argued that human beings had six senses instead of the usual five; in addition
to sight, hearing, taste, smell, and touch, humans also had a genital sense,
and this, like the other five, could be injured psychically as well as physically.
Thus people could be born sexually deficient, just as they could be born
deaf or blind; they could also be born with a predisposition to perversion,
just as others might be born with defective eyesight that required glasses.
Such a predisposition could be further provoked by particular environmental
conditions, but in any case it was purely pathological. Certain periods in
life were also more traumatic than others. Puberty and the approach of
senility were times of particular trauma for those predisposed to
homosexuality. People in hot climates, Moreau claimed, were more disposed
to lasciviousness than those in more temperate zones, and also were more
likely to fall victim to perversions. In his mind, pederasts, sodomites, sapphists
(lesbians), and others similarly labeled were a class separate and distinct
from the rest of humankind, forming a kind of intermediate category,

constituting a real link or union between reason and madness, the nature
and existence of which can most frequently be replaced only by one word:
heredity. . . . Not infrequently, under the influence of some vice or organism,
generally of heredity, the moral faculties may undergo alterations, which,
if they do not actually destroy the social relations of individuals, as happens
in case of declared insanity, yet modify them to a remarkable degree, and
certainly demand to be taken into account, when we have to estimate
the morality of these acts.[16]

This explanation led Moreau to conclude that aberrations of the sexual
sense were matters for the medical profession rather than for the courts,
and should be subject to therapeutic treatment rather than punishment. To
this end he urged that representatives of the medical faculty sit upon the
bench as advisers or assessors to deal with persons accused of outrages
against decency. Sexual inversion, in effect, was a symptom of hereditary
weakness, as were nymphomania, satyriasis, bestiality, and the profanation
of corpses. To save the victims of such illness from prison, it was essential
that they be delivered to an asylum.

The belief that the life cycle of the individual recapitulates the evolutionary development of the human species was used as further evidence
of the pathological nature of homosexuality. Since it was believed that organic
life had moved from the self-fertilizing to the bisexual to the heterosexual
stage, it was inevitable that homosexuality would be looked upon as a stage
of arrested development. The Italian psychiatrist and criminologist Cesare
Lombroso (1836–1909) put this in its most extreme form. He held that
humans represented an advanced stage of animal life, but in the process
of evolution some degenerate forms of humanity had been left at lower
levels. As evidence of this hypothesis, Lombroso pointed out that acts regarded
as criminal in civilized societies were natural among animals and common
among many primitive peoples. With the growth of society and civilization,
and as humans reached ever higher stages of evolution, the more advanced
of the species outgrew robbery, murder, promiscuity, and sexual "perversion."
Since, however, each child at birth had to repeat the evolution of society
to become civilized, it was inevitable that some would fail and become
criminals, sexual deviants, or mental defectives. These born criminals or
"perverts" were "morally insane," and were to be treated not by being punished
but by being sequestered in asylums and prevented from perpetuating their
species. In effect, they were a medical problem.[17]

Krafft-Ebing believed that, while sexuality was a powerful motivating force in society, it was absolutely necessary to restrain it. Religion, law, education, and morality had all cooperated to help bridle the animal lust potentially present in human beings.[18] In spite of this, individuals were ever in danger of sinking from the clear height of pure, chaste love into the mire of common sensuality. The retention of a person's morality involved a constant struggle; only those characters endowed with a strong will were able to emancipate themselves from sensuality and share in the pure love from which, Krafft-Ebing said, sprang "the noblest joys of human life."[19]

Krafft-Ebing took many of his ideas on homosexuality from Ulrichs, and though he subscribed in part to a biological cause, Krafft-Ebing also felt that certain behavior patterns, such as masturbation, also were crucial factors in its development. By the twelfth edition of his work, Krafft-Ebing had collected over two hundred cases of "abnormal" or "pathological" individuals, falling into the broad categories of fetishism, homosexuality, sadism, and masochism, but included as well were satyriasis, nymphomania, exhibitionism, voyeurism, and zoophilia. According to Krafft-Ebing, individuals who engaged in almost any kind of nonprocreative sex were afflicted with a "hereditary taint" or suffered from "moral degeneracy," and hence performed sexual acts of a psychopathic nature. Edward Brecher has gone so far as to argue that Krafft-Ebing made sex itself a loathsome disease[20]; however, Krafft-Ebing was only one of many physicians who worried about the dangers of nonprocreative sex. These men of medicine believed that by institutionalizing such individuals, they were helping them.

Both Magnus Hirschfeld and Havelock Ellis in the early twentieth century challenged Krafft-Ebing's concepts; both argued that homosexuality was but one aspect of being human. Hirschfeld still subscribed to a third sex theory,[21] while Ellis looked to multiple factors. Ellis felt that homosexuality could be both inborn and acquired, physical and psychological, and that such deviations from the norm could be harmless and perhaps even valuable.[22] Sigmund Freud (1856–1939), who, as much as anyone, has influenced twentieth-century attitudes about sex, regarded homosexuality as a variant pattern that was not necessarily pathological. It was nothing to be ashamed of, not a vice, not a degradation, not even an illness; moreover, many respectable individuals of the past and present had been and were homosexuals. When a mother wrote to Freud about her son, he told her that psychoanalysis probably would not "cure him" of his homosexuality; but if he was unhappy, torn by conflict, or neurotic, psychoanalysis might help him to come to terms with himself.[23]

In spite of Freud's position, the psychiatric community in the United

States looked upon homosexuality as an illness. In this, they were particularly influenced by Sandor Rado, who claimed Freud had made a fundamental error in his acceptance of potential bisexuality in humans, Rado went on to argue that homosexuality represented the dethroning of the normal heterosexual nature of human beings, something that could be brought about only by "schizophrenic disorganization."[24] To his mind, homosexuality was essentially a phobic response to members of the opposite sex, an interpretation that led Rado to adopt a more optimistic view of therapeutic "cure."

A number of psychoanalysts influenced by this view attempted to research homosexuality. One of the more ambitious attempts was carried out in the 1950s by the New York Society of Medical Psychoanalysts, which did a collaborative systematic study of a large number of their patients. Some seventy-seven psychiatrists contributed information on 106 homosexual and 100 heterosexual patients, the data on each being summarized in a 450-item questionnaire. The results were summarized by Irving Bieber, who reported that homosexuality was an adaption to "highly pathologic parent-child relationships and early life situations."[25] Particularly important in establishing such a pathological relationship was the mother-son relationship, which often inhibited the development of normal peer relationships with other boys and with the father. These boys were often effeminate, and did not relate well to their fathers. The fathers failed in turn to meet their sons' needs for affection and helped create a pathologic need which could only be satisfied through homosexuality.[26] Bieber also reported that a pattern of feminine behavior was often found in men who later became homosexual.

Bieber's findings describing the early pattern of gender nonconformity in homosexual men were ignored for a time as psychiatrists focused their attention on the illness model. The most extreme among them was Charles Socarides, who held that homosexuality was profoundly pathological. He argued that almost half of those who engage in homosexual practices have a concomitant schizophrenia, paranoia, a latent or pseudoneurotic schizophrenia, or are in the throes of a manic-depressive reaction. The rest were simply neurotic.[27] Socarides was much more combative than Bieber or others, as well as highly critical of psychotherapists who would help homosexuals adapt to their pathology.[28]

Such findings were based on wild generalizations and long-standing cultural prejudice. One of the difficulties was that psychiatry, as a client-oriented profession, was not well suited to research. Although Bieber made an attempt to go beyond his own practice by a collaborative study and an elaborate questionnaire, the members of the homosexual sample were all being treated by psychiatrists who were essentially committed to the belief that homosexuality could be successfully treated.

THE UNDERMINING OF THE PATHOLOGICAL MODEL

Even as the psychiatrists were carrying out their studies, their stand was being severely undermined by Alfred Kinsey, who in his studies found that homosexuality and lesbianism were not isolated phenomena, and that many people who later tended to lean toward heterosexuality, had experienced enjoyment with persons of their own sex. Kinsey's statistics indicated that 37 percent of the males in his sample had had same-sex experience to point of orgasm at some time in their lives. Among males who remained single past the age of thirty-five, half of the group reported overt homosexual experiences. Four percent of Kinsey's sample were labeled as exclusively homosexual.[29] Women were found to have had somewhat less homosexual experience than men. Only 28 percent reported homosexual arousal by age forty-five and only 13 percent had actually reached orgasm. Less than 3 percent were exclusively homosexual.[30]

The most recent survey, published in 1994, found somewhat lower figures but the authors raised doubts about their own findings. This is because though less than 3 percent of their sample identified as homosexual, they found that in the fifty largest cities the response rate was much higher, about 9 percent. Since such cities were underrepresented in their sample, the incidence overall probably begins to approach the Kinsey figure of 4 percent. Similarly the authors found lower incidences for females in their sample, less than 2 percent, although lesbians, while concentrated in the larger cities, were more evenly spread through the population. Probably the lesbian figures begin to approach the 3 percent found by Kinsey.[31] A major problem, however, remains in the sampling. The authors of the latest study wanted to more than double their present sample to get accurate data, but, since funding was not available to do so, they went with what they had. Also important is how the question is asked, and what is classified as homosexual conduct. This problem concerned the authors as well, and they are cautious in regarding any of their figures as final.

Also important in undermining the conceptualization of homosexuality as an illness was a study published in 1957 by Evelyn Hooker, a psychologist, who did a double-blind study of thirty male homosexuals with a nonhomosexual control group. She tested both groups using the projective psychological techniques that psychologists then used, and found that a panel of experts could not tell the homosexuals from the heterosexuals. They both appeared equally "normal."[32]

Martin Weinberg and Colin J. Williams, in their pioneering study of homosexuality in the United States, the Netherlands, and Denmark, found that most homosexuals passed in the everyday world as heterosexuals, and that many of the psychological problems associated with homosexuality were more the result of worrying about exposure and anticipating sanctions against them than with homosexuality itself.[33]

Probably the most comprehensive study of the social factors related to sexual preference was done in the 1970s by Alan Bell, Martin Weinberg, and Sue Hammersmith in San Francisco. Using path analysis they studied a sample of 979 homosexual men and women recruited from bars and steam baths, homosexual organizations, personal contact, mailing lists, and public advertising. These were compared with a random sample of 477 heterosexuals. Lesbians and gay men were more likely to report poor relationships with their fathers than heterosexual members of the study group, but it is not clear whether this separation was initiated by the father or the child, or whether it was a part of the causal sequence or a consequence of the child's failure to conform to gender norms. A common element in the childhoods of both men and women was a pattern of childhood gender nonconformity with lesbians fitting into a "tomboy" image and gay men going through a period of effeminate behavior. Homosexual preference usually developed in the teen years although there was no evidence that this was due to a lack of opportunity for heterosexual interaction.[34] Gay men were found to be less self-accepting and more lonely, depressed, and tense than heterosexual men, perhaps because societal pressure had helped make them so. Lesbians shared with other women the psychological difficulties of being female, although like their male counterparts they had lower self-esteem and more suicidal thoughts than did their heterosexual counterparts.[35] In spite of these generalizations there were great variations in childhood experiences and present lifestyles among the members of the study group. Because of this Weinberg and Bell argued that the term "homosexual" was misleading. Their first book describing the research was aptly titled, then, *Homosexualities* to emphasize the variations they found.

The findings related to the youthful patterns of gender nonconformity among lesbians and gays is interesting because it suggests a relationship between gender behavior and sexual preference. Although the folk wisdom has always held this to be true, the experts denied it for a time.[36] However, recent research documents the fact that both gay men and lesbians often go through a phase of gender nonconformity as children.[37] The most comprehensive longitudinal study was done by Richard Green who followed fifty feminine boys who had been referred to the University of California, Los Angeles, gender center. These boys had all started cross-dressing as girls very early (94 percent by age six); they played with dolls, preferred girl playmates, and indicated they wished they had been born girls.[38] When they reached their adult years three-fourths of the members of the sample who could be located indicated they were homosexual, with only one homosexual man in the fifty member-matched control group.[39] Another interesting facet of the studies of feminine boys is that although many or most of them are homosexual as adults, they are usually not overtly feminine. Most of them go through a defeminization process during adolescence. Joseph Harry points out that social class is a major factor in determining which of the feminine boys go through the transition to take on masculine demeanor, with working-class men more likely to remain feminine than those from a higher socioeconomic level.[40]

To date there has been no longitudinal study of girls who are tomboys, probably because cross-gender behavior in girls is considered less problematic. Frederick Whitam and Robin Mathy have, however, done retrospective studies of homosexual and heterosexual women in four societies: Brazil, Peru, the Philippines, and the United States. All four groups were volunteers located through clubs, bars, professional groups, student groups, or friendships. In all four societies lesbians were much more likely than heterosexual women to have been called tomboys, played with boy's toys, and played dress-up in men's clothing. The heterosexual women were more likely to have paid attention to women's fashions, and played dress-up in women's clothing. The authors consider these cross-gender childhood behaviors to be precursor patterns for women who later develop a lesbian lifestyle.[41]

The very early development of cross-gender behavior, and its link to later homosexual patterns, suggests the involvement of a genetic factor in the development of homosexuality. Also supporting the idea that there is a genetic factor is the fact that lesbians and gay men are more likely to have homosexual relatives than would occur by chance. This is particularly true among twins.[42] An early twin study was done in 1952 by Franz J. Kallman involving two sets of twins, one identical and one fraternal. In the 113 sets of twins, 100 percent of the monozygotic (single egg) twins were concordant for sexual orientation while only a third of the dizygotic (two egg) twins had the same sexual orientation.[43] An ongoing study started in 1980 by

Frederick L. Whitam, Milton Diamond, and James Martin includes sixty-one pairs of twins. The researchers sought out lesbians and gay men who were either identical or fraternal twins, to determine whether the other twin also had a same-sex preference. The identical twins were concordant for sexual preference 68 percent of the time while the fraternal twins had the same-sex pattern as their twin 30 percent of the time.[44] These high percentages of concordance, particularly among the monozygotic twins, is a powerful argument for a genetic factor in the causal sequence for homosexuality.[45]

The physiological mechanism by which the genetic influences on sex are translated into actual behavior is probably neurohormonal. This assumption is based on a vast and growing literature documenting the hormonal influence on gender behavior and the impact of prenatal hormones on the brain. The sex hormones are the messengers that cause bodily reactions interpreted as masculine and feminine. These hormones in turn exert influence on neural pathways and the neural endocrine axis (the link between the hypothalamus, the pituitary gland, and the other endocrine glands).[46] These neural pathways control future hormonal production and consequently influence sexual behavior.[47]

Human embryos of both sexes develop in an identical fashion for the first two months of gestation. Chromosomal sex, established at the time of conception, guides the process and directs the development of either ovaries or testes. If testes develop, their hormonal secretions direct the development of male secondary characteristics. Without the hormones from the testes, the embryo remains female. However, given the appropriate genetic message, slightly more than half of the embryos will secrete androgens which trigger and support differentiation into males.[48]

As the research continues and additional hormones and processes are identified, it becomes apparent that the prenatal course of development is complex and that variations in the pattern occur.[49] One type of research that is particularly relevant here is the studies by Anke Ehrhardt and Heino Meyer-Balburg of children with congenital adrenal hyperplasia, a genetic defect that prevents the adrenal cortex from synthesizing cortisone. Instead the cortex is stimulated to release excess adrenal androgens both before and after birth. If the child is a genetic female her external genitalia are masculinized. If the child is a genetic male his external genitalia are normal. Treatment is with cortisone, which suppresses the excess androgens. Studies of the girls who started treatment when they were born (so they would no longer be exposed to excess androgen) are of particular interest because they provide a natural experiment to assess the effect of prenatal male hormones on a female fetus. Ehrhardt and Meyer-Bahlburg report that these girls differ significantly from siblings and other controls. They enjoy rough-and-tumble play, associate with male peers, and they are identified by self and others as tomboys. They show low interest in role rehearsals for the wife and mother roles. The boys who had extra male hormones before birth exhibited higher energy expenditure in sports, and were somewhat more likely to initiate fights than their peers.[50] The fact that the masculinizing influence remains after the hormonal stimulation has ceased may mean that the neural pathways controlling masculinity and femininity have been affected.[51]

Biological processes are not, however, the final word. They are further influenced by the socialization process which shapes people into their assigned gender roles. While socialization takes place primarily in the small group settings such as the family and the peer group, the patterns for socialization tend to be provided by the broader culture. Sometimes the cultural patterns are outdated (cultural lag), but they remain powerful forces even when they may be dysfunctional to the goals of the society and the individual.

The findings described above suggest that a homosexual or lesbian identity is the result of a complex set of interacting variables including genetic, physiological, psychosocial, and cultural factors. No single microorganism or set of experiences can stand alone, so a model that looks upon the behavior as an illness to be treated is not very useful. This is probably the best reason for removing homosexuality from the list of psychiatric illnesses. However, logic does not always prevail; the change was probably due more to political factors, which are related to changing public opinion.

THE EFFECTS OF CHANGING PUBLIC ATTITUDES AND THE RISE OF GAY AND LESBIAN ORGANIZATIONS

A major factor in changing public attitudes was the growing militancy of the gays and lesbians themselves. Organizations struggling for the rights of homosexuals appeared late in the nineteenth century in Germany; Magnus Hirschfeld was particularly important in their organization. Hirschfeld also began publishing in 1904 the first journal devoted to the study of homosexuality. Other groups appeared in Europe, although their existence was often precarious. The oldest continuous group is that associated with the publication *Der Kreis* (*The Circle*) which started in Zurich in 1932. A Dutch organization, originally affiliated with Hirschfeld's Scientific Humanitarian

Committee in Berlin, had an older history but it disappeared with the Nazi occupation and was revived in new form after the end of the war. The Dutch group also began publishing *Vriendschap* in 1949 and, a short time later, *Lesbos,* a lesbian-oriented publication, one of the earliest to deal specifically with lesbian issues.

Progress was not easy, since even the most innocuous group could be made to sound sinister to a significant number of Europeans and Americans. This happened to the International Committee for Sexual Equality (ICSE) founded in Holland in 1951. The anti-homosexual writer R. E. L. Masters called the ICSE "by far the most powerful body in the history of homosexual organizations, one that may control to an extent of which few even dream the policies and organizational activities of homosexual groups throughout the world."[52] This was pure sensationalism not based on any real facts except that the ICSE did exist and did try to act as a sort of clearinghouse for the exchange of opinion and information.

In the United States most of the early homosexual organizations began under innocuous-sounding titles not only for their own protection but because they could do little. The telephone company, for example, refused to list any group with "homosexual" in its title until the late 1960s, and it was even later before the terms "gay," "lesbian," and "homosexuality" could be listed in any public directory or be the subject for discussion in a news story.

Real organizational activity in the United States appeared in the aftermath of World War II, much of it centered in Los Angeles. The most long-lasting of the groups to appear was the Mattachine Foundation, a semi-secret group founded by Harry Hay in 1950, and which, under a revised charter adopted in 1953, spread nationally. Some of those associated with the Mattachine group began publishing the magazine *One* in 1952. This was soon followed by other organizations and publications, including the Lesbian Daughters of Bilitis and its publication, the *Ladder.* Numerous other groups appeared all over the country as gay men and lesbians became more vocal and agitation for change mounted.

Other factors liberalizing attitudes were at work besides the findings of researchers in the field. There had been a basic shift in public opinion from pronatalism to a more neutral policy. Belatedly the realization was growing that the world was overpopulated and that natural resources were not inexhaustible. With the size of the average family declining, the availability of effective contraceptives and the legalization of abortion made it easier for a couple to limit the number of children. If reproduction is regarded as an individual option rather than a societal requirement, as it increasingly is, then it is possible for a couple to choose to be childless. At the same time there has been a more open acceptance of varied sexuality in our society. If procreation is not the aim, and sex is good, it seems a logical next step to accept nonprocreative sex between persons of the same sex.

Many religious and other groups began to question the traditional policy toward homosexuals. The American Civil Liberties Union (ACLU) in 1964 in its Los Angeles affiliate, and on a national level in 1965, came out for change in the laws dealing with homosexuality.[53] The American Friends Service Committee, also in 1964, argued that the quality of human relations was more important than the sex of one's partner.[54] A British parliamentary commission, known as the Wolfenden Commission, recommended that discrimination in employment against those labeled as homosexual be eliminated and that sexual behavior between consenting adults be decriminalized.[55] A similar recommendation was made by the American Law Institute and by the Ninth International Congress on Criminal Law. A special taskforce set up by the National Institute of Mental Health also urged that discrimination against homosexuals be eliminated and that sexual behavior between consenting adults be decriminalized.[56]

It was against this background of increasing activity that on June 27, 1969, the so-called Stonewall riots occurred in New York City. They resulted from a raid on a gay bar called the Stonewall which, unlike most previous raids, met with considerable resistance. A protest against the police action was organized for the next day and four days of confrontation followed. Out of this came the Gay Liberation Front. The importance of the Stonewall demonstrations was magnified in that they occurred in the media capital of the world, forcing the media at last to recognize and come to terms with homosexuality. In this sense they also marked a change in media attitude and ultimately in public attitudes, similar to that which followed the riots in the Watts district of Los Angeles in 1965. Also, the demonstrations marked the willingness of gays and lesbians to take a stand publicly. Once gays and lesbians recognized their potential power and increased freedom, it was found that they failed to conform to the pathological stereotypes so long proclaimed by the medical community and accepted by the public at large. Their numbers included liberals and conservatives, people who were flamboyant and those more reserved, lifelong companions and those who played the field. Organizations have proliferated to meet the needs of each. AIDS, and the early erroneous information about it, served as a further impetus to the gay and lesbian community; moreover, it made even the most uninformed of the general public aware that homosexuality and lesbianism existed and were widespread.

The example of gays and lesbians has not gone unnoticed by members of various other groups whose sexual behavior is stigmatized. Transvestites and transsexuals have set up their own organizations and have increasingly gone public. They have reached the point where homosexuality was in the late 1960s, out of the closet but not yet cognizant of their potential political clout.

CONCLUSION

As research into human sexuality progresses, we have become increasingly aware of how varied human sexual behavior is. Some forms, such as child molestation and rape, as well as some of the extreme versions of sadism, pose greater dangers to society than others, but individuals with variant sexual behavior can deal with their problems and function in society. Increasingly, behavior that has been stigmatized as pathological is no longer visualized in quite the same way. As society becomes freer in dealing with sexual behavior, and as past inhibitions are removed, an even wider range of sexual variants will manifest itself, at least temporarily, and organizations will grow up to lobby for various sexual causes. This raises a question: What kind of sexual behavior will continue to be stigmatized? Some undoubtedly will remain classified as pathological by the medical and psychiatric professions, until more evidence is accumulated to remove them from the list of diagnoses, but the number will surely decrease.

The question remains, however, whether behavior no longer considered pathological should be sanctioned by society at large. Probably society will have to make a conscious decision about what constitutes acceptable sexual behavior. The obvious rational basis for such a decision should be whether or not a particular behavior is harmful to others. When two or more persons are involved the answer also depends on whether each of them is mature enough to make a reasonable and voluntary decision. But the fact that behavior is nonprocreative or that it was once given a diagnostic label by an overzealous medical community should no longer constitute a reason for stigmatizing it.

NOTES

1. Richard von Krafft-Ebing, *Psychopathia Sexualis,* translated from the seventh enlarged and revised German edition by Gilbert Chaddock (Philadelphia: F. A. Davis, 1894), p. 1. The first edition appeared in 1887 and the twelfth in 1902. This statement remained more or less the same in each edition.

2. John Money, *Lovemaps: Clinical Concepts of Sexual/Erotic Health and Pathology, Paraphilia, and Gender Transposition in Childhood, Adolescence, and Maturity* (Amherst, N.Y.: Prometheus Books, 1986).

3. Havelock Ellis, *Erotic Symbolism, Studies in the Psychology of Sex,* 2 vols. in one (New York: Random House, 1936), 2, part 1: 57.

4. Howard S. Becker, *Outsiders; Studies in the Sociology of Deviance* (New York: The Free Press of Glencoe, 1963), p. 9.

5. Heinrich Kramer (Institoris) and James Sprenger, *The Malleus maleficarum,* translated by Montague Summers (reprint New York: Dover Publications, 1971).

6. A classic study of some of these societies can be found in Edward Sagarin, *Odd Man In: Societies of Deviants in America* (Chicago: Quadrangle Books, 1969).

7. E. Lasègue, "Les Exhibtionistes," *L'Union médicale,* May 1877.

8. Among the studies on incest we have consulted are Herbert Maische, *Incest,* translated by Colin Beame (New York: Stein and Day, 1972); R. E. L. Masters, *Patterns of Incest* (New York: Julian Press, 1963); Bernard J. Oliver, *Sexual Deviation in American Society* (New Haven: Yale University Press, 1967); Emile Durkheim, *Incest: The Nature and Origin of the Taboo,* translated by Edward Sagarin together with Albert Ellis in *The Origin and Development of the Incest Taboo* (New York: Lyle Stuart, 1963); Robin Fox, *The Red Lamp of Incest* (New York: Dutton, 1980); and W. Arens, *Original Sin: Incest and Its Meaning* (New York: Oxford University Press, 1986).

9. See S. Graham, *A Lecture on Epidemic Diseases Generally, and Particularly the Spasmodic Cholera* (Boston: C. H. Pierce, 1848), and S. Graham, *A Lecture to Young Men on Chastity, Intended also for the Serious Consideration of Parents and Guardians,* 10th ed. (Boston: D. Campbell, 1938).

10. M. [Claude-François] Lallemand, *On Involuntary Seminal Discharge,* translated by William Wood (Philadelphia: A. Waldier, 1839).

11. William Acton, *The Functions and Disorders of the Reproductive Organs in Childhood, Youth, Adult Age, and Advanced Life Considered in Their Physiological, Social, and Moral Relations,* 5th ed. (London: J. A. Churchill, 1871).

12. George M. Beard, *Sexual Neurasthenia, Its Hygiene, Causes, Symptoms, and Treatment with a Chapter on Diet for the Nervous,* edited by A. D. Rockwell (New York: E. B. Treat, 1884).

13. Karl Heinrich Ulrichs, *Forschungen über das Rätsel der mannmännlichen Liebe* (reprint Leipzig: Max Spohr, 1898). This was translated into English by Michael Lombardi-Nash as *The Riddle of "Man-Manly" Love: The Pioneering Work on Male Homosexuality,* 2 vols. (Amherst, N.Y.: Prometheus Books, 1994).

14. Karoly Maria Kertbeny published two anonymous pamphlets campaigning against the German laws on homosexuality. They were titled *143 des preussichsen Strafgesetbuchs und seine Aufrechterhaltung als 152 des Entwurfs eines Strafgesetzbuchs für den norddeutschen Bund* and *Das Gemeinschädliche des 143 des preussischen Strafgesetzbuches.* These were reprinted in *Jahrbuch für Sexual Zwischenstufen* 7 (1905): 3–66.

15. K. von Westphal, "Die konträre Sexualempfindung," *Archiven für Psychiatrie und Nervenkrankheiten* 2 (1869): 73–108.

16. Paul Moreau, *Des aberrations du sens génétique* Paris: Asslin & Houzeau, 1887).

17. Cesare Lombroso, *Criminal Man* (reprint Montclair, N.J.: Patterson Smith, 1972).

18. Krafft-Ebing, *Psychopathia Sexualis,* p. 1.

19. Ibid., p. 5.

20. Edward M. Brecher, *The Sex Researchers* (Boston: Little, Brown and Company, 1969), p. 21.

21. Magnus Hirschfeld, *Die Homosexualität des Mannes und des Weibes,* 2d ed. (Berlin: Louis Marcus Verlasgsbuchhandlung, 1920).

22. Havelock Ellis, *The Nature of Sexual Inversion,* in the *Psychology of Sex,* 2 vols. (reprint New York: Random House, 1936), 1: 347.

23. "Historical Notes: A Letter from Freud," *American Journal of Psychiatry,* 107 (April 1951): 786–87.

24. Sandor Rado, *Psychoanalysis of Behavior II* (New York: Grune & Stratton, 1962), p. 206.

25. Irving Bieber et al., *Homosexuality; A Psychoanalytic Study of Male Homosexuals* (New York: Basic Books, 1962), p. 173.

26. Ibid., pp. 79–80, 84, 114–15.

27. Charles Socarides, *The Overt Homosexual* (New York: Grune and Stratton, 1968), p. 90 and *passim.*

28. Charles Socarides, *Beyond Sexual Freedom* (New York: Quadrangle Books, 1975).

29. Alfred Kinsey, Wardell B. Pomeroy, and Clyde E. Martin, *Sexual Behavior in the Human Male* (Philadelphia: W. B. Saunders, 1948), pp. 651.

30. Alfred C. Kinsey, Wardell B. Pomeroy, Clyde E. Martin, and Paul H. Gebhard, *Sexual Behavior in the Human Female* (Philadelphia: W. B. Saunders, 1953), pp. 474–75.

31. Edward O. Laumann, John H. Gagnon, Robert T. Michael, and Stuart Michaels, *The Social Organization of Sexuality* (Chicago: University of Chicago Press, 1994).

32. Evelyn Hooker, "The Adjustment of the Male Overt Homosexual," *Journal of Projective Techniques* 21 (1957): 18–31, and reprinted, among other places, in Hendrik M. Ruitenbeek, ed., *The Problem of Homosexuality in Modern Society* (New York: E. P. Dutton, 1963), pp. 141–61.

33. Martin S. Weinberg and Colin J. Williams, *Male Homosexuals: Their Problems and Adaptations* (New York: Oxford University Press, 1974), pp. 267–71.

34. Alan P. Bell, Martin S. Weinberg, and Sue Kiefer Hammersmith, *Sexual Preference, Its Development in Men and Women* (Bloomington, Ind.: University of Indiana Press, 1981).

35. Alan P. Bell and Martin S. Weinberg, *Homosexualities* (New York: Simon and Schuster, 1978); see also Bell, Weinberg, and Hammersmith, *Sexual Preference.*

36. John Money and Anke Ehrhardt, *Man and Woman: Boy and Girl* (Baltimore: Johns Hopkins Press, 1972).

37. Bernard Zuger, "Effeminate Behavior Present in Boys from Childhood: Ten Additional Years of Follow-Up," *Comparative Psychiatry* 19 (1978): 363–69; Phil S. Lebovitz, "Feminine Behavior in Boys: Aspects of Its Outcome," *American Journal of Psychiatry* 128 (April 1972): 1283–89; Charles W. Davenport, "A Follow-Up Study of 10 Feminine Boys," *Archives of Sexual Behavior* 15 (1986): 1283–89.

38. Richard Green, "One Hundred-Ten Feminine and Masculine Boys: Behavior Contrasts and Demographic Similarities," *Archives of Sexual Behabior* 5 (1976): 425–46.

39. Richard Green, *The "Sissy Boy Syndrome" and the Development of Homosexuality* (New Haven: Yale University Press, 1987).

40. Joseph Harry, "Defeminization and Adult Psychological Well-Being among Male Homosexuals," *Archives of Sexual Behavior* 12 (1983): 1–19.

41. Frederick L. Whitam and Robin M. Mathy, "Childhood Cross-Gender Behavior of Homosexual Females in Brazil, Peru, The Philippines, and the United States," *Archives of Sexual Behavior* 20 (1991): 151–70.

42. Richard C. Pillard, Jeannette Poumadere, and Ruth A. Carretta, "Is Homosexuality Familial? A Review, Some Data and a Suggestion," *Archives of Sexual Behavior* 19 (1981): 465–75.

43. Franz J. Kallman, "Comparitive Twin Study of the Genetic Aspects of Male Homosexuality," *Journal of Nervous and Mental Disease* 115 (1952): 283–98.

44. Frederick L. Whitman, Milton Diamond, and James Martin, "Homosexual Orientation in Twins: A Report of 61 Pairs and Three Triplet Sets," *Archives of Sexual Behavior* 22 (1993): 187–206.

45. Judd Marmor, "Overview: The Multiple Roots of Homosexual Behavior," *Homosexual Behavior: A Modern Reappraisal* (New York: Basic Books, 1980): 3–22.

46. "News and Comment: Is Homosexuality Biological," *Science* 253 (August 30, 1991): 253, 257–59.

47. A. P. Arnold and R. A. Gorski, "Gonadal Steroid Induction of Structural Sex Differences in the Central Nervous System," *Annual Review of Neuroscience* 7 (1984): 413–22; John Bancroft, "The Relationship between Hormones and Sexual Behavior in Humans," in *Biological Determinants of Sexual Behavior,* edited by J. B. Hutchison (New York: John Wiley & Sons, 1978), pp. 494–519.

48. Jean D. Wilson, Frederick W. George, and James E. Griffin, "The Hormonal Control of Sexual Development," *Science* 211 (March 20, 1981): 1278–84.

49. Richard C. Pillard and James D. Weinrich, "The Periodic Table of the Gender Transpositions: Part I. A Theory Based on Masculinization and Defeminization of the Brain," *The Journal of Sex Research* 23 (November 1987): 425–54.

50. Anke A. Ehrhardt and Heino F. L. Meyer-Bahlburg, "Effects of Prenatal Sex Hormones on Gender-Related Behavior," *Science* 211 (March 1981): 1312–17.

51. Gunther Dorner, Wolfgang Rohde, Fritz Stahl, Lothar Krell, and Wolf-Gunther Masius, "A Neuroendocrine Predisposition for Homosexuality in Men," *Archives of Sexual Behavior* 4 (1975): 1–8.

52. R. E. L. Masters, *The Homosexual Revolution* (New York: Julian Press, 1962), p. 39. Master's books is a mixture of information and misinformation. Much more accurate is the doctoral dissertation of Edward Sagarin, "Structure and Ideology in an Association of Deviants" (unpublished Ph.D. dissertation, New York University, 1966). Particularly helpful is *Homosexuals Today: A Handbook of Organizations and Publications,* edited by Marvin Cutler (Los Angeles: One, Inc., 1956). See also John Lauritsen and David Thorstad, *The Early Homosexual Rights Movement (1869–1939)* (Albion, Calif.: Time-Change Press, 1974).

53. Vern L. Bullough, one of the authors of this book, wrote the ACLU policy of Southern California policy on the matter. See Vern L. Bullough, "Homosexuality and the American Civil Liberties Union," *Journal of Homosexuality* 13 (1986): 23–32.

54. *Towards a Quaker View of Sex* (London: Friends Home Service Committee, 1964).

55. *Report of the Committee on Homosexual Offenses and Prostitution,* Sir John Wolfenden, chair (London: Her Majesty's Stationery Office, 1957).

56. *National Institute of Mental Health Task Force on Homosexuality: Final Report and Background Papers,* edited by John M. Livingood (Rockville, Md.: National Institute of Mental Health, 1972). The publication of the report was delayed but versions of it appeared in the gay community long before it was published. One of great regrets is that we were asked to prepare a report for the committee on the history of homosexuality; but being overseas at the time, we could not meet the time commitment and so had to decline.

13

Sex in a Changing World

It is not only attitudes toward homosexuality that have changed, and it is not necessarily research that leads to challenges to traditional ideology. In this concluding chapter we will review changing attitudes toward a variety of sexual practices and how these changes reflect those in society at large.

NUDITY

We begin with nudity where attitudes have changed radically in the twentieth century, so much so that, beyond the voyeuristic attitudes often present in the first stages of nudism, some would claim that sexuality itself is not involved. Historically, however, nudity represents a case of conflicting attitudes in Western culture, with sexuality being very much part of this concern. Put simply, Judaism had been strongly opposed to nudity, while the Graeco-Roman tradition, with certain limitations, specifically in the case of women, had looked upon it favorably. In general, the Jewish tradition, which was incorporated into Christianity, became dominant in Western culture with the exception of the plastic arts, where the classical influence predominated. There was one notable difference, however, namely, the decided preference for the female nude over the male, particularly from the sixteenth century onward. Some have claimed that this occurred because the female contours offered greater interest and challenge to artists, but this seems doubtful. Others have argued that since the female genitalia were less visible than the male, they were less offensive, and since nursing mothers exposed their breasts for all to see, breasts were not so erotically charged as they later became. It is also possible that the homophobic attitudes of Western Christianity discouraged the depiction of male nudity on the grounds that such portrayals might somehow have homosexual connotations. On the other hand, since sculptors and their patrons were almost overwhelmingly male, the female nude might well have become dominant because patrons found the female figure more erotically stimulating than the more homosexually oriented Greeks had done. In short, we have no definitive answer to the question.

The attitude of the ancient Hebrews to nakedness is stated very early in Genesis, where it is emphasized that Adam and Eve in the Garden of Eden "were both naked . . . and were not ashamed."[1] Such innocence about sexual differences changed when the couple tasted the fruit of the tree of knowledge of good and evil and the "eyes of both of them were opened, and they knew that they were naked; and they sewed fig leaves together and made themselves aprons."[2] This revulsion over nudity became so deeply engrained among the early Hebrews that a lack of clothing came to be a sign of shame and humiliation. For example, a husband who discovered that his wife was unfaithful to him was allowed to strip her naked and turn her out to public gaze in vengeful humiliation.[3] In late rabbinic writing it became traditional for the bodies of executed criminals to be hung up naked for public viewing,[4] emphasizing their disgrace.

Although the Greeks of Homer's time had not looked upon nudity with favor, the climate of opinion had changed by the sixth century B.C.E. when the nude male began to be celebrated in life and art. Nudity in athletic contests, for example, was confined to males, with the Spartans being the exception. Gradually the female nude began to appear in sculpture in the fifth century B.C.E., but such representations remained rare.[5] Nudity in the male was regarded as godlike, with the unclothed Apollo representing the ideal proportions of man. Although the Romans initially were shocked by the nudity of Greek athletes, they soon adopted the Greek artistic models. As classical influence began to wane and Christian influence increase in the Graeco-Roman world, the concept of bodily perfection went into decline: the female nude disappeared in the second century C.E. and the male in the third.[6]

In its opposition to nudity, Christianity was not only influenced by Jewish scriptures, but was also reacting to the paganism of the Greeks and Romans, whose gods were often portrayed without clothing or only lightly draped. Christian attitudes likewise came under the spell of Platonic dualism, which we discussed in an earlier chapter. Nudity in this view was the ultimate material form emphasizing the degradation of the spiritual. Inevitably the body ceased to be the mirror of divine perfection and became an object of humiliation and shame. Still, matters are not so simple, and ambiguities remained if only because Christianity taught that Adam and Eve had been nude while in the state of innocence in the Garden of Eden; moreover, it was widely believed that humankind would appear naked in judgment before God. Thus throughout the medieval period there were often nude figures in art, although they were most often undergoing humiliation, martyrdom, or torture, or else suffering expulsion from Paradise.[7]

The belief in a nudity of innocence led to periodic outbursts among millennial cults such as the Adamites of the fourteenth century, who went naked in order to symbolize their association with Adam. Nakedness to them was essential to purity. They believed that only by going nude could the innocence of humans be restored.[8] But if nudity was associated with innocence among some heretical groups, it was more likely to be associated with sex in the public mind. In the medieval period the public baths, where individuals had to undress, were regarded as a beehive of prostitution. In spite of the attempts of authorities to insist on rigid seclusion of the sexes and periodic inspections, the reputation of such places is indicated by the fact that the terms "stew" and "bagnio" still remain euphemisms for brothels.[9]

Attitudes toward nudity in art shifted at the end of the medieval period, as classical influence regained some of its previous hegemony; by the sixteenth century, nude portraiture, particularly of the female, reached new heights. A brief reaction to nudity occurred during the seventeenth century, but only temporarily. The female nude soon made her appearance again, although there were relatively few male nudes. Interestingly enough, however, the nude appeared only in the art of certain European countries. In Spanish art, for example, only two portraits of nudes before the twentieth century are known to exist.[10]

Nudity in art is one thing, while nudity in real life is another. In all probability art did not reflect reality. That the medieval and early-modern periods regarded public nudity as something extraordinary is best indicated by the story of Lady Godiva, one of the best-known incidents of nudism in myth and legend. The story was first told by Roger of Wendover in the thirteenth century, some two hundred years after the event was supposed to have taken place. According to the story, Godiva had implored her husband to reduce the heavy taxes which he had imposed on Coventry. Her constant pleading with her husband on the subject led him to declare in exasperation that he would lower the taxes if his wife rode naked through the crowded marketplace, which she did. As the story was repeated by others new elements were added, including the legend of Peeping Tom, which became part of the story in the seventeenth century.[11]

There can also be observed some interesting double standards in nudity, since it was considered quite normal until well into the nineteenth century for men to swim in the nude at rivers or beaches provided they took reasonable care to be out of sight of women. No woman, however, would publicly expose herself in such a manner.

Modern nudism, sometimes called social nudity, made its appearance as a philosophical health movement. It is linked with the work of a young German intellectual, Richard Ungewitter, whose *Die Nacktheit* (*Nudity*) appeared in 1905. Unable to find a commercial publisher, Ungewitter initially issued the book on his own in order to inaugurate a utopian society where all persons would go without clothing, observe strict vegetarianism, and abstain from tobacco and alcohol. Nudism to Ungewitter was a panacea for the social problems afflicting modern civilization.[12] He had little scientific basis for his claims, although the simple act of getting the residents of the heavily industrialized cities into the countryside for fresh air and sunlight might well have had some therapeutic value. Ungewitter's book encouraged two fellow Germans with similar ideas to put his utopia into practice. Dr. Heinrich Pudor organized a nudist group called *Nackkultur,* publicizing his effort with a book by the same name (Berlin, 1906). Paul Zimmerman, another believer, opened the first nudist spa, the Freilichtparck, at Klingberg am See near Lübeck. From Germany, the movement spread into France and the Scandinavian countries, although its growth was slow until after World War I.

Early advocates of nudism put high on their list of goals the demystifying of the human body and the reintegration of the sex organs with the rest of the body. The emphasis, however, lay not so much on sexuality as on desexualization. Nudists of the time never tired of pointing out that the complete and unabashed practice of nudism was not an erotic experience; indeed, many went to almost puritanical lengths to make certain that no overt sexuality was associated with the movement. Most of the early nudist colonies refused to allow liquor, urged their members to follow health food diets, emphasized physical exercise in the open sunlight, and prohibited body contact between the sexes.

In the United States, nudism remained more or less underground until the 1930s, when newspapers discovered it and proceeded to sensationalize it. The *New York Times* initiated the media coverage in 1930 with a fairly accurate account of the French naturists, as they were called, which was soon followed by a series of articles on German nudists in the Scripps-Howard chain. Almost immediately the tabloid press began to exploit the subject, headlining "nudist cults" and "cavorting nudists" without offering much factual data.[13]

The first organizer of nudist activities in the United States was Kurt Barthel, a German immigrant, who had participated in nude groups in his homeland. Barthel, who established a nudist retreat in 1929, did not subscribe to all the dietary and athletic requirements associated with the German nudist movements. In part, as a result of Barthel's efforts and example, American nudism, as it began to spread, turned out to be more a social than a utopian movement. As publicity about nudist activities were sensationalized by the media, the nudist groups, especially concerned about charges of lewdness and indecency, turned to ever more stringent regulation of activities permitted on their grounds. Anything even indirectly sensual was prohibited for fear that a scandal might result. Touching became forbidden at most camps, and at some camps regulations were so strict that even married couples were forbidden to hold hands. Alcohol was prohibited, as was dancing in the nude, although several nudist camps allowed clothed dancing. Members called each other by their first names only, last names being kept secret. The result was a sexual denial far beyond that exercised by the culture at large. In fact, it became so important to deny a linkage between nudity and sex that the nudist movement came close to denying a link between nudism and life. This reign of sexual repression lasted until well into the 1960s, making nudists, in spite of their bodily exposure, much more repressive about sex than the general public. One English nudist, responding to a survey, felt enough was enough and was moved to complain:

> Please, please, please, let us be able to show some healthy affection for each other in front of our children—where one doesn't feel funny taking her husband's hand or holding him by the waist as we walk. This hands-off is so abnormal. Children see us hold hands at home, and when we come to camp we're ten feet away from each other and they wonder why! I'm sure this is a thing we married couples would not abuse and would use normally. . . .[14]

Undoubtedly one reason for their restriction on activities was that nudity was illegal in some states; even magazines depicting nudity were regarded as pornographic. *Sunshine and Health,* a magazine first published by nudists in America in 1933, fought a series of legal battles in which it finally emerged victorious in 1958. Ironically, once it had won, the magazine's circulation and influence dropped as it was being replaced by more stylishly produced publications that were taking advantage of the freedom it had won.[15]

Nudism itself changed as well, and many of the nudist groups that appeared in the post-World War II period emphasized touching and greater intimacy. Sexuality, which had so long been repressed in the nudist movement, began to play a more prominent role. Nude therapy was even encouraged, following the teaching of Abraham H. Maslow who held that

> nudism, simply going naked before a lot of other people, is itself a kind of therapy, especially if we can be conscious of it, that is, if there's a skilled person around to direct what's going on, to bring things to consciousness.[16]

Nude therapy became fashionable for a time, and several "growth centers" for nude encounter groups sprang up around the country. Nudists in turn began emphasizing their sense of emotional well-being instead of the physical well-being emphasized earlier. Many also took to painting and decorating their bodies.

In the 1980s organized nudism declined somewhat, although unorganized nudism continued to grow with the establishment of nude beaches in many areas of the country—not only on both coasts but along lakes and rivers. What had seemed revolutionary and obscene earlier was now increasingly accepted. Although organized nudism had to fight some important legal battles, the change in public attitudes seemed to be more reflective of the greater openness to and acceptance of sexuality per se, and in this the nudists themselves changed. Whether nudism is good for the health or the psyche seems to be something that each individual has to decide for himself or herself.

SADOMASOCHISM

Another area of change is the case of sadomasochism. Until diagnosed in the late nineteenth century, it received little attention and was not even classified as a sin. In fact, Christianity has always tolerated if not encouraged masochistic conduct, since many of its followers have tried to enact the suffering of Jesus by scourging themselves. Fasting, isolation, and all kinds of self-punishment were common among the early saints. Many deliberately sought martyrdom in order to demonstrate the strength of their faith. The belief in the need to suffer in turn led to the necessity of imposing punishment and suffering, and ultimately to sadism itself.[17] The suffering Jesus with the crown of thorns so often represented in art and sculpture can arouse both sadistic and masochistic responses.

Sadism derives its name from Louis Donatien François Alphonse de Sade (1740–1814), who several times during his life was arrested for acts of debauchery and violence, and at one time was sentenced to death in absentia. His reputation as a sadist, however, derives more from his novels than from his life. Most of these were written in prison or other institutions where de Sade spent nearly thirty years. Among his most famous novels are *Justine, Juliette,* and *120 Days of Sodom.* In them he attempted to systematically describe all forms of sexual diversion. Philosophically de Sade believed that pain excited the nerves more than joy and hence awakened a more lively thrill. He also believed that women had much greater potential for cruelty than men, because of the greater sensitivity of their sexual organs. Thus he often portrayed scenes in which a person found sexual pleasure in causing other people pain, or forcing them to submit to various forms of degrading behavior.[18] Other French writers followed de Sade's example, although to a lesser extent. Inevitably, Richard von Krafft-Ebing turned to French fiction to describe sadism as the "impulse to cruel and violent treatment of the opposite sex, and the coloring of the idea of such acts with lustful feelings."[19]

Usually paired with sadism is masochism, a term also coined by Krafft-Ebing to mean a desire to suffer pain and be subjected to force, a condition in which the affected individual's feeling and thought are "controlled by the idea of being completely and unconditionally subject to the will of a person of the opposite sex or being treated by this person as by a master—humiliated and abused."[20] Though nineteenth-century pornographic fiction is full of bondage stories that would fall into this category, Krafft-Ebing took his term from the name of the German novelist Leopold von Sacher-Masoch (1836–1895), whose personal life and novels, particularly his *Venus in Furs,* were full of incidents of men being whipped and punished by women.[21]

While psychiatrists and other medical professionals were hesitant to use these two terms because they did not "follow the usual rules of scientific terminology," they quickly become well established in the popular imagination. We often refer to guards and others in police authority as sadistic, and to people who seem unable to stand up for themselves as masochistic. This is not exactly what Krafft-Ebing had in mind in his diagnosis; therefore, in order to separate popular imagery from scientific discussion, many professionals have adopted the terms "algolagnia" or "algolagny" coined by A. von Schrenk-Notzing from two Greek words, *algos* (pain) and *lagnos* (lascivious, lustful).[22]

Many individuals who would be classed as sadomasochists by Krafft-Ebing, however, have challenged the definition of their behavior as a psychiatric abnormality. Today there are clubs and organizations devoted to S/M, as it is often called, and they issue and publish fantasy literature. This behavior might be called social sadomasochism because the masochist being punished is actually the person in control of the situation, while the sadist or dominant responds to key signals given by the submissive partner. Since S/M culturally reflects the dominance-submission pattern inculcated by the gender roles of society itself, much of social sadomaoschism involves a reversal of traditional gender roles in which the woman assumes the role of the dominatrix while the man plays the submissive. Many in such situations obtain temporary relief from expectations imposed by social tradition upon them, and enjoy a kind of symbolic restitution.

S/M groups exist not only in heterosexual society but also in gay and lesbian circles. In most gay and lesbian S/M groups the wearing of leather garments, together with chains and other accroutements, is common. Such apparel is often the focus of fetishistic attachment as well, and serves to emphasize the element of theater and performance present in some S/M circles. In addition to flagellation, genital torture, use of hot wax, and similar activities, S/M scenes include "water sports" (urinating on the masochist or causing him or her to swallow urine). Much less common is the ingestion of feces. Handballing or fist fucking, in which the hand or even the lower arm is inserted into the anal passage, was common in some gay S/M groups, although in the aftermath of the AIDS epidemic this has declined. Often used are sexual toys such as handcuffs, tit-clamps, and whips, although there is usually an avoidance of any activity that would lead to permanent marking or bodily harm. There also exists a vast bondage fantasy literature aimed at both heterosexuals and homosexuals.[23] Interestingly, such sadomasochistic subcultures are most often confined to urban-industrial societies where (1) dominance-submission relationships are embedded in the culture and aggression is socially valued; (2) there is a well-developed and unequal distribution of power between social categories which may make the temporary illusion of its reversal erotically stimulating; (3) there is sufficient affluence enjoyed by at least some segments of the population to enable them to experience leisure-time activities; and (4) imagination and creativity are encouraged and valued assets, as evidenced by the importance of scripts and fantasy in sadomasochism.[24]

RAPE

Just as redefinition takes place in nudism or sadomasochism, modifying traditional ideas, the same thing occurs in other areas of sexual contact. Rape is a most obvious case. Traditionally rape was regarded as a crime against property, the daughter and wife being envisioned the property of the father and husband, or else the brother or some other male relative. This attitude ultimately changed as rape was redefined as a particular kind of assault; however, it differed from traditional assault in that the victim often had to prove she (or sometimes he) was a victim. That is, the victim was often seen as inviting rape by dressing or acting provocatively or by being in places where women (men) should not go. A victim was supposed to struggle to prevent rape; if she (or he) failed to do so, their very passivity was taken as consent. If a woman had been sexually active before (unless she was a respectable mother with children), charges of rape were usually not accepted. In many jurisdictions penetration and ejaculation of semen into the vagina had to occur before rape could be charged. Different standards, however, were used depending upon the respective social classes of the victim and the accused. In some areas of the American South, even in the twentieth century, a black man could be charged with rape for "being overfriendly" with a white woman who became upset at his approach. Most male rapes traditionally occurred in prisons, and authorities usually refused to intervene. And although it is difficult for some to believe, a man can also be raped by a woman, i.e., forced to have intercourse under duress.

American states (and legislative bodies in many other countries) began redefining their rape laws in the 1960s and 1970s following the rise of the second wave of feminism. One of the major changes was to pay more attention to the victim, usually a woman, and to give her the psychological support to help overcome the trauma that a violation of her person often caused. Past sexual history of the victim was downplayed, with the growing recognition that a sexual partner had the right to say no and that sexual intercourse was an act of mutual consent. Even a woman who had had sex earlier with the man she now accused of raping her had a right to be heard. This led to the inclusion of marital rape and "date rape" in the overall category, and renewed emphasis on the fact that approximately 80 percent of all rapes involve individuals who are acquainted with each other.[25] Although most rapes remain unreported, 51 percent of those reported in 1994 involved females younger than eighteen. Girls younger than twelve were victims in 16 percent of the reported rapes, and one in five of these had been raped by their fathers; most of the others had been raped by family members. The percentage of rapes by strangers increased as the age of the victims increased.[26]

If feminist insights have led to rape being redefined more in light of the view of the victim, as most crimes in fact are, sexual harassment is a new term which first entered into public consciousness in 1975 at a speakout held on the Cornell University campus in Ithaca, New York. The term was defined at that time by the Working Women's Institute as

> any sexual attention on the job which makes a woman uncomfortable, affects her ability to do her work, or interferes with her employment opportunities. It includes degrading attitudes, looks, touches, jokes, innuendoes, gestures, and direct propositions. It can come from supervisors, co-workers, clients and customers.[27]

The concept of sexual harassment caught on rapidly. This original definition is similar to the one that by 1980 had been adopted by the Equal Employment Opportunity Commission (EEOC), which had been authorized under the Civil Rights Act of 1964 to eliminate gender discrimination. This moved the subject from one merely of discussion to a matter of law. Sexual harassment was defined as "unwelcome sexual advances, requests for sexual favors, and other verbal or physical conduct of a sexual nature."[28] Ironically, the EEOC was later headed by Clarence Thomas, who was charged with harassment by Anita Hill in hearings preceding his confirmation as a U.S. Supreme Court Justice in 1991.

Inevitably, the redefinition of rape to include date and marital rape, and the developing concept of sexual harassment, have led to an examination of the socialization of males and females. A pioneer investigator into this topic was Donald Mosher, who reported that males often looked upon sexual coercion as an instrument of power. He defined a cult of macho men, afflicted by hypermasculinity, whose attitudes were often reinforced by the mass media. He found that traditional male socialization has often included the belief that women are not particularly interested in sex, but with enough persuasion and seductive power, they can be "awakened" sexually.[29] This idea led some feminists to argue that gender role rigidity for males and sexual assault or violence were correlated. They sought sources for such gender rigidity, and one result was the attack on male reading material such as *Playboy* and *Penthouse* (discussed earlier in the chapter on pornography). More importantly, however, there was an effort to challenge some of the cultural assumptions which seemed to leave women so vulnerable, thus leading to an emphasis on assertiveness training for women. Obviously harassment involves a complex of issues that can be solved only by changed power relationships and better communication between the sexes.

Just as the first wave of feminism at the end of the nineteenth century led to a greater legislative concern for children, so has the second wave of feminism. Unfortunately, however, it has not led to a greater understanding of childhood sexuality. One reason for this failure is our hesitation to investigate such a forbidden topic. Although we have done developmental studies of children which referred in passing to the sexual stages,[30] studies of actual childhood sexual behavior have depended mostly on recollections by adults. Questioning of children themselves was simply not permitted. The major exception to this rule has been a major longitudinal study published in English in 1994 and conducted by the Austrian sex researcher Ernest Borneman.[31] Even though long past retirement age when his study was published, Borneman was accused by some critics of being a pedophile because he had asked children eight years old about their sexual development.

In fact, obtaining and disseminating information about sexuality in both adults and children is not an easy task. Even medical researchers ran into difficulty. Richard von Krafft-Ebing, whose *Psychopathia Sexualis* has often been mentioned in this book, ran into considerable hostility from his professional colleagues. The *British Medical Journal* in 1893 editorialized about the English translation of Krafft-Ebing's work:

> We have considered at length whether we should notice this book or not, but we deem the importance of the subject and the position of the author makes it necessary to refer to it in consideration of the feelings with which it has been discussed by the public. We have questioned whether it should have been translated into English at all. Those concerned could have gone to the original. Better if it had been written entirely in Latin, and thus veiled in the decent obscurity of a dead language.[32]

Havelock Ellis, who followed the path blazed by Krafft-Ebing, likewise experienced considerable difficulty in getting his information to the public. Magnus Hirschfeld, a contemporary of Ellis, had his library and his research notes destroyed by the Nazis. Even when publication became easier, as it had by the middle of the twentieth century, researchers had problems in gathering data. A physician could report on his patients but these were a highly selective group. Krafft-Ebing also researched court cases, while Ellis turned to historical examples and primitive tribes, as well as his numerous correspondents for information. Hirschfeld went more public and sought out people to give him information, but the result was a self-selected (hence scientifically questionable) sample. One possible solution was to gather quantified sexual data. Although there were several attempts in this direction made in the first half of this century,[33] Alfred Kinsey was the man who, more than anyone else, set the stage for modern sex research. He collected detailed sexual histories on some twelve thousand Americans of both sexes, married and unmarried, drawn from every state and every educational and socioeconomic level.[34]

Even though Kinsey's sample was not a truly random one, it was nonetheless representative and his data were invaluable. One of his valuable assets, as well as a liability, was his ability to look at sex with what might be called scientific detachment. Kinsey determined neither to condemn nor to define what was natural or unnatural, but to find what kind of practices people engaged in. This made his work controversial, and ultimately cost him his funding. Kinsey had, however, made the task easier for others.

Two of the major beneficiaries of Kinsey's trailblazing research were William H. Masters and Virginia Johnson, who began their studies into sexual physiology by using prostitutes (both female and male), but soon found they could extend it to nonprostitutes. For their initial study, 382 women and 312 men, a total of 694 participants, experienced a total of 10,000 orgasms under laboratory conditions. Volunteers engaged in masturbation, either with their hands or with mechanical vibrators, or else with a transparent probe that was electronically controlled; they also engaged in sexual intercourse with various kinds of instruments attached. These volunteers' efforts enabled Masters and Johnson to answer many of the questions associated with the physiology of the sex act. They found that in women the clitoral and vaginal orgasms were physiologically indistinguishable; they also found that, while the clitoris played a major role in female orgasm during intercourse, the penis rarely if ever made contact with it. Instead body movement during intercourse stimulated the clitoral glands and the friction on the clitoris came from the movement of its own hood in contact with the labia. Masters and Johnson were also able to bring effective relief to those men who suffered from premature ejaculation or impotence, or to women who were unable to have orgasm. They set up a counseling center to help couples with their problems, and their example was soon followed by others, many of whom had been trained by them.[35] Although initial success everywhere was high, as discussed in an earlier chapter, once the easy cases had been dealt with, success rates declined in part because there were many more physiological factors connected with impotency than at first realized.

Additional studies into sex and gender by John Money and others also mentioned earlier in this book likewise challenged traditional ideas, and often resulted in changes. While we might be closer to a better understanding of some of the variables involved in homosexuality or other sexual behaviors, we do not now, and probably never will, have final answers on many sexual topics. We do not even know why some of us seem more content with monogamy while others are dissatisfied. Moreover, in spite of our new knowledge, the old fallacies, some of them dating from the time of the Greeks, continue to have their followers. Sex mythology and misinformation take a long time to die, and many of our assumptions about sex continue to depend upon past mythology that has been handed down from one generation to another, perhaps since humans first began to think about sex.

Obviously things are changing, as any observer of the popular television and radio talk shows can testify. Oprah Winfrey, Sally Jessy Raphael, Phil Donahue, Ruth Westheimer, and others bring information about varieties of sexual conduct which many people never knew existed before. Popular magazines run articles which a few years ago would have been called pornographic. In a sense our society is becoming much more open about and accepting of sexuality; in the process many of our traditional assumptions about human sexual activity have been undermined. In many ways the current sexual revolution is more threatening to past traditions and assumptions than the Copernican revolution in astronomy or the Darwinian revolution in biology.

PREDICTIONS FOR THE FUTURE

Ongoing research has challenged traditional assumptions about premarital and extramarital sex, as well as attitudes toward nonprocreative sex which past societies have stigmatized as being deviant or unnatural. The research has also indicated that people in the past, particularly those in the West, have sought to keep themselves uncomfortable and full of anxiety by emphasizing the sinful nature or the inherent sickness of those who engaged in an active sex life.

While we do not claim to be prophets, we suspect that this revolution in sexual thinking, like other revolutions that have preceded it, will eventually be accepted. After an initial period, during which the foundations of society appear to be undermined, this revolution's findings will be reinforced by a new ideology. Old institutions will be modified and reinvigorated, and society will continue, albeit in a slightly different form. Any social revolution, however, is attended by great unrest and anxiety; people are confused over whether they should follow the old norms or look to the new. This is especially hard on the young. To work through this period of confusion we must examine the assumptions of the past in order to understand our current situation. In looking at those past assumptions we need to make some conscious decisions about what should be discarded, and what should be preserved and applied to today's issues. This has been the purpose of our discussion.

If we are in any way pathfinders for the new morality in sexual behavior, we argue that the basis of what should or should not be permitted is whether or not a particular sexual behavior harms others or society at large. Any kind of sexual behavior that forces participation should continue to be stigmatized. Any behavior, however, which presupposes that those who engage in it are of age, and desire or want it, and which does not result in great harm probably should be permitted. It is essential, however, that the conduct be consensual and that the persons consenting be of age and have the freedom to consent. Such a qualification allows for charges of sexual harassment to be made and for laws against date rape or marital rape to remain on the books. It also protects children. The fact that the behavior is nonprocreative is certainly no longer a reasonable basis for stigmatizing it; nor is the fact that some medical authority attached a name to it reason enough for denying others the right to engage in a sexual activity, even if it causes pain, as often happens in S/M groups.

By implication, if these ideas are adopted, traditional institutions such as marriage and the family will also be affected, at least in the short run. These institutions are already under attack by other forces, and the concept of the family as it once was in either its nuclear or extended form is becoming less common and less the expected standard in Western countries. What we label traditional family patterns were formed in periods without effective contraceptives or consciousness of the dangers of overpopulation, when the subordination of women to men was accepted and women had no other alternative, and when there was a general denial of the pleasures of sex. Moreover, many of the tasks once carried out by the family—such as the care of the sick, economic aid to the depressed, succor to the needy, education of children, and recreation and entertainment for its members—are now handled by other institutions. Still, two basic functions of the family continue to exist, namely, the emotional support of its members and the primary socialization of its children. The family should be assisted in every way possible to carry out these aims.

In light of these changing norms and the narrowed scope of the family's function, people are clearly reassessing their own need for forming and sustaining families. The average family size is shrinking. The divorce rate has increased and serial monogramy has become a reality for large segments of the population. Delayed marriages and delayed childbearing patterns are also becoming the norm as the modern world demands two wage earners in a family. Many couples have reconceptualized the marriage contract as a temporary rather than a lifelong commitment. We actually heard a young woman about to be married say she thought that the man she was going to marry would be a good *first* husband. While the family as an institution will survive because there are still those, probably the majority, who want to raise children and who prefer a contractual relationship to less formal ones, the concept of the family will inevitably undergo some change. Sociologists who study families are faced with two alternatives. One is to redefine the term "family" to include units not previously accepted as families, such as purposely childless couples, groups of three or more adults who are not blood relatives, gay or lesbian couples, single-parent families, temporary liaisons, and perhaps even single adults. The other alternative is to conceptualize families in the traditional fashion while accepting the fact that this is no longer the only or even the dominant living arrangement. A traditional couple ourselves, we have been married for nearly fifty years and have raised a family. We have watched our own relationship change over the years, but somehow we have kept together, growing with each other. Many of our friends, however, have not.

Obviously society needs to seriously reevaluate its past attitudes toward sexuality. If this book has a message, it is that Western society has felt uncomfortable about its sexuality, and Western men and women have been filled with shame, anxiety, and fear about it. In retrospect it seems that we have almost consciously adopted attitudes toward sex that have kept us unhappy, frustrated, and hostile. It is hoped, as we come to terms with our own sexuality, that this cause of frustration will be eliminated. The changes will not come easily, since any new approach to sexuality undermines many of our most established and revered assumptions. Moreover, a better understanding of sexuality will itself not lead to any panacea. We do not yet know what the family of the future will be but it will continue to exist, although probably in a somewhat different form from what we now have or which we often fantasize we have.

NOTES

1. Gen. 2:25.

2. Gen. 3:7.

3. There are a number of passages indicating shame and revulsion. See, for example, Isa, 3:17, 47:3; Hos. 2:3, 9–10; Jer. 13:26; and Ezek. 23:26.

4. Louis M. Epstein, *Sex Laws and Customs in Judaism* (reprint New York: Ktav Publishing House, Inc., 1967), p. 26.

5. Kenneth Clark, *The Nude: A Study in Ideal Form,* Bollingen Series, XXXV, 2 (New York: Pantheon Books, 1956), p. 75.

6. Ibid., pp. 52–53, 93.

7. Ibid., pp. 310–19.

8. For the brief description, see Jeffrey Burton Russell, *Witchcraft in the Middle Ages* (Ithaca: Cornell University Press, 1972), pp. 224–25.

9. Vern L. Bullough and Bonnie Bullough, *Women and Prostitution* (Amherst, N.Y.: Prometheus Books, 1987).

10. See Jean Cassou and Geoffrey Grison, *The Female Form in Painting* (New York: Harcourt, Brace, and Company, 1953).

11. For a discussion see Frederick R. Burbide, *Old Coventry and Lady Godiva* (Birmingham: Cornish Brothers, 1952).

12. Richard Ungewitter, *Die Nacktheit* (Stuttgart: Strecker & Schröder, 1907).

13. Frances and Mason Merrill, *Nudism Comes to America* (New York: Alfred A. Knopf, 1932).

14. Quoted by Peter Fryer, *Mrs. Grundy: Studies in English Prudery* (New York: London House and Maxwell, 1964), p. 200.

15. William Hartman, Marilyn Fithian, and Donald Johnson, *Nudist Society* (New York: Crown, 1970), pp. 216–24.

16. Abraham H. Maslow, *Eupsychian Management* (Homewood, Ill., Irwin-Dorsey Press, 1965), p. 160.

17. This concept has been developed at great length in Vern L. Bullough, Dwight Dixon, and Joan Dixon, "Sadomasochism in the Western Tradition," in *Sexual Knowledge, Sexual Science,* edited by Roy Porter and Mikulas Teich (Cambridge: Cambridge University Press, 1994), pp. 47–63.

18. There is a vast literature on de Sade. His novels, after being banned for much of the twentieth century, are now in print in English versions. See Simone de Beauvoir, *Must We Burn de Sade,* translated by Annette Michelson (London: Peter Nevill, 1953); Geoffrey Gore, *The Revolutionary Ideas of the Marquis de*

Sade (London: Wishhart & Company, 1934); Iwan Bloch, *Marquis de Sade: His Life and Work,* translated by James Bruce (New York: Brittainy Press, n.d.); James Cleugh, *The Marquis and the Chevalier* (London: Andrew Melrose, 1951); and Gilbert Lely, *The Marquis de Sade,* translated by Alec Brown (New York: Grove Press, 1961).

19. Krafft-Ebing, *Psychopathia Sexualis,* p. 60.

20. Ibid., p. 89.

21. There are also many translation of his novels now available. See also Cleugh, *The Marquis,* and Cleugh, *The First Masochist* (London: Anthony Blond, 1967).

22. A. von Schrenk-Notzing, *Therapeutic Suggestion in* Psychopathia Sexualis, translated by Charles Gilbert Chaddock (Philadelphia: F. A. Davis, 1895), p. 121.

23. Michael Grumley and Ed Gallucci, *Hard Corps: Studies in Leather & Sadomasochism* (New York: Dutton, 1977); Thomas S. Weinberg and G. W. Levi Kamel, eds., *S and M* (Amherst, N.Y.: Prometheus Books, 1983); Andreas Spengler, *Sadomasochisten und ihre Subculturen* (Frankfurt am Main: Campus Verlag, 1979); Thomas S. Weinberg, "Sadomasochism in the United States: A Review of Recent Sociological Literature," *Journal of Sex Research* 23 (February 1987): 50–69; and R. F. Baumeister, "Masochism as Escape from Self," *Journal of Sex Research* 25 (1988): 28–59.

24. Paul Gebhard, "Fetishism and Sadomasochism," in J. H. Masserman, ed., *Dynamics of Deviant Sexuality* (New York: Grune and Stratton, 1969), and Thomas S. Weinberg, "Masochism" and "Sadism," in *Human Sexuality: An Encyclopedia,* edited by Vern L. Bullough and Bonnie Bullough (New York: Garland Publishers, 1994), pp. 377–79, 527–28.

25. Susan Bond, "Rape," in *Human Sexuality: An Encyclopedia,* pp. 511–14. There has been a large number of studies on rape in recent years. Among them, Menachem Amir, *Patterns in Forcible Rape* (Chicago: University of Chicago Press, 1971); Susan Brownmiller, *Against Our Will: Men, Women and Rape* (New York, 1975); Lee Ellis, *Theories of Rape* (New York: Hemisphere Publishing [Taylor and Francis], 1989); Susan Estrich, *Real Rape* (Cambridge: Harvard University Press, 1987); Carolyn J. Hursch, *The Trouble with Rape* (Chicago: Nelson-Hall, 1977); Judith Rowland, *Rape: The Ultimate Violation* (New York: Doubleday, 1985); and *Rape: An Historical and Social Enquiry,* edited by Sylvana Tomaselli and Roy Porter (Oxford: Blackwell, 1986).

26. See the *Los Angeles Times,* June 23, 1994, A12.

27. M. Dawn McCaghy, *Sexual Harassment: A Guide to Resources* (Boston: Hall, 1985).

28. D. R. Ledgerwood and S. Johnson-Dietz, "The EEOC's Foray into Sexual Harassment: Interpreting the New Guidlines for Employer Liability," *Labor Law Journal* 31, no. 4 (1980): 741–44.

29. D. L. Mosher, "Sex Callousness toward Women," *Technical Reports of the Commission on Obscenity and Pornography,* No. 8 (Washington, D.C.: U.S.

Government Printing Office, 1970), pp. 313–25; Mosher, *Scripting the Macho Man: Theory, Research, and Measurement of Hypermasculinity* (New York: Guilfrod, 1992); D. L. Mosher and S. S. Tomkin, "Scripting the Macho Man: Hypermascline Socilization and Enculturation," *Journal of Sex Research* 25 (1988): 60–84.

30. For example, Erik Erikson, *Childhood and Society,* rev ed. (New York: Norton, 1968); Erikson, *Identity, Youth, and Crisis* (New York: Norton, 1986); and an ongoing study by June M. Reinisch, Leonard A. Rosenblum, Donald B. Rubin, and M. Fini Schulsinger, on over 9,000 Danish children, but only partial data are available. See the article by Reinisch, Rosenblum, Rubin, and Schulsinger, "Sex Differences in Developmental Milestones during the First Year of Life," *Journal of Psychology and Human Sexuality* 4, no. 2 (1991): 19–36.

31. Ernest Bornemann, *Reifungsphasen der Kindheit,* translated as *Developmental Phases of Childhood* by Michael Lombardi-Nash (Amherst, N.Y.: Prometheus Books, 1994).

32. This is quoted in the introduction to the translation of the twelfth edition of *Psychopathia Sexualis,* translated by Franklin S. Klaff (New York: Bell Publishing, 1965), p. xi.

33. See Vern L. Bullough, *Science in the Bedroom: A History of Sex Research* (New York: Basic Books, 1994), for many examples.

34. Alfred Kinsey, Wardell B. Pomeroy, and Clyde E. Martin, *Sexual Behavior in the Human Male* (Philadelphia: W. B. Saunders, 1948), and Kinsey, Pomeroy, Martin, and Paul H. Gebhard, *Sexual Behavior in the Human Female* (Philadelphia: W. B. Saunders, 1953).

35. William E. Masters and Virginia E. Johnson, *Human Sexual Response* Boston: Little, Brown and Company, 1966) and Masters and Johnson, *Human Sexual Inadequacy* (Boston: Little Brown and Company, 1970).

Index

Abortion, 131, 147–56
Abraham, 160, 205–206
Abraham, Karl, 218
Abstinence, 37
Acton, William, 72, 233
Adam, 17, 107, 112, 203, 252–53
Adamites, 253
Adepts, 22–23, 37
Adolescence, 118
Adoption, 178
Against Naera, 185
AIDS (Acquired Immune Deficiency Syndrome), 133, 141, 208, 213, 222, 245, 258
Albertus Magnus, 55, 163
Albina, Leontina Espinosa, 125
Alcithous, King, 209
Alexander, Pope, 189
Allah, 38–39
Allen, Edgar, 169
Alternate views (of sexual activity), 29–42
Ambrose, 91
American Academy of Arts and Sciences, 113
American Academy of Pediatrics, 78
American Civil Liberties Union (ACLU), 153, 245
American College of Obstetricians and Gynecologists, 78
American Eugenics Society, 131

American Friends Service Committee, 245
American Journal of Obstetrics, 112
American Law Institute, 151–52, 245
American Medical Association (AMA), 8
American Psychiatric Association, 246
American Social Hygiene Association, 216
Amniocentesis, 154
Anańga Rańga, 34
Anatomie of Abuses, The, 207
Anatomy, 7, 164
Anemia, 111
Anonymous Insemination Donor (AID), 170
Anovulatory cycle, 110
Apollo, 252
Apuleius, 185
Aquinas, Thomas, 55–56, 91, 148, 206
Arcand, Bernard, 198–99
Archbishop of Canterbury, 172
Aretino, Pietro, 186–88
Aristotle, 14, 48, 147–48, 161, 163, 165
Aristotle's Masterpiece, 112
Arkell-Smith, Lieutenant Harold, 95
Arkell-Smith, Valerie, 95
Artificial Insemination, 159–78
Artificial Insemination Husband (AIH), 170
Art of Love, The, 185
Asceticism, 37
Ashanti Tribe, 126

Atharva Veda, 34
Athena, 12
Athenaeus, 185
Auditors, 22–23
Augustine, 21–23, 50–51, 53–55, 69, 206
Augustus the Strong, 125
Avicenna, 163

Bacchic rites, 12
Baer, Karl Ernst von, 165
Bailey, Derrick Sherwin, 49
Barbach, Lonny, 80
Barker, Colonel Victor, 95–96. *See also* Arkell-Smith, Valerie
Barr, Murray L., 98
Barry, James, Inspector General of Hospitals, 95, 102
Bart, Pauline, 120
Barthel, Kurt, 255
Battle Creek Sanitarium, 75
Baulie, Étienne-Émile, 153
Beard, George M., 234
Beaumont, Charles Geneviève-Louis-Augusta-André-Timothée d'Éon, 93–94
Becker, Howard, 230
Behn, Aphra, 191–92
Bell, Alan, 240
Bell, Ralcy Husted, 78
Bem, Sandra, 86
Benjamin, Harry, 96
Benkert, Karoly Maria, 235
Ben-wa, 67
Berman, Edgar, 120
Bertram, E. G., 98
Besant, Annie, 194
Bestiality, 53, 55, 59, 73, 185
Bieber, Irving, 238
Bikini condom, 133
Billings, Evelyn, 140
Billings, John, 140
Birth Control, 125, 156

Bisexuality, 101
Bishop, Joel Pretiss, 59
Blackstone, William, 57–58
Blank, Joanni, 198
Blue Boy, 87
Boccaccio, Giovanni, 188
Bodysex Workshop, 80
Borden, Lizzy, 108
Borneman, Ernest, 261
Book of Ezekiel, 49
Booth, General William, 214
Bowdler, Dr. Thomas, 9, 192
Bradlaugh, Charles, 194
Bramacharya, 37
Brecher, Edward, 237
Brinkley, John J., 167
British Home Secretary, 196
British Medical Journal, 172, 261
British Vigilance Society, 215
Brown, Dr. Isaac Baker, 77
Brownmiller, Susan, 197–98
Brown-Séquard, Charles Édouard, 167
Bryn Mawr College, 118
Buddhism, 29
Buggery, 56–58
Burton, Sir Richard, 194
Bush, George, 153
Butler, Mrs. Josephine, 214

Campbell, Lord Chief Justice, 192
Candida albicans, 213
Canon law, 47, 54, 60, 69, 185, 207, 232
Caprio, Frank, 218
Carrington, Charles, 194
Cassianus, Julius, 20
Castrati, 92, 97
Catamenial week, 114
Catherine the Great, 93
Cauldwell, D. O., 96
Celibacy, 23, 33, 37, 48, 56, 126, 149
Celsus, 16

Censorship, 188, 194–95, 198
Cervical caps, 133–35
Chamberlain, Lord, 108
Charms, 34
Chastity girdles, 76
Chaucer, Geoffrey, 185
China, 29–33
Ching (divine element), 31
Chlamydia, 133, 176, 211–12
Choise of Valentines, 187
Choisy, Maryse, 218
Choisy, Abbé François-Timoleon de, 92–94, 102
Christian Mission, the, 214
Christianity, 11, 14, 18–23, 29, 38–41, 47, 69, 90–92, 185
Chromatin test, 98
Chromosomes, 98–99
Church Fathers, 48, 50, 53, 60, 69, 71, 92, 107
Circumcision, 77–78, 80
Civil law, 60
Civil Rights Act, 260
Civil War, 8
Clarke, Edward H., 113–18
Cleland, John, 189
Clement of Alexandria, 19
Clinton, William, 153
Clouston, T. S., 116
Cockburn, Chief Justice, 193
Coitus *in ano,* 53
 in femoribus, 53
 in manu, 53
 in os, 73
 inter femora, 73
 interruptus, 53, 68–69, 73
 reservatus, 31, 33
Coitus Training Apparatus, 176
Coke, Sir Edward, 57
College of Urologists, 78
Columbus, Christopher, 209
Combination pills, 137–38

Commentaries on the Laws of England, 57
Commentaries on the Laws of Statutory Crimes, 59
Committee for Research in the Problems of Sex, 169
Committee for Theraputic Abortion, 152
Committee on Obscenity and Film Censorship, 196
Commission on Pornography, 196
Comstock, Anthony, 8–9, 131, 195
Concordia discordantium canonum, 54
Condom, 129, 132–33, 135, 141, 149, 222
Condom, Dr., 132
Confessional Unmasked, The, 193
Confucianism, 29
Constans, 51
Constantius, 51
Continence, 127
Contraception, 125–42, 147, 151, 155–56
Cook County Hospital, 73
Cornell University, 260
Creditors, 108
Crimes against nature, 47, 57–60
Crisis of infertility, 177
Cross-dressing, 89–90, 93–97, 101–102, 241
Cunnilingus, 33
Curel, Edmund, 188–89
Curse of Eve, the, 107
Cynics, 16
Cystitis, 134

Dalcon Shield, 139
Danwei, 150–51
Darwin, Charles, 130
Davis, F. A., 195
Decameron, 188
Decretals, 54
Deipnosophists, 185
De medicina, 16
Demeter, 12
Democritus, 15

Demosthenes, 185
D'Éon, Chevalier, 90
Depo-Provera, 138, 142
Deutsch, Helene, 218–19
Deviancy, 230–31, 236, 246, 263
Devil, the, 12, 21–22, 163. *See also* Hades,
    Satan
Dewey, John, 116
Dialogues of the Courtesans, 185
Diaphragm, 132–35
Dickinson, Robert L., 168
Didascalia, 50
Diethylstilbestrol (DES), 153
Diogenes, 16
Dionysus, 11–12
Disadvantaged, 155
Divorce, 39
Djerassi, Carl, 136
Docter, Richard, 101
Dodds, E. R., 13
Dodson, Betty, 79–80
Dog of Early Autumn, 32
Doisy, Edward, 169
Donahue, Phil, 263
Donor insemination, 170–71, 173
D'Orléans, Philippe, 93
Down's Syndrome, 111
Drysdale, George, 130
Dualistic ideas, 11, 14, 17, 19, 22, 29, 30
Dworkin, Andrea, 197–98
Dysmenorrhea, 110–11, 120, 136

Edwards, Robert, 174
Ehrhardt, Anke, 242–43
Elbe, Lili, 97
Elements of Social Science, 130
Elephantiasis, 208
Elizabeth I (queen of England), 192
Ellis, Havelock, 78, 90, 93, 194–95, 218,
    230, 237, 261
Embryology, 164
Empedocles, 13

Encratites, 21
Endometriosis, 110
Endometrium, 109
English Common Law, 148
English Eugenics Society, 131
Enslin, Morton, 11
Enovid®, 136
Eonism, 90
Epicurean School, 15–16
Epicurus, 15
Equal Employment Opportunity Com-
    mission (EEOC), 260
Er (husband of Tamar), 203
Erectile dysfunction, 175, 178
Ergotamine, 147
Eros, 12
Erroneous assumptions, 7–9
L'Escholle des filles, or *The School of
    Venus,* 187
Eskimo, 126
Essay on Man, 189
Essay on the Principle of Population, An,
    129
Essay on Woman, An, 189
Estrogen, 112, 136–37, 153
    replacement therapy (ERT), 112
Estrous cycle, 162
Etymology, 67
Eucharist, 20
Eugenics, 130
Eunuch, 97
Eurydice, 12
Eustachio, Bartolomeo, 164
Eve, 17, 107, 112, 203, 252–53
Exhibitionism, 232
Explicit sexual material, 196–97, 199

Fallopio, Gabriele, 164
Fallopius, 132
Fang Chung, 32
*Fanny Hill, or Memoirs of a Woman of
    Pleasure,* 189

Feminine Mystique, The, 151
Fennel v. *State,* 58
Fetishist, 101
Fifteen Plagues of Maidenhood, The, 188
Finkbine, Sherri, 151
First Amendment, 197
Fithian, Marilyn, 80
Flagyl, 212
Fol, Hermann, 165
Follicle-stimulating hormone (FSH), 177
Food and Drug Administration (FDA),
    133–34, 136, 138–39, 151, 153–54
Foote, Edward Bliss, 110, 131
Fourth Lateran Council, 54
Fracastoro, Girolamo, 208
Franco, Niccolo, 186
Frazier v. *State,* 58
Frelichtparck, the, 254
French Revolution, the, 94
Freud, Sigmund, 218, 237–38
Friedan, Betty, 151
Fruits of Philosophy, 130, 194
Functional factors, 175
Furies, 13

Gaea, 12
Gainesborough, Thomas, 87
Galen, 19, 69–70, 162, 165, 208
Galloping Steed, 32
Gallup polls, 155
Galton, Francis, 130
Gandhi, Mohandas, 37
Garden of Eden, 252–53
Gardnerella, 213
Gay Liberation Front, 245
Gender confusion, 98–102
    identity, 87–89, 98, 101–102
    role, 87–88
Genesis, 68
George III (king of England), 94, 189
Glover, Edward, 218–19
Gnosticism, 18–22, 41

God, 14, 17, 19–21, 24, 38, 41, 47, 49,
    51–52, 54–56, 58, 90–91, 112, 159,
    172, 204–206, 233, 253
Gomorrah, 40, 48–49, 51
Gonorrhea, 112, 127, 133, 176, 208–209,
    211–212
Good Housekeeping, 86
Goodman, John, 116
Good Vibrations Bookstore, 198
Gospel According to the Egyptians, 20
Graaf, Regnier de, 165
Graafenberg, Ernst, 138
Graafian follicle, 165
Graham, Sylvester, 233
Granville, Earl of, 189
Gratian, 54
Green, Richard, 241
Greenwald, Harold, 219
Gummata, 210

Hades, 12, 21–22, 163. *See also* the Devil,
    Satan
Hagar, 160
Hagenbach, Allen W., 73
Hall, G. Stanley, 118–19
Ham, Johan, 165
Hammersmith, Sue, 240
Hampson, Joan, 88
Hampson, John, 88
Hand, Judge Learned, 193
Harlotry, 69
Harry, Joseph, 241
Hartman, C. G., 169
Hartman, William, 80
Harvard University, 113, 115
Harvey, William, 164–65
Hasse, C., 133–34
Hay, Harry, 244
Haynes, William, 192
Helmreich, Robert, 86
Henry VIII (king of England), 56
Herpes, 133, 212

Hertwig, Oscar, 165
Hesiod, 12
Hexagrams, 30
He-yin-yang-fang, 32
Hicklin, Justice Benjamin, 193–94
Hill, Anita, 260
Hinduism, 35, 37–38
Hippocrates, 128, 160
Hippocratic Corpus, 160–61
Hirschfeld, Magnus, 89–90, 96, 237, 243, 261–62
Hirschfeld's Scientific Humanitarian Committee, 243–44
Hitchcock, Alfred, 73
Hite, Shere, 80
Hitler, Adolf, 131, 198
Hoffman, Eric, 209
Hollingworth, Leta Stetter, 119
Home, Everard, 167
Homer, 12, 252
Homosexualities, 240
Homosexuality, 33, 39, 40, 51, 55, 69, 73, 88, 90, 101–102, 127, 185, 195, 218, 225, 229–46, 251, 263
Hooker, Evelyn, 239
Hostility toward sex, 11–24
Hot flash, 111
House of Lords, 189
Howard, Elfrida, 96
Howe, Joseph W., 73
Huang ching, 31–32
Huang-ti, 32
Human papilloma virus, 133
Humphrey, Hubert H., 120
Hunter, John, 167–68
Hutterites, 125–26
Hypertonic saline solution, 154
Hysterotomy, 154

Ibuprofen, 111
I Ching, 29–30
Illustrations and Proofs of the Principles of Population, 129
Imperator-McGinley, Julianne, 88
Impotence, 159–78, 221
Incantations, 34
Incest, 232
Index librorum prohibitorum, 188
India, 33–38
Infertility, 159–78
In flagrante delicto, 39
Intercourse, extramarital, 263
    marital, 23
    premarital, 79, 263
    promiscuous, 37
Intrauterine device (IUD), 138–39, 154–55, 176
In vitro fertilization, 174, 177
Ishimpo, 32
Islam, 38–42
Ismail, Moulay, Emperor of Morocco, 125
International Committee for Sexual Equality (ICSE), 244
Ivanov, Ilyra Ivanovich, 168
Ivo, Bishop of Chartres, 53–54

Jacobi, Abraham, 73
Jacobs, Arleta, 134
Jacobson, Cecil B., 173
Jehovah, 160, 204
Jericho, 204
Jerome, 91
Jesus, 14, 19–21, 38, 160, 204–205, 256–57
John, the Apostle, 160
John the Baptist, 38
John Hopkins University, 8, 97
John Paul II, Pope, 172
Johnson, Lyndon B., 196
Johnson, Virginia, 80, 175, 262
Jones, D. Gareth, 173
Jorgensen, Christine, 96–97, 102
Journal of the American Medical Association, 171

Joyce, James, 195
Judah, 69, 203–204
Judaism, 38
Justinian (emperor of Rome), 52, 207
Juvenal, 185

Kai Kā'ūs ibn Iskander, 40
Kallman, Franz J., 241
Kāmāsutra, 34
K'an (water, clouds, or woman), 30
Kaplan, Helen Singer, 80
Kaposi's sarcoma, 213
Katharsis, 13
Kellogg, John Harvey, 75, 116–17
Kelly, Howard, 8–9
Kimberly-Clark, 108
King, A. F. A., 112
Kingdom of Darkness, 22
of Light, 22
Kinsey, Alfred, 239, 262
Kinsey Group, the, 79, 126, 149, 220
Kisch, Heinrich, 109
Klinefelter's syndrome, 99
Knaus, H., 169
Kneeland, George, 217
Knowlton, Charles, 130, 194
Konträre Sexualempfindung, 235
Kotex®, 108–109
Krafft-Ebing, Richard von, 73–74, 218,
    230, 236–37, 257–58, 261
Kramer, Heinrich, 231
Kreis, Der, 243
Krishna, 41
Kronos, 12
Ku Klux Klan, 198
Kuttani-mata, 34
Labia majora, 100
    minora, 100
Ladder (a lesbian publication), 244
Ladies Home Journal, 109
Lady Godiva, 253
Lallemand, Claude-François, 233

Landon, Alfred M., 167
Lawrence, Sir Thomas, 87
Leeuwenhoeck, Anton van, 165
Legitimation League, 194–95
Leo IX, Pope, 53
Leprosy, 208
Lesbian Daughters of Bilitis, 244
Lesbos, 244
Levan, A., 98
Levirate Law, 203
Leviticus, 68
Lewis, Denslow, 8
Li (fire, light, or man), 30
Lice, 213
Licensing Act, 188
Lippes, Jack, 139
Livingston, Edward, 58
Lombard, Peter, 54–55
Lombroso, Cesare, 218, 236
London Committee, the, 215
London Surgical House, 77
LoPiccolo, Joseph, 80
Lot, 39, 48–49
Louis XIV (king of France), 93
Louis XV (king of France), 93–94
Louis XVI (king of France), 94
Love, 14–16
Low-dose pills, 137
Lucian, 185
Lucretius, 16
Lunar cycle, 107
Luteinizing Hormone (LH), 177
Luther, Martin, 207

McCormick, Katherine Dexter, 136
MacKinnon, Catherine, 197–98
McLeod, Charles (Charlotte), 97
Magdalene, Mary, 204–206
"Maiden Tribute of Modern Babylon,
    The," 215
Malamatis, 41
Malleus maleficarum, 231

Malpighi, Marcello, 165
Malthus, Reverend Thomas Robert, 129
Manichaeism, 21–23, 41, 56
Mani, 22–23
Mann Act, 216
Marcionites, 19
Marcion, 19–20
Marriage, 16–17, 19–24, 37, 40, 50–51, 59, 74, 110, 127, 151, 160, 171, 173, 232, 264–65
Martyr, Justin, 14, 20–21
Mary the Egyptian, 206
Mary (mother of Jesus), 20
Masters, William, 80, 175, 262
Massachusetts Labor Bureau, 116
Masturbation, 67–81
Maslow, Abraham H., 256
Masters, R. E. L., 244
Material (forces), 11–12, 16, 18–19, 22, 29, 41, 48, 50, 91
Mathy, Robin, 241
Mattachine Foundation, the, 244
Matter, 13–14
Maudsley, Henry, 116
Ma-wang-tui Hans Tomb, 32
Meese, General Edwin, 196
Mein Kampf, 198
Memoirs of a Coxcomb, The, 189
Menarche, 109–10, 118
Menopause, 111, 139
Mensigna diaphragm, 133
Mensigna, Wilhelm P. J., 133–34
Menses, 108–12, 114, 138, 140, 160
Menstruation, 107–20, 161
Meyer-Balburg, Heino, 242–43
Meyer, Robert, 169
Midwife, 148, 160
Mindell, Fania, 132
Mini-pill, 137
Mink, Patsy, 120
Minneapolis City Council, 197
Mithraism, 22

Model Penal Code, 151
Molluscum contagiosum, 213
Money, John, 86, 88, 230, 263
Montgomery Ward, 109
Moodie, John, 76
Moral philosophy, 129
Morbus gallicus, 208
Moreau, Paul, 235–36
Morning-after pill, 153
Mosaicism, 99
Mosher, Celia, 119
Mosher, Donald, 260
Motherhood, 189, 191
Müllerian-inhibiting substance, 100
Muhābiyāh, 41
Muhammad, 38
Murray, Fanny, 189
Musonius Rufus, 16
Mut'a, 39

Nackkultur, 254
Nacktheit, Die, 254
Nagara-Sarasva, 34
Nashe, Thomas, 187
National Abortion Rights Action League (NARAL), 153
National Association for the Repeal of Abortion Laws, 152
National Committee of Maternal Health, 133
National Fascisti, 96
National Institute of Mental Health, 245
National Organization for Women (NOW), 152
National Research Council, 169
Natural family planning, 126, 139–40, 151, 156, 169
Natural history, 107
Neisser, Albert, 211
Neoplatonists, 22
Neurosyphilis, 211
New Testament, 11, 18

New York Academy of Medicine, 96
New York Federal Court of Appeals, 195
New York Medical Journal, 117
New York Society of Medical Psycho-
analysts, 238
New York Times, 254
Nicholas, Thomas L., 72
Ninth International Congress on Crim-
inal Law, 245
Noble, Elizabeth, 172
Nonoxynol-9, 135
Noonan, John T., 19
Norplant®, 138
Nudity, 251–56, 259
Numantius, Numa. *See* Ulrichs, Karl
Heinrich
Nun in Her Smock, The, 188
Nurse practitioner, 120, 134

Obscene Publications Act, 192–93
Obscenity, 183–99
O'Donovan, Oliver, 173
Ogino, K., 169
Old Testament, 11
Olympic Games, 98
Onan, 56, 68–69, 203–204
*L'Onanisme, dissertation sur les maladies
produites par la masturbation,* 71
Onanuth, 69
One magazine, 244
120 Days of Sodom, 257
Oral contraceptives, 136–37, 141, 151, 153
Oregon Medical Society, 117
Orford v. *Orford,* 170
Organic factors, 175
Orpheus, 12
Orphic religion, 11–13
Osteoporosis, 112
Ota, Tenrei, 138
Othello, 9
Ovid, 185
Owens, Robert Dale, 129–30

Paired Dance of the Female Phoenix, 32
Palestinian Pseudepigrapha, 49
Pall Mall Gazette, 215
Pānchasāyaka, 34
Pandora, 203
Parent-Duchatelet, A. J. B., 216
Party Congress, 151
Parsons, Dr. Ralph W., 117
Paul VI, Pope, 172
Pauline Epistle, 47
Pearce-Crouch, Ernest, 95
Pearson, Karl, 130–31
Peeping Tom, 253
Pelagia, 92
Pelagius, 92
Pelvic inflammatory disease (PID), 176
Penitential literature, 47, 52–54, 69
Penthouse magazine, 260
Pepys, Samuel, 187
Peritoneum, 110
Persephone, 12
Personal Attributes Questionnaire, 86
Pessaries, 133
Peter, the Apostle, 160
Peter Damian, 53
Petronius, 185
Pflüger, E. F. W., 113
Phaedrus, 15
Pharisees, 204
Philo, 17, 48, 91
Pincus, Gregory, 136
Pinkie, 87
Pius IX, Pope, 148, 156
Pius XII, Pope, 172
Place, Francis, 129
Plain Facts for Old and Young, 116
Planned Parenthood, 132, 136, 153
Plato, 13–15, 17–18, 147
Playboy Foundation, 79
Playboy magazine, 260
Pliny the Elder, 107
Plotinus, 17–18

Plumptre, James, 9
Pneumocystitis carinii, 213
Poggio Bracciolini, 185
Polygamy, 125, 127
Pomeroy, Wardell, 220
Popular Mechanics, 86
Popular Science Monthly, 116
Population Council, 154
Pornography, 161, 183–99
Porphyry, 18
Poseidon, 12
Prahanana, 36
Prajapati, 33
Pratt, Dr. E. H., 77
Preface of St. Gildas on Penance, 52
Premenstrual syndrome (PMS), 111, 120
President's Commission on Obscenity and Pornography, 196
Presumptions of legitimacy, 171
Prince, Virginia, 101
Pristine innocence, 8
"Pro-Choice" slogan, 153
Procreation, 22–24, 35, 48–52, 55, 58, 60, 72, 234, 245
Progesterone, 136, 153, 169
Progestin, 100, 112, 136–39
Prostaglandin, 154
Prudishness, 8
Psychogenic factors, 175
Pychopathia Sexualis, 230, 261
Psychology of Sex, 194
Pudor, Dr. Heinrich, 254
Putana errante, La, 186
Pythagoras, 13–14
Pythagoreans, 13, 20, 22, 41

Qābūs-nāma, 40

Radcliffe College, 115
Rādhā (consort of the god Krishna), 41
Rado, Sandor, 238
Raimondi, Marcantonio, 186–87

Rape, 259–63
    date, 259–60, 264
    marital, 259–60, 264
Raphael, Sally Jessy, 263
Rati Mānjarī, 34
Rati-rahasya, 34
Rati-ratna-Pradīpakā, 34
Read, James, 188
Reagan, Ronald, 152
Reality® vaginal pouch, 133
Red light district, 216
Réglementation, 213, 216, 223
Rehab the Harlot, 204–205
Reproductive freedom, 153
Rhea, 12
Rhythm method, 139, 169
Ricord, Philippe, 209
"Right to Life" movement, 152–54
Rockefeller Foundation, 135, 169
Roe, H. V., 132
Roe v. *Wade,* 53
Romano, Giulio, 186–87
Roosevelt, Franklin D., 167
Roth v. *United States,* 195
Roussel-Uclaf, 153
RU-486, 141, 153–54
Rush, Benjamin, 71–72
Russell v. *Russell,* 171
Russell, William Oldnall, 59

Sacher-Masoch, Leopold von, 257
Sade, Marquis de, 230, 257
Sadism, 230, 246
Sadomasochism, 232, 237, 256–59, 264
Salvation, 13
Salvation Army, 214–15
Samaya-mātrika, 34
Sanger, Ethyl, 132
Sanger, Margaret, 131–32, 134, 136, 141
Sanger, Dr. William, 216–17
Sanitary napkin, 107
Sarah (the wife of Abraham), 160

Satan, 12, 21–22, 163. *See also* the Devil, Hades

Satyricon, 185

Scabies, 213

Schaudin, Fritz, 209

Schrenk-Notzing, A. von, 258

Scott, Henry, 193

Scott, James Foster, 73

Scott, Sir Walter, 191

Scripps-Howard chain of newspapers, 254

Scully, Diane, 120

Sects, 37–38, 41

Semele (mother of Dionysus), 12

Semen, 161–62, 164, 168, 170–71

Seneca, 16

Seven Years War, 94

Sex Education: or, A Fair Chance for Girls, 113

Sex and gender, 85–102

Sex labeling, 229–46

Sex role inventory, 86

Sexual dysfunction, 178

Sexual harassment, 260–61, 264

Sexual inversion, 194–95

Sexual positions, 34, 36

Sexual surrogate, 221

Sexually transmitted diseases (STDs), 141, 176, 208–25

Sexology, 74

Shakespeare, William, 9, 192

Shelah (son of Judah), 204

Sherente tribe, 198–99

Shi-wan, 32

Shifting Turning Dragon, 32

Shroeder, Robert, 169

Sickness model, 9

Sims, Marion, 168

Sin, 7, 9, 23, 47–56, 60, 68, 71, 80, 107, 156, 206, 229, 232–33, 256

Sioux Indians, 126

Sirius, 209

Smith, Mary Roberts, 118

Socarides, Charles, 238

Society for the Suppression of Vice, 131

Sodom, 48–49, 51, 54, 60
    sin of, 39

Sodomy, 52–60, 207

Song of Songs, 184

Soranus of Ephesus, 147

Soul, 13–14, 18–19, 41, 91

Spallanzani, Lazzaro, 165, 167

Spells, 34

Spence, Janet, 86

Sperm, 163, 165–66, 168, 171–72, 174, 176–77

Spermicide, 133, 135, 222

Spiritual forces, 11–12, 19, 29

Spirochaeta pallida, 209

Spitz, R. A., 77

Sprenger, Jakob, 231

Stalin, Joseph, 150

Stanford University, 97

Stead, W. T., 215

Stein, Martha L., 220–21

Steinach, Eugen, 166–67

Stephen, Sir James Fitzjames, 59

Steptoe, Patrick, 174

Stereotypes, 85

Stewart, Potter, 183

Stigmatized behavior, 229–46

Stoicism, 16, 48

Stonewall Riots, 245

Stopes, Dr. Marie, 132

Stritantra, 35

Stubbes, Philip, 207

Studies on the Psychology of Sex, 78

Subincision, 128

Suetonius, 185

Sufism, 41

Sunshine and Health, 255

Swinburne, Algernon Charles, 192

Symonds, John Addington, 194

Syntex laboratories, 136

Syphilis, 133, 176, 208–11
Syphilis sive morbus gallicus, 208
System of Penal Law for the United States, A, 58

Tamar, 203–204
Tampon, 107, 154
Taoism, 29, 31–32
Tatian, 21
Tertullian, 21
Thalidomide, 151
Thaumaturgus, Gregory, 205
Third Lateran Council, 54
Thomas, Clarence, 260
Thomas, Martha Carey, 118–19
Thousand Nights and a Night, 194
Trigrams, 30
Tian-xian-zhi-tao-tam, 32
Tijjio, J. H., 98
Tissot, S. A. D., 71, 74, 80, 190, 233
Titans, 12
Today® spermicidal sponge, 135
Toxic shock syndrome, 134
Transsexualism, 88, 96–98, 101–102, 229, 246
Transvestism, 88–96, 98, 101, 229, 232, 246
Transvestiten, Die, 89
Treatise on Crimes and Misdemeanors, A, 59
Treatise on the Criminal Law of the United States, A, 58
Trichomoniasis, 212
Triphasic pills, 137
Tubectomy, 140
Tuberculosis, 213
Turner's syndrome, 99
Twain, Mark, 192

Ulrichs, Karl Heinrich, 234, 237
Ulysses case, 195
Ungewitter, Richard, 254

United States Patent Office, 76
United States Post Office, 8
United States Supreme Court, 152–53, 195, 197
University of California, Los Angeles, 241
University of Chicago, 81
University of Edinburgh, 95
University of London, 130
University of Oxford, 173
Unnatural sex, 47–60
Uranos, 12
Urninge (male homosexuals), 234
Urninginnen (female homosexuals), 235

Vaginal sponge, 129
Van Dyke, F. W., 117
Vasectomy, 140, 166
Vassar, 114
Vassilyev, Feodor, 125
Vātsāyana, 34, 36
Venereal disease, 127, 133, 208, 223
Venereal warts, 212–213
Venus (goddess of love), 208
Venus in the Cloister, 188
Venus in Furs, 257
Vesalius, Andreas, 164
Vibrator, 68
Victoria (queen of England), 191
Virginity, 23
Volpar® (phenylmercuric acid), 135
Voronoff, Serge, 166–67
Vriendschup (pioneering Dutch gay publication), 244

Wagner, Einar, 97
Watch and Ward Society, 131
Webster v. Reproductive Health Services, 153
Weinberg, Martin, 240
Wendover, Roger of, 253
Westheimer, Dr. Ruth, 263
Westphal, Karl, 235

Wharton, Francis, 58–59
Whitam, Frederick, 241–42
"White slave" trade, 214–16
Wilkes, John, 189
Williams, Colin J., 240
Williams Committee, 196
Willard, Mrs. Elizabeth Osgood Good-
    rich, 74–75
Winfrey, Oprah, 263
Witchcraft, 163, 231
Wolfenden Commission, 245
Wolffian ducts, 100
Woman Plain, 32
    Profound, 32–33
    Selective, 32
Women Against Pornography, 197–98
Women of the Streets, 219
Woolsey, John M., 195

Woolworth, F. W., 109
Working Women's Institute, 260
World War I, 95, 108, 169, 216, 254
World War II, 195, 244, 256

Yahweh, 49
Yang, 30–33
Yasuyori, Tamba, 32
Yin, 30–33
Yoni, 36
Young, Merle, 132
Young Rubber Company, 133

Zimmerman, Paul, 254
Zeno, 16
Zeus, 12
Zoroastrianism, 22
Zosimus, 206